BEYOND HEALTH AND NORMALITY:

Explorations of Exceptional Psychological Well-being

BEYOND HEALTH AND NORMALITY:

Explorations of Exceptional Psychological Well-being

Edited by

Roger Walsh, M.B., Ph.D., MRANZCP
Department of Psychiatry and Human Behavior
California College of Medicine
University of California at Irvine
Irvine, California

Deane H. Shapiro, Jr., Ph.D.
Department of Psychiatry and Human Behavior
California College of Medicine
University of California at Irvine Medical Center
Orange, California

VNR VAN NOSTRAND REINHOLD COMPANY
NEW YORK CINCINNATI TORONTO LONDON MELBOURNE

Manufactured in the United States of America

Published by Van Nostrand Reinhold Company Inc.
135 West 50th Street, New York, N.Y. 10020

Van Nostrand Reinhold Publishing
1410 Birchmount Road
Scarborough, Ontario MIP 2E7, Canada

Van Nostrand Reinhold
480 Latrobe Street
Melbourne, Victoria 3000, Australia

Van Nostrand Reinhold Company Limited
Molly Millars Lane
Wokingham, Berkshire, England

15 14 13 12 11 10 9 8 7 6 5 4 3 2 1

Library of Congress Cataloging in Publication Data

Main entry under title:

Beyond health and normality.

    Includes index.
    1. Mental health.   2. Psychology—Philosophy.
I. Walsh, Roger N.   II. Shapiro, Deane H.
RA790.B487 1982   150'.1   82-8321
ISBN 0-442-29173-6   AACR2

To Frances Vaughan
Whose loving kindness, gentle humor, and clear wisdom have contributed so much to wellbeing.

ROGER WALSH

To my family of origin:

My father—for his toughness and his hugs, and for providing a "strong" male model for me;
My mother—for her love and her confidence, and for instilling in me an unquenchable desire for learning;
My brother, Tom—for providing a true male friend—from lifting weights and football to sharing music and Las Vegas;
My sister, Nancy—for being a loving and caring woman—with deep appreciation, and congratulations on becoming a doctor and having a new child, Evan, at the same time.

And to my colleague Gordon Globus for his support, caring, and generosity, as well as for providing a model of a true scholar.

DEANE H. SHAPIRO, JR.

The exploration of the highest reaches of human nature and of its ultimate possibilities ... has involved for me the continuous destruction of cherished axioms, the perpetual coping with seeming paradoxes, contradictions, and vaguenesses, and the occasional collapse around my ears of long-established, firmly believed in, and seemingly unassailable laws of psychology.

Abraham Maslow, 1968

List of Contributors

Ken Anbender
  Werner Erhard and Associates, San Francisco, California
Arthur Deikman, M.D.
  Associate Clinical Professor, Department of Psychiatry, University of California Medical School, San Francisco, California
Mark Epstein
  Department of Psychiatry, New York Hospital, New York, New York
Werner Erhard
  Werner Erhard and Associates, San Francisco, California
Victor Gioscia
  Werner Erhard and Associates, San Francisco, California
Gordon Globus
  Department of Psychiatry, University of California, Orange, California
Maria Globus,
  Laguna Beach, California
Daniel Goleman, Ph.D.
  Senior Editor, *Psychology Today,* New York, New York
Douglas Heath, Ph.D.
  Psychology Department, Haverford College, Haverford, Pennsylvania
Jack Kornfield
  Insight Meditation Center, Barre, Massachusetts
Deane H. Shapiro, Jr., Ph.D.
  Department of Psychiatry and Human Behavior, California College of Medicine, University of California at Irvine Medical Center, Orange, California

Johanna Shapiro, Ph.D.
Department of Family Medicine, University of California at Irvine Medical School, Orange, California.

Huston Smith
Professor of Religion and Adjunct Professor of Philosophy, Syracuse University Syracuse, New York

Frances Vaughan, Ph.D.
California Institute of Transpersonal Psychology, Menlo Park, California

Roger Walsh, Ph.D.
Psychiatry and Human Behavior, University of California Medical School at Irvine, Irvine, California

Ken Wilber
Editor, *Revision,* Cambridge, Massachusetts

Acknowledgments

The editors would like to acknowledge and thank the many people who assisted in the preparation of *Beyond Health and Normality*. The following warrant special mention.

The authors for the quality of their contributions and their patience.

The editors of Van Nostrand Reinhold, Susan Munger and Ashak Rawji, for their guidance, encouragement, and patience.

Sonja Hays for her excellent and good-natured assistance with editing and typing, and her unswerving support, assurance, friendship, and "therapy."

Susan Fontana for again pitching in at the eleventh hour!

Ken Wilber for sharing his knowledge and expertise.

Frances Vaughan for her love, support, and editorial assistance.

Our families for their unfailing love and support.

All those who have ever attempted to understand and actualize psychological well-being, for their contribution to us all.

The authors would like to thank the following publishers and authors for permission to reprint: *Cutting through Spiritual Materialism,* by Chögyam Trungpa. Copyright © 1973 by Chögyam Trungpa. Reprinted by special arrangement with the publisher, Shambhala Publications, 1920 Thirteenth Street, Boulder, Colorado 80302; *The Experience of Insight,* by Joseph Goldstein. Copyright © 1976. Reprinted by permission of the publisher, Unity Press, Santa Cruz, California; *Living Buddhist Masters,* by Jack Kornfield. Copyright © 1977. Reprinted by permission of the publisher, Unity Press, Santa Cruz, California; *The Life of Milarepa,* by L.P. Lhalungpa. Copyright © 1977 by Far West Translations. Reprinted by permission of the publisher, E.P. Dutton, New York; *Listen Humanity,* by Meher Baba. Copyright © 1967. All rights reserved. Reprinted by permission of the publisher, Harper & Row, New York; *Something Beautiful for God,* by M. Muggeridge. Copyright © 1971. All rights reserved. Reprinted by permission of the publisher, Harper & Row, New York; *The Teachings of Ramana Maharshi,* by A. Osborne. Copyright © 1962. Reprinted by permission of the publisher, Samuel Weiser, New York; *The Zen Teachings of Rinzai,* by Rinzai. Translated from the Chinese by Irmgard Schloegl. Copyright © 1975 by Irmgard Schloegl. Reprinted by special arrangement with Shambhala Publications, 1920 Thirteenth Street, Boulder, Colorado 80302; *I Am That,* by Sri Nisargadata Maharaj. Copyright © 1973. Reprinted by permission of the publisher, Chetana Publishers, Bombay, India; *Zen Mind, Beginner Mind,* by R. Suzuki. Copyright © 1970. Reprinted by permission of the publisher, John Weatherhill, Inc. New York. The consciousness disciplines and the behavioral sciences, by R. Walsh. Copyright © 1980. Updated and expanded by permission of the American Journal of Psychiatry, Washington, D.C.

Contents

IV. Integrations among Perspectives

V. Epilogue/493

I
INTRODUCTION

1

In Search of a Healthy Person

Roger Walsh and Deane H. Shapiro, Jr., Ph.D.

When the wren and cicada were told that there are birds which can fly hundreds of miles without stopping they quickly agreed that such a thing was obviously impossible. "You and I know very well," they said, "that the furthest one can ever get even by the most tremendous effort is that elm tree over there. . . . All these stories about flying hundreds of miles at a stretch are sheer nonsense."

Arthur Waley[1]

Are we all that we can be? Or are there greater heights and depths of psychological capacity within us, undreamed of by most, glimpsed by some, and nurtured and brought to fruition by but a few?

If such capacities exist, then what is their nature, how can they be recognized, how can we learn about them, and how can they best be cultivated?

This book was born out of a search for the answers to these questions.

THE SEARCH FOR SOMETHING MORE

The assumption that there are unexplored reaches of the human potential has been a theme expressed across cultures and millennia. Goaded from behind by an existential cry in the face of human suffering and limitations, drawn forward by a sense of something "more"—fueled by myth, legend, and occasional experience—individuals from all walks of life, on different continents, across centuries, have left the safety and comforts of home,

3

family, and security; have endured every conceivable natural and human-made hardship; have tempered and trained every aspect of mind and body; and have followed both the most degrading and the most uplifting of disciplines and leaders: all in an effort to reach or attain—what? That so many have endured so much speaks eloquently of the power that the desire for this "more" can assume.

This desire can be consciously cultivated. In several psychologies, such as humanistic psychology in the West and Hindu in the East, human motivation is seen as hierarchically organized, and the desire to actualize one's full potential and transcend our customary limitations is viewed as the peak of this hierarchy. Many psychologies which aim at actualizing this "more" regard the "purification" of the desire for it, both by cultivating the desire itself and by paring away competing pulls, as a central component of their training. They claim that a major, perhaps the major, prerequisite for attaining the very highest levels of psychological maturity and well-being, is that the desire to do so should be the central motive of one's life. For them, as for Kierkegaard, "Purity of heart is to will one thing."

For most people, such single-mindedness and intensity of interest are foreign, even incomprehensible. Yet almost all of us have some experience of this same pull, this same desire and curiosity to know and be all that we might become. Who among us has not puzzled over perennial questions such as, Who am I? What am I? Is this all there is to me—to life? and How do I fit into it all? Who has not made some tentative explorations, either theoretical or practical, external or internal, intellectual or experiential? And who has not found such questions uncomfortably disturbing, forcing us to reflect on the "unconscious" assumptions and habits which govern us and yet usually remain hidden from awareness beneath the busyness and routine of our daily lives? The search, and the means for avoiding it, can and do take many forms. This book attempts to explore the nature of this "more" and the paths which point towards it.

WHY HAS THERE BEEN SO LITTLE STUDY OF WELL-BEING?

One of the primary reasons for the existence of Western psychiatry and psychology would seem to be to contribute to our understanding of psychological well-being and to enhance our ability to realize it. Yet, paradoxically, there has been extraordinarily little research and thinking about the nature of psychological health. Rather, our Western clinical psychologies have been almost entirely pathology oriented. Why might this be so?

As a relatively young discipline born around the turn of the century, psychology sought to establish its respectability by emphasizing objectivity and hard-nosed empirical criteria. In this it has been relatively successful, but the price has been a neglect of more subtle, subjective, and difficult areas which do not lend themselves as readily to objective measurement and criteria. Yet these areas include some of the most basic questions such as the nature of consciousness and of well-being. Joseph Royce[2] commented that in psychology some of "the most important issues go begging. I have a rough rule of thumb which says the more important the problem, the less we know about it."

For a number of reasons, the major emphasis has been on the understanding and treatment of psychopathology. This is hardly surprising since much psychopathology is obvious, readily observable and measurable, and so clearly associated with enormous suffering that its understanding and alleviation are obvious pressing needs, needs supported to some degree by most societies.

By comparison, the study of exceptional health, which faces a number of difficulties above and beyond those involved in the study of pathology, has been neglected. Perhaps the most fundamental of these difficulties are questions of definition, identification, and measurement of healthy people. If we don't know what psychological well-being is, then how do we recognize and measure it? The psychologically healthy do not wear name tags proclaiming their status. In fact, some traditions suggest they may tend to seek anonymity. Further, they are not thrust together in hospitals or outpatient clinics, and their sense of well-being may be manifested in relatively subtle changes which are hard to measure. Yet, in order to research the nature of well-being, we first need to ḳnow what it is; and in order to know what it is, we need to find subjects; and in order to find subjects, we need to know what qualities we are looking for. Thus, we may become caught in a catch-22.

Most observation and theorizing have therefore been on disturbed individuals with only occasional extrapolations to the healthy. Thus our major psychological models, which until relatively recently have been almost entirely psychoanalytic and behavioral, have been largely based on pathology. For example, the index to Freud's complete works contains over 400 references to neurosis and none to health.

The fact that our major psychological models have tended in the past to be pathology-based has a number of important and self-prophetic consequences because of the nature of models. For what is being increasingly recognized is that our models are powerful determiners of the ways in which we perceive and interpret our world and ourselves. They tend to act as filters, determining the ways in which we select, observe, analyze, and interpret phenomena, and it seems that they do so in self-fulfilling, self-prophetic ways. In short, we tend to see what is consistent with our models and to overlook or misinterpret what is not.

Consider the implications then, of the fact that our traditional psychological models focus primarily on pathology. Might they not tend then to overlook, or even to misinterpret and pathologize, well-being?

Such indeed seems to be the case. Consider, for example, the way in which psychoanalysis, which was for a long time our major personality theory, has viewed suggestions of "higher needs" such as the pull towards self-actualization and self-transcendence, and reports of practices designed to induce advanced states of consciousness and well-being. Recall that in the psychoanalytic model, the major human motive has been viewed as sexual and that psychodynamic conflict has been seen as a given, to be reduced but never fully relieved. From such a perspective, motives such as self-actualization and self-transcendence cannot be accorded independent validity but must be interpreted and diagnosed in terms of defenses against "real" drives. Here we begin to see a general principle: namely, that what lies outside the range of a model may tend to be pathologized and diagnosed away by it.

Thus, for example, mystical experiences have been interpreted as "neurotic regressions to union with the breast,"[3] ecstatic states seen as narcissistic neurosis,[3] yoga and Zen dismissed as artificial catatonias,[4] and enlightenment diagnosed as regression to intrauterine stages.[5] Thus some of our traditional psychological models, though having contributed much to our understanding of psychopathology and human nature, may have limited in some ways our ability to appreciate and understand well-being.

Another possible constraint lies in the personality, experience, and maturity of the investigators. It is an interesting question to what degree we can perceive and understand levels of well-being beyond our own. Our own psychological maturity might well set the limit to that which we can appreciate in others. Maslow's[6] concept of the "Jonah complex," the fear of our own and others' potential and greatness, may be relevant here. If, as Maslow and others[7,8] have suggested, we actively defend against our own higher aspects as well as the lower, then we may be incapable of seeing beyond our own level of development, partly at least, because we are unwilling to. We see what we look for. Eastern traditions offer a particularly powerful metaphor for this, saying that a pickpocket who meets a saint sees only pockets.

Cultural factors are also probably involved. For example, the success of science and technology has been so great in their fields that science has been termed the religion of our time. For most of us, well-being and "liberation" are assumed to be found externally through technological manipulation and mastery of the environment rather than mastery of our minds and ourselves.

In addition, many of the prevailing cultural values, goals, and myths are so clearly inconsistent with true well-being as to be culturally and individually damaging. To a sizable portion of the population, perhaps the majority, the material triumvirate of wealth, power, and prestige seems the dominant life goal, a goal symbolized by Hollywood stars and the super-rich, and fanned by a media which often caters to and cultivates the lowest and most powerful common denominators of greed and fear.[9] Much in our culture seems not only inconsistent with, but positively damaging to, the exploration and realization of true well-being.

WHY STUDY WELL-BEING?

Why study well-being? One reason is that speculation and extrapolation from the less healthy may not be capable of providing a complete picture of the human potential. Even healthier specimens do not necessarily show us the limits of full development since there always remains the possibility of further latent potentials.

This is not to deny that studies of psychological disorder can be valuable and suggestive. The error comes when we fail to recognize the possibility that the psychologically healthy may display capacities, ways of being, modes and depths of experiencing, interests, values, and motives that do not show up at all in the unhealthy. In addition, the very healthy may not do some things which are so widespread in the culture as to have been accepted as universal and intrinsic to human nature.

Indeed it is an interesting question to consider to what extent a truly mature individual might be recognized and understood by the rest of us, and to what extent he or she might appear, by our cultural norms, eccentric, irrational, and perhaps at times even disturbed. As the translators of Patanjali's yoga, one of the best known of all yoga teachings, remarked,

> The behavior of a saint is often very hard for us to understand; it seems strange, arbitrary, or capricious, precisely because it is not subject to our familiar compulsions.[10]

Only by direct study of such people can we find out if this is so. Probably no amount of theorizing from the study of psychological disability can give us a full picture of potential capability. Psychological well-being may therefore hold quite a few surprises for us.

Examining the very healthy should also give us some insights into not only what they are like, but also how they got there, why the rest of us didn't, and how, if we wish, we can begin to move in the directions they reveal to us. Let us list some basic questions which we feel need to be addressed.

For example, how do the very healthy achieve and express their well-being? What attitudes, values, and beliefs do they hold, what qualities do they cultivate, what habits do they have, what emotions predominate, how do they interact with others, whom do they prefer to spend time with, and what types of relationships do they seek?

How did they get there? What family and social backgrounds and environments did they spring from and what can we learn from them about what Maslow[6] called "eupsychic" factors, i.e., factors which facilitate psychological well-being? What education, training, and disciplines, if any, appear to be necessary or effective in eliciting exceptional development?

What impact do the very healthy have on the rest of us, both personally and socially, and how can we best learn from them and use them?

How have the rest of us limited ourselves? Do we carry limiting beliefs and assumptions, recognized or unrecognized, about who and what we are and must be to function, succeed, and be happy? What cultural values, norms, and expectations have we adopted which are detrimental and limiting rather than, as we believe, helpful? How could our interactions and relationships foster rather than hinder the well-being of all participants? These are just some of the very practical questions which spring to mind when we consider a direct examination of positive health.

The study of psychological health may also lead to a productive cross-fertilization between traditional psychologies and those which have emphasized the study of well-being, such as humanistic and transpersonal psychologies in the West, and Buddhist and Sufi psychologies in the East. This is a useful antidote to our usual assumption that one psychological model, usually our own, must be correct and others necessarily wrong. Rather what is becoming apparent is that *any* model, including any psychology, is necessarily partial and selective, and that different psychologies may be partially correct and complementary rather than necessarily antagonistic.

An examination of other models and psychologies necessarily points us back to a fresh examination of our own. So many of our own hypotheses slip into unconscious assumptions and hence become filters from which we examine the world. The awareness of other perspectives and models helps us raise our own assumptions back into awareness and forces us to acknowledge the possibility that they are partial, and culturally and temporally relative, rather than being universal descriptions of human nature. Furthermore, with a deeper understanding of multiple psychologies and models, rather than just the one with which we are most familiar, it becomes possible to see commonalities and begin to build conceptual bridges from one to another.

In addition to the development of broader psychological theory, the study of the farther reaches of human development may well bring with it a deeper exploration and understanding of the practices which aim to induce it, for example, meditation. In recent years, as mental health professionals have begun to practice and research these disciplines, they have begun to be at least partially understood in Western psychological terms. Goleman and Epstein provide one such interpretation in their excellent chapter on Buddhist meditation (see Chapter 9). There is now a rapidly expanding research literature which, although only in its early stages, does lend some support to ancient claims that meditation is a practice capable of eliciting a range of altered states of consciousness and enhancing psychological and psychosomatic health.[11,12] This seems to represent a fertile meeting place for Eastern practice and Western science.

SOCIAL IMPLICATIONS OF THE STUDY OF WELL-BEING

It has been frequently observed, and almost as often forgotten, that there exists a subtle and pervasive dialectical interaction between psychological systems and the individuals and societies in which they arise.[13,14] We would suggest that psychological assumptions and logics may be derived from, and may then feed back into and reinforce, the beliefs and cosmologies of the larger culture in which they originate. Cultural beliefs shape individuals and their self-images, including those of mental health professionals. They in turn may crystallize their own beliefs as formal models, and then project and look for support for these models in the individuals and culture from which they were derived. The crystallization and reification of cultural beliefs in the form of psychological theories may in turn tend to permeate back into the larger culture, thus effectively constructing and concretizing a social reality. Those aspects of formal psychological models which resonate, either immediately or eventually, with cultural beliefs may become accepted as reality and submerge into and as the cultural paradigm. At this stage the beliefs seem to be largely unrecognized for what they are, and people tend to accept them unconsciously and unquestioningly as statements of truth.

For example, it is probably difficult for any of us to appreciate the full extent of the influence of Freudian psychology on our culture and ourselves. So many of the tenets of psychoanalysis are taken for granted as truths by so many of us that it comes as a shock to realize that they are only beliefs, only one way of looking at things, only one possible perspective and model, and that other equally valid perspectives exist. For example, most people in our culture would probably accept almost without question the psychoanalytic hypotheses that the unconscious is largely driven by brutal id forces, locked in perpetual conflict, which can never be fully resolved or transcended; that motivation is largely or primarily sexually derived; and that defenses and some degree of continuous vigilance are essential in order to control and manage the forces of the id. Furthermore, terms such as defenses, repression, projection, and unconscious, have become part of our everyday vocabulary.

In short, Freudian psychology seems to have played a significant but largely unrecognized role in shaping our individual and cultural beliefs about who and what we are and can be. On the other hand, other psychologies suggest very different views of human nature.

Now if everything we do, think, and say is a function of who and what we think we are then the question of the cultural acceptance of one view of human nature over another becomes extraordinarily important. If our prevailing cultural and psychological models have underestimated what we are and what we can become, then perhaps we have set up a self-fulfilling, self-limiting prophecy. In such a case, the exploration of extreme psychological well-being, and the permeation of that knowledge into psychology and the larger culture, becomes a particularly important undertaking. Indeed it may even be that shifting our self-concept may be one of the most strategic interventions for personal and cultural transformation. What is envisaged as possible may become a compelling vision and attraction.

THE VISION OF THIS BOOK

Several years ago when we first became interested in psychological well-being we were astonished at just how little was actually know about it and how little it was discussed in Western psychology. For although implicit and often unrecognized beliefs abounded, indeed whole schools of psychology and psychotherapy appeared to be based on them, there were few explicit models and statements, and even fewer hard facts. Therefore it seemed to us that the first task was to bring together the most advanced thinking on this subject and see what could be learned from examining and comparing a range of descriptions from the world's major psychological systems.

We were particularly interested in looking at the extremes of psychological growth, the farthest reaches, the greatest heights, the most stirring visions of human potential and realization. From these we hoped to extract and integrate general principles which would hold across traditions and cultures. Also we hoped that we might obtain an overview of current thinking and use this to point towards the future, seeing the most fruitful avenues for personal and social investigation and application.

With this vision in mind, several issues arose. The first of these was which disciplines to represent. Should we include all the major psychological systems or limit ourselves selectively? Our choice was to emphasize those which addressed themselves specifically to the nature of exceptional psychological well-being.

Prominent among such disciplines are various non-Western psychologies, and this raised the question of how best to introduce and incorporate them. Although attitudes are rapidly changing, for many of us in the West such systems have traditionally been viewed with suspicion. It is only in recent years that we have begun to recognize that certain of the non-Western systems may be psychologies which, in their own but quite different ways, represent conceptual frameworks as sophisticated as our own. Only with the recognition of phenomena such as paradigm clash and state dependency have we begun to be able to appreciate alternate models based on different assumptive frameworks. Therefore we felt it important to include a description (Chapter 3) of the nature of various non-Western psychologies in order to dispel many of these misunderstandings, as well as to demonstrate how theoretical clashes and inappropriate pathologizing interpretations can result if we are not aware of the biasing effects which our own beliefs and models exert on us.

Buddhist, Hindu, Sufi, and shamanistic perspectives are presented in subsequent chapters. These are complemented by Western views on relationships, empirical research, and the development of consciousness, and by personal accounts of the experience of well-being described by noted masters. Because these maps and guides have remained largely separated from one another over the centuries, divided by language, culture, and parochial claims of superiority, it has been little appreciated how closely some of them converge in their deepest levels, displaying at their core tendencies towards a "transcendent unity" which Schuon[15] and others[7,8] have suggested as one of the hallmarks of the world's great psychological-religious systems. Holding these maps within the pages of a single book encourages us to look more closely beneath surface differences to extract the commonalities and parallels which run more deeply. Integrative chapters by Wilber, Shapiro, Walsh and Vaughan are devoted to just that task.

A statement which we encountered repeatedly in various disciplines was that intellectual understanding of them was dependent upon some degree of direct personal experience. This obviously limited the range of potential authors considerably. Few people indeed could meet the criteria of both intellectual and experiential expertise. Thus we found ourselves choosing from a small, in fact a very small, pool of people who were skilled communicators and had also attempted to live the disciplines they were describing. The authors of this book meet these two demanding criteria.

Here then is a collection of descriptions from many of the world's major accounts of the nature of the human potential. From this vision of who and what we might become may come the motivation to actualize it at personal and cultural levels and to expand our psychologies to describe and facilitate the emergence of this larger Self. The study of the psychologically healthy may well swell their numbers. Such is our hope and the reason for this book.

The world partly . . . comes to be how it is imagined.

Gregory Bateson[16]

REFERENCES

1. Smith, H. *The Religions of Man*. New York: Harper & Row, 1958.
2. Royce, J. Psychology is multi-: Methodological, variate, epistemic, world view, systemic, paradigmatic, theoretic, and disciplinary. In *Nebraska Symposium on Motivation, 1975: Conceptual Foundations of Psychology*. Lincoln, Nebr.: University of Nebraska Press, 1976, pp. 1–64.
3. Lewin, B. *The Psychoanalysis of Elation*. New York: Psychoanalytic Quarterly, 1961.
4. Alexander, F.G. and Selesnich, S.T. *The History of Psychiatry*. New York: The New American Library, 1966, p. 457.
5. Alexander, F. In *The Psychology of Religion* (O. Strunk, Ed.). New York: Abingdon, 1959, p. 59.
6. Maslow, A.H. *The Farther Reaches of Human Nature*. New York: Viking Press, 1971.
7. Wilber, K. *The Atman Project*. Wheaton, Ill.: Quest, 1980.
8. Wilber, K. *Up From Eden*. New York: Doubleday, 1981.
9. Elgin, D. *Voluntary Simplicity*. New York: Morrow, 1981.
10. Prabhavananda and Isherwood, C. (translators) *How to Know God: Yoga Aphorisms of Patanjali*. New York: Signet, 1969.
11. Shapiro, D. *Meditation: Self Regulation Strategy and Altered States of Consciousness*. New York: Aldine, 1980.
12. Shapiro, D. and Walsh, R. (Eds.). *The Science of Meditation: Research, Theory, and Experience*. New York, Aldine, 1982.
13. Berger, P. and Luckman, T. *The Social Construction of Reality: A Treatise on the Sociology of Knowledge*. New York: Anchor Books, 1966.
14. Wilber, K. *The Spectrum of Consciousness*. Wheaton, Ill.: Quest, 1977.
15. Schuon, F. *The Transcendent Unity of Religions*. New York: Harper & Row, 1975.
16. Bateson, G. *Mind and Nature: A Necessary Unity*. New York: Dutton, 1979.

One of the prime functions of a book like Beyond Health and Normality *is to posit descriptions of exceptional health which may provide guideposts and models for individuals. An important question which this task raises, however, is the line between religious sermonizing and scientific verification.*

In this chapter Deane Shapiro attempts to provide a framework from which to examine the descriptions of exceptional psychological health given by both Eastern and Western traditions, and notes some of the difficulties that both East and West may have in perceiving the other accurately. Arguing from the perspective of science, he suggests the potential problems and dangers of positing unexamined values and ennobling visions. Arguing from the perspective of values, he discusses the advantages and importance of a view of exceptional psychological health, and suggests potential limitations of a strictly scientific approach. Finally, the article explores the question of if, where, and to what extent there might be a wedding between values and science.

Deane H. Shapiro, Jr., Ph.D. is currently on the faculty of the Department of Psychiatry and Human Behavior, California College of Medicine, and Director of the Outpatient Psychiatry Clinic, Adult Services, University of California Irvine Medical Center. Previously he served on the clinical faculty of the Department of Psychiatry and Behavioral Sciences, Stanford University Medical School, and as Dean of Academic Affairs at Pacific Graduate School of Psychology. He has lived and studied in Asia, and is the author or co-editor of three books and several dozen articles on positive health, stress, meditation, and Eastern and Western self-control strategies.

2

Science or Sermon: Values, Beliefs, and an Expanded Vision of Psychological Health

Deane H. Shapiro, Jr., Ph.D.

The known is finite, the unknown infinite; intellectually we stand on an islet in the midst of an illimitable ocean of inexplicability. Our business in every generation is to reclaim a little more land.

A. Huxley

Today we have discovered a powerful and elegant way to understand the universe, a method called science.

Carl Sagan[1]

On these issues (as to how people should live their lives, childrearing, sex, duty, guilt, sin, self-indulgence, etc.) psychology and psychiatry cannot yet claim to be truly scientific and thus have special reasons for modesty and caution in undermining traditional (religious) belief systems.

Donald Campbell[2]

The role of science in understanding human nature, and science's relationship to religion, philosophy, and the humanities is complex. It involves questions of the process by which knowledge is best arrived at, as well as questions about the nature of the knowledge itself. This chapter does not presume to tackle in depth the intricate and myriad subtleties involved; rather it attempts to provide an overview of the differences, disagreements, and interface between a values tradition (secular and nonsecular) and the scientific tradition. In so doing, I hope to help counter what Maslow described as two particularly dangerous attitudes being developed in our culture with regard to science.[3] One attitude rejects the scientific approach altogether and confuses impulsiveness with spontaneity. The other attitude is a belief in an amoral, value-free technological science.

Since we all bring our own biases to a book like *Beyond Health and Normality* and a discussion of values and science, this chapter first examines specifically the issue of understanding our biases. Then, in Part I, arguing from the perspective of science, suggests potential problems and dangers of positing unexamined values and ennobling visions. Part II, arguing from the perspective of values, discusses the advantages of positing ennobling visions, and suggests potential limitations of a scientific approach. Finally, Part III addresses the question of if, where, and to what extent there might be a wedding between values and science. In other words, is the vision of an integrated, complementary science which is clinically relevant, experientially and morally based, and yet maintains a rigorous, empirically oriented research framework, a possibility, or a mere pipe dream?

The Importance of Understanding Our Biases

There is an often-told story about an opinionated, loquacious professor from the West who traveled to Asia in order to learn about Zen. The story goes as follows:

> Nanin, a Japanese tea master during the Meiji era, received a university professor who came to inquire about Zen. Nanin served tea. He poured the visitor's cup full, and then kept on pouring. The professor watched the overflow until he could restrain himself no longer. "It is overfull, no more will go in," he cried. "Like this cup," Nanin responded, "you are full of your own opinions and speculations. How can I show you Zen unless you first empty your cup?"[4]

Many of us would probably sit back and chuckle at the story of Nanin and the one-sided simplicity of our Western professor who is not aware of his own biases. Although there may be a few rare individuals who have totally removed all bias from their life and world view, I would suggest that most of us do have filters through which we see the world, and that an important task for all of us is to try to be as precise and as careful as possible in understanding what those filters are.

Although some of the chapters in this book will attempt to point out problems and biases with both Eastern and Western schools, the majority of them, like Nanin, attempt to show Westerners their blinders in viewing the East. Unless we understand this perspective of the book, and try to look carefully at our own preconceptions *before* reading this book, we may end up trading one set of limiting biases which are unacknowledged for another set which are also unacknowledged.

The task, however, as we shall see, is not a simple one. Part of the problem comes from the blurring (and polarizing) of distinctions between science and religion which is occurring in our culture. On the one hand, because of the time of moral confusion in which we live—the zeitgeist of the so-called death of God movement—the boundaries between religion, science, psychotherapy, and healing are beginning to blur. In this book, Deikman refers to Sufism as a science, and Smith and Goleman talk about the psychological cores of Buddhist religion. Psychotherapy is often being referred to as a new religion, and scientists and psychotherapists as the new gurus. In addition, many Western therapeutic systems are looking to religions, Near and Far Eastern, as well as our own Judeo-Christian heritage, for insights into the fundamental nature of healing.

Insofar as religious systems represent an attempt at healing both the mental and the physical distress of the individual, and insofar as "spiritual beliefs" create mental and physical well-being, then this is important information for the health sciences. However, if religions can heal, if psychotherapists and scientists are the new gurus, then we move into a perplexing gray amalgam—where does religious healing leave off and scientific/psychotherapeutic healing begin?[5]

To make matters even more difficult, we are also faced with a plethora of psychotherapeutic approaches, and new ones seem to be springing up with regularity. There are the new-age psychotherapies (versus the "old-age" ones?); the holistic ones (as opposed to the segmental ones?); the uplifting, ennobling ones (as opposed to the degrading, debasing ones?). Sometimes one may feel lost in a large convention hall of detergent manufacturers, where each one explains how his *new* product will do a whiter, cleaner, better job of cleansing our minds, bodies, and/or souls.

Who is against ennobling visions, or against trying to develop the full range of their human potential? Pushing new frontiers, whether geographic, stellar, or intrapsychic, may be seen as part of our pioneering human spirit—as American as apple pie, motherhood, and Kansas wheat. Thus, a book which argues for extreme psychological health, love, compassion, and sensitivity clearly has to be on the side of the angels.

Nevertheless, a question which must be asked is, How does a book like this differ from a religious sermon? Are we merely missionaries proselytizing a new world view, expressing revelations with an evangelical spirit? Do the values and beliefs of expanded psychological health expressed in this book have anything to do with our scientific tradition? What, if any, is the overlap between science and sermon, research and revelation, evangelism and empiricism?

A trial in California in 1981, *Seagraves* v. *California,* a so-called Second Monkey Trial, or Scopes II, cuts to the heart of these issues. This trial raised the question of whether the teaching of evolution in California schools must include a belief that the biblical account of creation has equal merit with scientific findings. One of the witnesses for the defense, Dr. Richard Dickerson, a professor of physical chemistry at California Institute of Technology, said the following:

> Science is not a dogma or a body of belief; it is a process by which accurate knowledge about our world can be obtained. The role of the scientist is to learn, not to justify. A person who unconsciously works toward a predetermined conclusion is a poor scientist, and one who consciously works toward a predetermined conclusion is no scientist at all.[6]

How would Dickerson evaluate our statement about this book which appeared at the end of the first chapter?

> Here then is a collection of descriptions from many of the world's major accounts of the nature of the human potential. From this vision of who and what we might become may come the motivation to actualize it at personal and cultural levels and to expand our psychologies to describe and facilitate the emergence of this larger Self. The study of the psychologically healthy may well swell their numbers. . . . such is our hope. . . . [7]

Are we being scientific; are we sermonizing? Are we stating beliefs and hopes; and/or are we doing some combination of all of the above? Do we need to make an absolute distinction between ideal health as a *state* versus ideal health as a motive?[8] As a reader, where would your bias be on this science/sermon debate? Is it enough just to put out a vision, which may motivate individuals? Do you believe that it is nonscience to work toward a predetermined conclusion? Do you believe that science never has a belief system? Do you believe that religious values need to be verified for their "truth"?

At another level, what is your bias in terms of human nature? At a "gut" level, quite apart from research data or claims of scientific truth, what view of our human nature is most satisfying to you as a belief? What view of our human potential? Please take a few moments and think about that question, think about how you view other people—at their core.

In terms of how we acquire our knowledge, do you believe that it is best arrived at intuitively and holistically; or through piecemeal, segmental understanding? If you were to choose which is most important to you, would you choose seeing the world as dichotomous, or seeing the oneness and harmony of existence? Being or doing? Analyzing and interpreting reality, or being able to flow with and accept without interpretation, without preconceptions?

There are no right or wrong answers in the above questions, and many of you may feel that your bias, in some cases, was to choose both alternatives. All of us have biases, and these biases color our perceptions of reality. Although there is nothing wrong with biases per se, it is when we are unaware of them that we sometimes get into trouble.

Therefore, if we are to be successful in moving toward and developing new, larger, and more visionary paradigms of exceptional psychological health (which is indeed a bias and hope of this book), I believe that we need to do it with sophistication, and with a careful examination of our own biases. If not, the following parable may someday apply all too well to us:

> Dr. Jack Johnson, a university professor during the 1980s, received a disciple of a patriarch of an esteemed spiritual discipline, who came to learn about science. The professor stood before the blackboard, writing with his right hand, and with a bucket and cloth, erasing with his left hand everything he wrote. Finally, with great patience, the disciple said, "When will you begin?" "Like this blackboard," the professor replied, "you are full of your own emptiness. How can I teach you science unless you first empty your holistic cup?"

PARAMETERS OF THE SCIENCE/SERMON DEBATE

The phrase *values tradition* is used to apply to those schools of thought which are involved in the development and promulgation of precepts of "morality," "how to live," "optimum well-being." This includes most religious and many philosophical traditions, consciousness disciplines, and some branches of psychology.[9] The phrase *scientific tradition* applies to those schools of thought which utilize an empirical/analytical approach, hypothetical/deductive reasoning in order to arrive at knowledge about the world. Within this tradition, there are again many schools.[10]

By utilizing the phrases "values tradition" and "scientific tradition," and covering so many diverse schools under single umbrellas, there is, of course, a danger of oversimplification. The following discussion attempts to avoid setting up "straw men" within either tradition, and tries only to clarify similarities and differences between traditions by extracting those principles of high relevance. This simplification of issues is not intended to cloud the complexity and multifacetedness of the topics, but only to help highlight them at a broad, overview level.

Clearly, there are individuals who take extreme positions in either the values tradition or the scientific tradition, and sometimes it seems that there are more differences within traditions than between them. There are extreme positions in either tradition—those who have unquestioning faith in their respective approaches—whether scientism (narrow-based, insular science arguing for itself) or cultish religion (religious evangelicalism unquestioningly arguing only for itself). To only critique these extreme positions would be creating "straw men". My belief, however, is that these views are not uncommon, and therefore do need to be examined. However, mere examination of the extreme positions does not seem sufficient, and I will also attempt to examine where a creative interface may lie between the two positions. In the following discussion, we would do well to follow Donald Campbell's advice on the need for epistemic humility. Campbell notes:

> The epistemic arrogance of behavioral and social scientists is perhaps as much an obstacle to understanding . . . as is the epistemic arrogance which traditional religionists exhibit in their claims of revelation and absolute certainty. A kind of literalism on the part of scientists when looking at religious matters matches the biblical literalism of the fundamentalist as a hinderance to communication.[11]

Assuming as a shared belief that both extremes of our scientific/values debate needs softening, let us look at what the issues are which need attention, how the extremist's position can be softened, and what the critical parameters relevant to different traditions are.

PART I: THE SCIENTIFIC TRADITION

Ideally, science is not a fact, but an approach. It is a method of studying reality. It is self-correcting;[1] it is open-ended.[6] As Sagan notes, "Science looks for order in the universe. Laws of nature are the foundations for science."[1] Some would argue, however, that when science comes to believe that its methods are objective, factual, truthful, and better than other approaches, and that there are "right" and "wrong" methods for looking for order in the universe, then science moves away from its ideal and becomes bad science. Kuhn,[12] Kessler,[13] Popper,[14] Polanyi,[15] and Tart,[16] among others, have stressed the subjective hunches and intuitive personal understandings that are brought to scientific progress. As Campbell again notes,

> We are being convinced . . . of the message of Hume and Kant: All scientific knowing is indirect, presumptive, obliquely and incompletely cor-

roborated at best. The language of science is subjective, provincial, approximate, and metaphoric, never the language of reality itself.[2] (p. 1120)

Within these scientific traditions in general, and the behavioral sciences in particular, there is often fundamental disagreement about the nature of research strategies needed to understand reality. Thus, many of the criticisms which follow, and are made of the values tradition, could in some cases be applied just as easily to extreme scientific positions. Further, the criticisms should be seen not as absolute pronouncements applied to all of the values traditions, but rather as cautions to help keep us from falling into unacknowledged traps on either end of the continuum.

From the perspective of the scientific tradition (or at least my view of a traditional scientific establishment position), the following would be issues raised for consideration. First, there would be critical attention to the issue of the *orientation as a demand characteristic*.

In scientific pursuits, the orientation, model, or paradigm which is utilized creates a framework within which to order the world, test hypotheses, and evaluate information. An orientation of a psychotherapeutic school, or a religious training organization, is a similar belief system, and creates a certain demand on the client, patient, student, or follower. These demand characteristics postulate, implicitly or explicitly, a vision for the student or patient, and a belief that if the person practices and learns correctly, positive consequences will follow.[17]

These demand characteristics may have both positive and negative aspects. On the one hand, the belief by the therapist or religious organization in the efficacy of its own treatment strategy or orientations, appears to be an important factor in therapeutic success.[18] Further, the transmission of this belief to the client and the client's belief in its credibility are also important factors.[19] However, adverse effects of these "demands" arise when the therapist or organization holds them so strongly as to be unwilling to question them and/or have them altered by invalidating evidence. This applies to both the traditional and the new-age psychotherapeutic approaches as well as to the religious traditions. For if there is unwillingness to question one's own assumptions, the orientation, rather than being a useful method for organizing information and hypotheses about the world, becomes a blinder to new information and may cause a type of evangelical fervor in order to convince others of the correctness of one's views.

To help us understand and make explicit the "demand characteristics and orientation" of the authors of this book, and thereby to minimize some of the potential adverse effects, the reader is referred to Table 2-1. Neither scientists, psychotherapists, nor religious leaders are immune to the potential problems of the adverse effects of demand characteristics. This in no way

TABLE 2-1. Implicit and Explicit Global Biases of the Articles in the Book.

PART I

Shapiro	To make biases explicit is important; analysis is critical, in addition to "holism"; both can be "higher" at different times.
Walsh	Eastern "awareness" can be/allows for higher; consciousness disciplines are "higher," more encompassing.

PART II

Wilber	Eastern spiritual is higher on spectrum of consciousness.
Erhard, Gioscia, and Anbender	Eastern and Western are both good and bad; more than "bits and pieces of each" are needed. Calls for a new "paradigm" of paradigms.
Heath	Utilizes a scientific approach primarily which also acknowledges need to look to religious traditions for values.
Shapiro and Shapiro	Relationship is posited as an important value, and its centrality, at times, as a major context, is stressed.

PART III

Walsh	Eastern psychologies are a "gold mine."
Goleman and Epstein	Eastern Buddhist approaches provide highest levels of health.
Shapiro	Zen is poetic and offers an elegant metaphor of health and well-being.
Smith	The sacred unconscious and spiritual level is the highest realm; "more" ultimate.
Deikman	Western science is problematic; Sufis claim a more highly developed science.
Globus and Globus	There is no ultimate spiritual reality; *nagual* (altered state) offers extraordinary dimension but needs to be balanced by *tonal* (ordinary awareness).
Kornfield	Spiritual realms are most important.

PART IV

Wilber	Spiritual consciousness is more evolved developmentally, is larger than, and includes, other forms; Chinese box.
Shapiro	Control is a critical construct; analysis of when to use different types of control is important; balance is value.
Walsh and Vaughan	Eastern/spiritual consciousness is higher; ordinary reality, perceptions, identification create problems.

mitigates the fact that individuals who argue for ennobling visions, whether included in this book or not, argue from a heartfelt place. I believe they are earnestly and conscientiously making an effort to develop visions in the service of humanity. However, the question we must ask is whether a new vision, a new demand characteristic, no matter how poetic and elegant it may sound, is accurate and "truthful." As Michael Scriven, a philosopher, noted on an American Psychological Association Task Force on Ethics and Psychotherapy,

If psychotherapy were a drug, it would be banned by the FDA based on its outcome effectiveness.[20]

He went on to say that honest and heartfelt belief by the therapist in his or her treatment did not make it any more effective than honest and heartfelt belief in snake oil treatment. Thus, one of the primary premises of this discussion is that all systems—scientific and religious—need to be rigorously evaluated for their efficacy.* Therefore, I would like to caution the reader, in reviewing the chapters in this book, to keep a sense of personal responsibility and openness to the ideas expressed. Ennobling beliefs are fine, but we need to be careful of unquestioned acceptance and of those who preach—whether in science or in religion—with too great an evangelical fervor.

One of the hallmarks and primary advantages of the scientific approach is the evaluation of information to test hypotheses, and the reporting of procedures used so that others may replicate the experiment. Beliefs, stated as scientific theory, may be a necessary first step, but are insufficient. Follow-up evaluation is necessary in order to insure that beliefs are not merely ungrounded speculation.

For some, scientific analysis of poetic visions may seem useless at best, or destructive at worst. On the other hand, without some framework for evaluation how will we know if the implications of the ennobling vision are ever brought to reality? Do these ennobling visions ever cause harm, albeit inadvertently? How do we know either way? Arguing from a scientific position, I would suggest the need for grounded hypotheses and research which can test the visions of psychological maturity and health cited in this book. Although I would not argue for any one "type" of research (e.g., phenomenological versus objective, etc.), I would hope, as much as possible, that the research be done with an open mind and not with predetermined conclusions.

Where adequate research has not yet been done or it appears difficult to compare specific positions, either through problems of paradigm clash[21] or radical translations,[22] we must be careful to try to avoid resolving competing values by rhetorical debate in the marketplace. As Erhard et al. note, "The West argues for itself, and the East does the same." Thus, as indicated in Table 2-1, the reader should try to remain as sensitive as possible to the demand characteristics of the authors in the book (as well as authors in general) to try to separate out belief systems and values from supported facts.

For example, Rajneesh, utilizing very strong demand characteristics, says,

---

* I am ducking the question here of "how" this evaluation can best be executed. Although it's a topic I've addressed at length elsewhere (40), I still don't believe there are any simple or final answers.

"God is very destructive. If you don't go rightly, you will be destroyed—because God is fire! Many people go mad if they don't move rightly; if they don't move under the right guidance.... "[23] At this point, I'm not questioning whether or not Rajneesh is right, but I am trying to point out the very strong pressure that may be placed on the followers: the fear of not going along with what the master says, may make them mad. For some individuals, who can come from a place of conscious choice and full responsibility, full surrender may be possible and advantageous. However, as experiences such as Jonestown have suggested, some individuals may be drawn to religious practices and cults seeking an external figure to "take care of them"—a master to whom one can unquestioningly yield and accept everything that is said. Here, there may be potential danger of what Erich Fromm called escape from freedom.[24,25] The ability to maintain personal integrity against peer group or authority pressures is an equally important issue whether in scientific experiments,[26] in the political arena, or in the religious tradition.

Again, we come back to the issue of evaluation. Rajneesh says, "I am not interested at all in the outsider's understanding of it. It is a very esoteric game. It is only for insiders, it is only for mad people ... only they have the attitude of being in which understanding becomes impossible."[23] Unfortunately, a view which is not interested in having itself evaluated by outsiders, is not a tenable position from the scientific perspective. This is just as true for religious and value-oriented ennobling visions as it is for psychotherapeutic practices.

Openness to self-scrutiny and critical analysis of the new visions seem essential. If Dostoevski's Grand Inquisitor created a compelling, ennobling vision that people wanted to believe, does that mean it is true? Or good science? Or merely a strong demand characteristic?

Summary

The scientific tradition would suggest that several caveats are in order when we approach the values tradition. It is important, first, to label values as beliefs—and not as facts—and, further, to beware of proselytizing those beliefs as facts. Issues of demand characteristics of the orientation need to be looked at, acknowledged, and made explicit. We need to be aware of the possibility of an anti-intellectual bias which may create ennobling visions, but may be unwilling to evaluate them. This can lead to a position which is antiscientific at worst or, without careful scrutiny, pseudoscience. Finally, where there is as yet no compelling evidence to determine the "truth" of a belief system, we need to be careful of rhetorical debates which may be nothing more than power struggles to gain a larger foothold in the marketplace.

PART II: THE VALUES TRADITION

In a recent senate subcommittee meeting on abortion, Dr. Leon Rosenburg, chairman of the Yale Medical School Department of Human Genetics, said,

> Science doesn't deal with the complex quality called "humanness" any more than it does with such complex concepts as love, faith, or trust.[27]

Rosenburg added that philosophers and theologians had to make those definitions.

Where does science leave off, and where do values begin? At a time when rapid technological breakthroughs are occurring in fields ranging from molecular biology and genetic engineering to nuclear armament, what is the role of values and science? Does the person who has the knowledge to make a technological breakthrough have no responsibility to posit values or look at the consequences of those breakthroughs? Fundamentally, the question becomes whether an individual can claim that he or she is taking a stance of scientific noninvolvement and objective observation. According to this view, nature follows certain orderly laws and the task of the scientist is merely understanding.

The critics of this view, both in this book and elsewhere, express strong concerns and reservations about this particular scientific attitude. For example, Deikman notes that science needs to address the question of "what is the function of the healthy person" and "what is the purpose of human life." He says that the scientific community has consistently dodged this question by saying that it is outside the view of science or that the question is false because the human race has developed by chance in a random universe. Deikman comments that these answers are not sufficient and that,

> "Science's penchant for objective measurement, control, and stilted non-teleological description". . . . and scientific world view of an orderly, mechanical, indifferent universe in which human beings exist as an interesting biochemical phenomenon—barren of purpose. . . . [cause our] therapies and theories . . . [to] share the fundamental limiting assumptions about man that are basic to our culture. [This] hinders the development of the higher capacities . . . [and] perpetuates the endemic illness of meaninglessness and arrested human development.[28]

These critics of science argue that a more intuitive, nonreductionistic approach is necessary for understanding the human process and creating an ennobling vision. They further suggest that science not only will not, but perhaps cannot, provide it. For example, Wilber says that when the scientific community tries to understand these ennobling visions, to absorb them, it ends up misusing them. He says of "narrow based" science:

Those transpersonalists who exegetically embrace the paradigm of personalistic psychology (behavioristic self-regulation, mechanistic psychology, etc.) in an attempt to gain acceptance by their orthodox peers, simply run the risk of not only violating the phenomenology of their own field by reducing it to personalistic dimensions, but also leading orthodox psychologies to think that transpersonal concerns could be absorbed (and thus dismissed) by its own personalistic paradigm. This has already happened with the physiological approaches and with behavior modification approaches.[29]

A third issue involves the question of noninvolvement and objectivity. As Heath notes,

Behavioral scientists disagree about the possibility of ever achieving such value neutrality when studying complex behaviors like intelligence and mental health.[30]

Particularly in the social and behavioral sciences, if individuals try to assume an "objective" posture, they may become mere evaluators of "what is." In so doing, they may allow current social mores to become, by fiat, the value and vision. As Nolan noted,[31] "We need to be careful of applying social standards as a guideline for health. Otherwise the techniques may come to determine the vision, rather than a vision determining the purpose of the scientific techniques." Therefore, from a values viewpoint and an existential perspective, to act as if one can be an amoral scientist is already making a moral decision, for one's evaluation may de facto perpetuate the status quo, or one's scientific advance may create technology that can either hurt or help humankind.

Further, it may be that objectivity of observation is in fact impossible. For example, research is quite convincing that our values and expectations influence what we are studying.[32] Thus, we might suggest that science not only cannot be value free, but that even if it could, it shouldn't. Scientists in general, and behavioral scientists in particular, may need to take responsibility for assessing very carefully their own assumptions, and to see how their beliefs (including beliefs in objectivity and noninvolvement) may influence the reality they are studying.

A final criticism of scientific tradition is that it may tend to avoid and/or pathologize that which does not seem to fit into its paradigmatic view. Thus, ennobling visions or spiritual disciplines may be conveniently absorbed in a reductionistic way or given pathological interpretations. For example, Freud[33] dismissed oceanic experiences as reflective of infantile helplessness. The noted psychoanalyst Franz Alexander[34] called these types of experiences delusional, psychotic, and catatonia-like, and a recent report from the group for the Advancement of Psychiatry[35] also explains away many of these experiences as "epiphenomena" not worthy of consideration or as examples of regression.

Summary

A values tradition, as a critic of scientific tradition, suggests that the scientific viewpoint needs to be careful of its own potential biases. These biases include an effort to reduce all experience to objective laws of "cause and effect," reductionistic understanding of the universe, and cutting the "stream of consciousness" into pieces. Further, the scientific viewpoint may be unduly pathologically based, and therefore barren of hope for individuals. As Deikman notes,

> Freud's model of man as an organism seeking relief from tension, forced to negotiate a compromise between instinct, reason, and society, leaves even the most successful negotiator in a position of impoverishment as pathological, in its own way, as any illness listed in the diagnostic manual.[28]

In addition, science may (inappropriately) believe that an amoral position is tenable, and may perpetuate an "illusory" view that noninvolved, objective observation is possible. Finally, when scientists do study disciplines which have different world views, they may avoid, pathologize, and/or reduce those viewpoints to fit within their own world view.

PART III: TOWARD A CONSTRUCTIVE INTERFACE BETWEEN VALUES AND SCIENCE

Is the reduction of religious experience to a matter of organic molecules acting at brain synapses a sufficiently ennobling vision? What about the higher emotions of the human spirit that the religious and values traditions talk about and the comfort that their world view can offer? On the other hand, is an ennobling vision anything more than soft pseudoscience, an area of the void where absence of precise knowledge leads to mystical speculation? Can the two ever meet? Is a moral science possible? Can we expand the vision of science or are we merely sermonizing? Where do values and personal biases begin, and where does science end? Can science and religious vision meet?

Or are there radical translations between the two that make their interface on certain dimensions impossible?

This section seeks to articulate a process vision—an approach suggesting where science and values might interface.

As a beginning, let us look at the following three statements:

1. People are compassionate.
2. People should be compassionate.
3. People can be compassionate.

"People are compassionate" may be a belief, a value, or a theory, but it is stated as a fact. There would need to be some support and research to validate the theory, and to determine, quite precisely, whether people are compassionate across different situations, with different individuals, etc. The second sentence, "People should be compassionate," is a value. One can't argue with a person's values, nor can a value be proved. However, one can look precisely at the functionality of compassion and look at the criteria of "why" people should be compassionate. The final statement, "People can be compassionate," is testable. We can operationalize our term "compassion" and suggest whether people can learn these skills. Whether we would want to teach them those skills becomes a value question.

Science cannot disprove religious views per se (e.g., the world is teleologically planned), but it can seek to confirm alternative hypotheses (the Bible versus evolution). Further, it can look at the effect beliefs have on people (e.g., are those who believe in the Bible, or Buddhism, or Sufism, nicer, gentler, kinder, better contributors to humanity, etc.?). It can also determine which beliefs are "more comforting" to individuals and what effect that has on them. Thus, we can see that there can be overlap as well as separate areas between issues of values and science. As Maslow has noted, there is a point at which the issue of what is fact and what is value becomes fused,[36] and Wilber has pointed out that one cannot determine values through empirical/analytical efforts.[37]

Further, when describing religion and science, or Eastern and Western psychologies, the different contexts in which the traditions developed, the different views of the value of the intellect, and the different approaches utilized to understand reality may make it easy for each to misunderstand and misinterpret the other. For example, in fourth century China, Lao-tzu, the principal advocate of what may be referred to as Taoism, or a holistic view of the world, proclaimed that names implied differentiation and loss of the original state of Tao. His disciple Chuang-tzu noted, "Banish wisdom, discard knowledge, and people shall profit a hundred fold.[38] Lao-tzu suggested that we are not free as long as we are *bound by* labels and words, as long as we need to seek to exclusively understand cause and effect. The seasons come and go, whether or not we understand them. The free person is one who has learned to let go of analysis, yield, and follow the way of the water.

Confucius, on the other hand, believed that problems in human beings stemmed from the fact that people didn't have accurate enough names and labels. To restore harmony and order to living, he felt we needed more and better rules of conduct. In a sense, the contemporary content of Confucius' viewpoint can be seen in science in general, with an emphasis on precise labeling of experience and a sequential analysis of causality.

Thus, clashes between traditions may be inevitable and, in the case of the two traditions we are discussing, may reflect different views on the role of concepts, language, and analysis.

It is critical to acknowledge that both science and religion are based upon belief systems and faith in them. While acknowledging that religion is based on quite a strong belief system (i.e., faith), scientists are often less willing to acknowledge their own preconceptions—paradigms of the world.[11,12] These scientific beliefs (concepts, models, paradigms) may affect not only the content of what is observed, but also the process by which it is observed and interpreted. They may act as self-fulfilling filters to the acquisition of knowledge and its interpretation.

Science has primarily attempted to gain conceptual knowledge of phenomena by setting up hypotheses, hypothetical/deductive reasoning, empirical testing, and evaluation of results. From this process we gain a map, primarily in linguistic or symbolic form. The meditative traditions point out the critical difference between conceptual and experiential knowledge and the danger of confusing them or of obliterating the experiential by the conceptual. They state that only through direct experience can "true" reality be understood. As D.T. Suzuki noted, "True understanding involves a special transmission outside the scriptures: No dependence on words or letters."[39] Lao-tzu observed, "Those who know do not talk, those who talk do not know."[38]

The type of approach represented by Lao-tzu, Suzuki, and the meditation traditions in general, is a scientist's nightmare. How can we form testable hypotheses about experiences which cannot be conceptualized or talked about and in which the practitioners themselves say that any attempt to analyze it will cause the nature of the experience to change? This is a real dilemma. Unfortunately, scientists have often reacted by simply dismissing these experiences.[40]

On the other hand, the mystical traditions have, for the most part, eschewed formal scientific analysis and, therefore, have no formal empirical frame of reference for evaluating the efficacy of their hypotheses and practices.*

Scientists are expected to use the data from their research to evaluate the veracity of their hypotheses and, when data do not accord with belief, to change their beliefs. *Those who believe only on faith* use data (whether confirming or negating their belief) as a means of strengthening what they already believe.

Given the difficulties of attempting an interface, it is not surprising to find a paucity of previous efforts trying to wed values and science. Certainly, we need to look at the pioneering work of Robert Kantor on the implications of a moral science.[41] Further, we owe an important historical debt to the contributions of Abraham Maslow's[42] self-actualization and Jung's individuated self,[43] as well as to the developmental models of Erikson,[44] Kohlberg,[45] and more recently Vaillant[46] and Levinson,[47] in terms of higher phases of moral, cognitive, and personal growth. We also can find an interface in the cognitive sciences, particularly the work on the healing effect of placebo and belief systems, including the efforts of Benson,[48] Frank,[49] and Ellis[50] among others. Finally, we need to look to the social psychological literature where it has been shown that expectations often determine outcome.[51]

In this book, both Heath and Deikman have suggested areas of overlap between values and science. Deikman says that there may be a fundamental significance to certain values and that "missing from our culture are the bases whereby the concept of virtue can be seen to have a functional, rather than a moral, significance."[28] For example, he suggests that humility is not a moral virtue per se, or one that earns credit in a heavenly bank account, but that humility serves an imperative formula: "It is the attitude required for learning. Humility is the acceptance of the possibility that someone else or something else has something to teach you which you do not already know." By framing the question as he does, he makes it a researchable question: i.e., whether certain attitudes (e.g., humility) in fact create higher learning outcomes. Heath[30] theorizes that values of the great religious traditions have a survival role (i.e., to help societies function with a higher probability of survival).

If anything has been clear from the foregoing discussion, it should be that

---

*To some extent, the above statements, though accurate, are an oversimplification. The mystical traditions would argue, and with some truth, that they are highly empirical but utilize a personal and contemplative science rather than a physicalistic one. However, this contemplative approach does not deal with "expectation effects, demand characteristics, etc." Similarly, some in the scientific tradition would suggest that they also use intuition in formulating hypotheses.[13]

both traditions, religious and scientific, need to be careful about what they call facts. For example, Loren Eiseley, the noted archaeologist, said,

> No one should object to the elucidation of scientific principles in clear, unornamental prose. What concerns us is the fact that there are some scientists not representing the very great in science who would confine us entirely to this diet. Once again, there is revealed a curious and unappetizing puritanism that attaches itself all too readily to those who, without grace or humor, have found their salvation in "facts."

Those facts, said Eiseley, are "dwarfed by the unseen potential of the abyss where a science stops."[52]

In mathematics, physics, and astronomy, scientific "facts" themselves are being called into question. For example, the mathematician Kline[53] has suggested that laws of logic are no longer sufficient or infallible in mathematics. In physics, quantum and relativity theories have destroyed the Newtonian dream that scientists one day would reduce the material universe to invisible "elementary" particles. As Neil Bohr said, "Isolated material particles are abstractions, their properties being definable and observable only through other particles."[54] The idea became common among physicists, including Einstein, that subatomic particles were less particles than "perturbations" in the energy fields in which they existed.[55]

Facts, then, are not independent according to these views, and there is a dynamic interconnectedness of all things. Certain astronomers, for example, are convinced that the existence of physical laws as we know them is dependent upon the universe being exactly as it is, and that if the solar system existed in isolation from the rest of the universe, it would not exist at all, at least not in any recognizable form. Again, this is similar to the Eastern religious view of the dynamic interconnectedness of all things—the total ecological dependence of all that exists upon all else that exists. As Huston Smith notes, "Modern astronomical time and space, which irrevocably smashed the West's previous world view, slip into the folds of Buddhist cosmology with scarcely a ripple."[56]

Summary: On the Values ⟶ Scientific Side of the Equation

From the values sector—poets, philosophers, theologians, and some mental health professionals—there has been a cry, almost a plea, for the development of ennobling visions. These visions can help provide what Joseph Campbell[57] referred to as "myths to live by," symbols of excellence and cooperation, new possibilities and paradigms for the positive evolution of human nature. This vision of humanity, which goes beyond mere physical survival and cultural adaptation, can become a self-fulfilling prophecy, lifting individuals, society, and culture to new realms of cooperation, understanding, and peace. As Gordon Allport said,

> By their own theories of human nature, psychologists have the power of elevating or debasing that same nature. Debasing assumptions debase human beings; generous assumptions exalt them.[58]

Thus, one of the primary tasks of the values camp in general, and this book in particular, may be in a sense to be evangelical, to stir up as many people as possible to pursue the exploration of the further reaches of their human potential. There may be a self-fulfilling prophecy in this. If we *believe* in ourselves as innately self-actualizing, we may be more willing to trust ourselves. If we believe that other people have a Buddha nature in them and are delicate and lovely human beings innately, then we may act toward them in that way and create a self-fulfilling prophecy interpersonally. For example, when a Rogerian therapist acts toward a client with love, caring, acceptance, and with a belief in that client's essential worth, these may be imparted to the client.

Thus, *Beyond Health and Normality* is written largely from the perspective of the values tradition. One of its prime tasks is to begin to provide models and visions from which we, as individuals, whether scientists or not, can begin to formulate our own self-chosen realities. The visions can provide a values context and vision for science, and may serve as self-fulfilling prophecies moving us individually and collectively toward heights of "something more." Further, this tradition can point out the limitations of a strictly "rational" scientific approach, including when it pathologizes, reduces, or avoids that which doesn't precisely fit into its paradigm. It can provide an alternative theory to a strictly barren world view (i.e., our evolution from globular matter versus a teleological, ennobling vision). Further, the values camp, insofar as it reflects a critique of the scientific tradition, may suggest that those who don't have a holistic or intuitive sense, and yet are attracted to the order of science, may end up becoming mere technicians and fact finders. Further, even when intuition and precision are more in balance, it still may be necessary to have a context of values. Finally, this can assist us in pointing out that a scientific approach is an *approach* and that scientific facts are merely stepping stones until new facts are discovered. Therefore science, too, rests upon a belief system and paradigmatic assumptions.

On the Scientific ⟶ Values Side of the Equation

On the other hand, it is suggested that when reading this book, we be cautious to separate out beliefs and theories from assertions of fact. We in the West may have a halo which we place on all things ennobling, Eastern, holistic, spiritual. Thus we have to be very careful, I would suggest, when we look to the East with excitement and exaltation. Evangelical words are used throughout this book (e.g., gold mine of information), and as noted in Table 2-1, there is often the suggestion that things Eastern and spiritual are exalting. We need to be careful that we don't apply less skepticism and scientific rigor to these traditions than we would apply to our own religious beliefs. For example, nowhere in this book is the Judeo-Christian heritage called a gold mine, and extreme caution would be used in ever describing a new scientific *theory* as a gold mine.

Another example of the problem of imprecise labeling of theory, and of belief versus fact, may be seen in the assertion made by Maslow, "If you deliberately plan to be less than you are capable of being, then I warn you that you will be deeply unhappy for the rest of your life."[59] How does Maslow know this? How is his statement different from a religious sermon? In fact, it isn't. He is expressing his personally felt beliefs, just as theologians and philosophers for centuries before him have done. We need to make sure that assertions, no matter how deeply felt, are not taken as scientific fact, based solely on strength of conviction.

Similarly, in this book when there are statements that there are no limits to the capacity of the mind, this may be an excellent motivator. However, it may be bad science. It may be a value to encourage people to develop themselves to their fullest potential, but it also may make people believe that they have more capabilities than they in fact do. Again, the area of overlap between values and science needs to be looked at very precisely. Therefore, in the realm of vision and morality, the values tradition may be far ahead of the Western scientific approach, but from the perspective of being an empirical science, the values tradition may not be on such sophisticated ground.

Concluding Remarks

I am suggesting that we need to utilize both values and a scientific approach to the study of human behavior. I believe we need efforts to develop a new vision, but that we need to do this within a context which does not negate our scientific tradition. Therefore, although certain chapters of the book will be somewhat evangelical in tone and have an intent to share a new vision of possibilities, I believe this must be balanced by attempts to ground the vision, to show scientific problems in the study of the healthy person, and to point the way for future research.

Although I'm not sure of the exact way to achieve this balance, I'm really suggesting that at least two hats be worn. One hat is that of the academician or scientist. This hat would like, as much as possible, beliefs tied to data. No statements would be made as fact unless there was sufficient empirical research to justify its conclusion. This is an important position, for once we leave the data, we are in the realm of speculation and educated guesses. There may be a tendency, amidst the excitement of new thoughts, new integrations, new visions of wellness and extreme psychological health, to speak in hyperbole. We may be creating a vision like that of Teilhard de Chardin, a vision of the omega point as an evolution toward higher and higher consciousness. Although elegant as a belief, it may cause us to have blinders to some of the problems and our own lack of skills that need to be developed. Beliefs need to be stated as beliefs and hopes.

The other hat that many of us wear is that of clinicians and educators who are on the front line, who see people every day. We need to present our clients and patients with the best, most up-to-date skills and knowledge possible. In a sense, as noted earlier, we become preachers in a secular age. Individuals' concerns won't wait for final empirical findings. So, we go with our best, albeit an incompletely documented, effort. We try to be honest with ourselves and acknowledge the intuitive seat-of-the-pants speculation that is often used in our efforts. At the same time, we need to be honest in evaluating the effectiveness of our effort.

Thus, our task is to work on two levels. To say which one is right or truer is really to pose a chicken-and-egg question which may not be able to be answered. On the one level, our task is speculative, heuristic, and visionary. We need to create the framework for the information that we will subsequently research. Yet we need to look at our research data and go beyond that to create the new vision. Once we have revised and refined our vision, our next task is to see if we can't develop additional skills and means for reaching it, and then to honestly assess our efficacy in so doing. In formulating the vision, we need also to acknowledge where cognitive, analytical skills are not enough and where there are ineffable experiences which are part of the vision, even though they cannot be adequately conceptualized.

If I were to make a tentative beginning formulation about ennobling visions, it would be as follows:

1. We cannot escape models and visions.
2. I would suggest that ennobling visions may be functional and have many positive purposes.
3. I believe the vision should give us a sense of hope and purpose.
4. I believe that a purposive vision should not attempt to proselytize, and that beliefs should be stated as beliefs.

5. I believe the vision should also see the distress in life and not see transcendence too simply. Otherwise I believe transcendence may become an avoidance of honestly focusing on the suffering that occurs.
6. I believe we need to remain ethically and personally responsible for our choice of beliefs.
7. I believe that we need to be able to use an open-ended scientific approach in trying to understand and evaluate the efficacy of our beliefs, and that we should not stop in our attempts at evaluation even though there may be limits and problems in so doing.
8. I believe the ennobling belief should be a process of attainment rather than a final ideal state.
9. I believe, as much as possible, that we should try to look at both (all) sides of the science/values/ennobling belief issue.

The behavioral sciences, psychology, psychiatry, and the mental health professions are currently undergoing a revolution in thinking and conceptualizing. There is an openness in these fields, a breaking down of the traditional scientific paradigms. Although this makes for a confusing time in a scientific discipline, it can also make for an exciting time, for there is the opportunity for new approaches and new paths to be explored. The twin lions at the Eastern temple gates are sometimes said to represent confusion and paradox, and the person who would have true wisdom must be willing to pass between both. Somehow, it seems important to be able to maintain a paradox of holding an open mind while challenging ourselves with a fully disciplined consciousness to go for the highest possible potential; to have a full belief in the possibility of our vision, and at the same time not be guilty of simplistic naiveté. It seems we need to free ourselves, to give ourselves permission for this exploration; in addition, we need to take the time to verify the results of our exploration. Again, I concur with the sentiments expressed by Donald Campbell who noted, "The issues are so complex, and the data available so uncompelling. . . ∴ that this article needs to be seen as a challenge rather than as established conclusions."[2]

It is in this spirit of open inquiry and searching on both personal and professional levels, that I am writing this chapter and that we are editing this book. The challenge awaits.

ACKNOWLEDGMENTS

I wish to thank Dr. Gordon Globus, Dr. Robert Kantor and Dr. Johanna Shapiro for their comments on previous drafts of this manuscript.

REFERENCES

1. Sagan, C. *Cosmos*. New York: Random House, 1980.
2. Campbell, D. D. On the conflict between biological and social evolution and between psychology and moral tradition. *American Psychologist*, 1975, 1103–1126.
3. Maslow, A. *The Psychology of Science: A Reconnaissance*. New York: Harper & Row, 1966.
4. From Reps, P. *Zen Flesh, Zen Bones*. Rutland, Vt.: Charles Tuttle, 1958, p. 5.
5. See for example Benson, H. *The Mind/Body Effect*. New York: Simon and Schuster, 1979; Franks, J. *Persuasion and Healing*. New York: Schocken Books, 1963.
6. Dickerson, R. E. Scopes II: A threat to the value of science. *Los Angeles Times*, March 13, 1981, Part II, p. 11.
7. Walsh, R. and Shapiro, D. H. In search of a healthy person. This book.
8. Dubos, R. J. *Man Adapting*. New Haven, Conn.: Yale University Press, 1965.
9. Walsh, R. N. The consciousness disciplines and the behavioral sciences: Questions of comparison and assessment. *American Journal of Psychiatry* 1980, 137(6) 663–673.
10. Simon, H. A. The behavioral and social sciences. *Science*, 1980, *209*(4), 72–78.
11. Campbell, D. D. Op. cit., p. 1120.
12. Kuhn, T. *The Structure of Scientific Revolutions*. Chicago: University of Chicago Press, 1971.
13. Koestler, A. *The Act of Creation*. London: Hutchinson, 1964.
14. See Popper, K. R. *The Logic of Scientific Discovery*. New York: Basic Books, 1959; and Popper, K. R. *Objective Knowledge: An Evolutionary Approach*. Oxford: Clarendon, 1972.
15. Polanyi, M. *Personal Knowledge: Toward a Post-Critical Philosophy*. London: Routledge and Kegan, Paul, 1958.
16. Tart, C. States of consciousness and state specific sciences. *Science*, 1972, *186*, 1203–10.
17. Orne, M. T. On the social psychology of the psychological experiment: With particular reference to demand characteristics and their implications. *American Psychologist*, 1962, *17*(10) 776–83.
18. McReynolds, W. T., Barnes, A. R., Brooks, S. et al. The role of attention placebo influences in the efficacy of systematic desensitization. *Journal of Consulting and Clinical Psychology*, 1973, *41*, 86–92.
19. Smith, J. Psychotherapeutic effects of TM with controls for expectations of relief and daily sitting. *Journal of Consulting and Clinical Psychology*, 1976, *44*(4), 630–7.
20. Scriven, M. Comments on the APA task force on ethics. *American Psychological Association Monitor*, 1978.
21. Walsh, R. N. The psychologies of East and West. This book.
22. Globus, G. Personal communication, January 1981.
23. Rajneesh, S. B. op. cit.
24. Fromm, E. *Escape from Freedom*. New York: Reinhart, 1941.
25. See for example the newsletter on cults, *Psychologists for Social Action*, March 30, 1980, Vol. I, Issue II.
26. See the experiments of Milgrim, S. Behavioral study of obedience. *Journal of Abnormal and Social Psychology*, 1963, *67*, 371–378.
27. Cited in the *Los Angeles Times*, April 25, 1981, Part I, p. 4.
28. Deikman, A. Sufism and the mental health sciences. This book.
29. Wilber, K. The evolution of consciousness. This book.
30. See for example Heath, D. The maturing person. This book; also Smith, M. B. Mental

health reconsidered: A special case of the problem of values in psychology. *American Psychologist*, 1961, *16*, 299–306.

31. Nolan, J. D. Freedom and dignity: A functional analysis. *American Psychologist,* 1974, *29,* 157–160.
32. Rosenthal, R., Persinger, G. and Fode, K. Experimenter bias, anxiety, and social desirability. *Perceptual and Motor Skills,* 1962, *15*(1), 73–4.
33. Freud, S. *Civilization and Its Discontents.* New York: Norton, 1962.
34. Alexander, F. Buddhist training as an artificial catatonia. *Psychoanalytic Review,* 1931, *18,* 129–45.
35. Group for the Advancement of Psychiatry. *Mysticism: Spiritual Quest or Psychic Disorder?* Washington D.C.: Group for the Advancement of Psychiatry, 1977.
36. Maslow, A. Fusions of facts and values. *American Journal of Psychoanalysis,* 1963, *23,* 117–131.
37. Wilber, K. Reflections on the new age paradigm. *Revision,* 1981, *4,* 53–74.
38. Lao-tzu. *Tao Ching* (A. Waley, translator). London: George Allen and Unwin, Ltd., 1936; see also Chuang-tzu, *Basic Writings* (B. Watson, translator). New York: Columbia University Press, 1964.
39. Suzuki, D. T. *Manual of Zen Buddhism.* London: Rider, 1956.
40. Shapiro, D. *Meditation: Self-regulation Strategy and Altered State of Consciousness.* New York: Aldine, 1980.
41. Kantor, R. E. *Implications of a Moral Science.* Menlo Park: Stanford Research Institute, 1971.
42. Maslow, A. *Motivation and Personality.* New York: Harper & Row, 1970.
43. Jung, C. G. The structure and dynamics of the psyche. In *Collected Works,* Vol. 8. Princeton: Princeton University Press, 1960.
44. Erickson, E. *Childhood and Society.* New York: Norton, 1963.
45. Kohlberg, L. The development of children's orientations toward a moral order. *Vita Humana,* 1963, *6,* 11–33.
46. Vaillant, G. E. and Milofsky, E. Natural history of male psychological health: Empirical evidence for Erickson's model of the lifecycle. *American Journal of Psychiatry,* 1980, *137*(11), 1348–1359.
47. Levinson, D. J. *The Seasons of a Man's Life.* New York: Knopf, 1978.
48–50. See for example the early works of Ellis, A. *Reason and Emotion in Psychotherapy.* New York: Lyle Stewart and Citadel Press, 1962; Ellis, A. The place of meditation and cognitive behavior therapy in rational emotive therapy. In *The Science of Meditation* (D. H. Shapiro and R. N. Walsh, Eds.). New York: Aldine (in press); the works of Franks, J. and Benson, H. cited in reference 5.
51. See for example references 17 and 32.
52. Cited by Richard Gilluly, editorial writer of the *Baltimore Sun,* in the *Los Angeles Times.*
53. Kline, M. *Mathematics: The Loss of Certainty.* New York: Oxford Press, 1980.
54. Bohr, N. *Atomic Theory in Human Knowledge.* New York: Wylie, 1958.
55. Capra, F. *The Tao of Physics.* Berkeley: Shambala, 1975; see also Zukav, G. *The Dancing Wu Li Masters.* New York: Bantam, 1980.
56. Smith, H. The sacred unconscious. This book; see also Smith, H. *Forgotten Truth: The Primordial Tradition.* New York: Harper & Row, 1980.
57. Campbell, J. *Myths to Live By.* New York: Bantam, 1973.
58. Allport, G. Cited in Walsh and Vaughan, this book.
59. Maslow, A. *The Farther Reaches of Human Nature.* New York: Viking, 1971, p. 36.

If you deliberately plan to be less than you are capable of being, then I warn you that you'll be deeply unhappy for the rest of your life.

Abraham Maslow

Until very recently Western mental health professionals and behavioral scientists usually assumed that our own psychologies were the only ones worthy of serious consideration and that those of other cultures amounted to little more than primitive superstitions. Like the British envoy to India who made himself famous at the end of his career by remarking that he had never felt the need to learn the native language because he knew the Indians had nothing worthwhile to say, we in the West have usually dismissed non-Western psychologies on the basis of ignorance rather than informed opinion.

Recently, however, there has been a dramatic increase in interest in these non-Western systems. In part this reflects a widespread cultural interest in the East. However, it also stems from the fact that certain advances in Western psychology and science have rendered some of the non-Western claims more comprehensible. In addition, an increasing number of Western professionals have experimented with non-Western practices such as meditation and have found, often to their surprise, that they have proved valuable in understanding both themselves and the psychologies from which they are derived.

In "The Psychologies of East and West," Roger Walsh points out that recent developments in our understanding of such things as models, paradigm clash, and state dependency have suggested that our assumptions and models may have acted as perceptual filters, reducing our ability to appreciate psychological systems other than our own. In addition, studies from areas as diverse as altered states of consciousness, peak experiences, meditation outcome research, psychedelics, and quantum physics have begun to lend convergent support to some of the claims of certain Eastern psychologies. Certain of these psychologies, it seems, may complement our traditional Western models.

Roger Walsh's interests in the nature of psychological well-being began as a result of his experiences in psychotherapy and meditation. Finding these to be of considerable personal benefit, he began a personal and experimental investigation of psychologies and practices which emphasized the study of

37

well-being. These explorations took him into fields such as meditation, humanistic, transpersonal, and non-western psychologies, and the psychology of religion. He is the author of Towards an Ecology of Brain *and* The Universe Within Us: Contemporary Perspectives on Religion and Buddhist Psychology *(In Press), and coeditor of* Beyond Ego: Transpersonal Dimensions in Psychology. *He was formerly an acrobat in Wirth-Coles Circus.*

3

The Psychologies of East and West: Contrasting Views of the Human Condition and Potential

Roger Walsh

The history of science is rich in the example of the fruitfulness of bringing two sets of techniques, two sets of ideas, developed in separate contexts for the pursuit of truth, in contact with each other.

Oppenheimer[1]

Western psychology and psychiatry are little more than a century old yet in that brief span of historical time have made extraordinary progress. This progress is largely a result of their embracing a rigorous empirical approach which lifted them beyond their philosophical and applied medical backgrounds and transformed them into a multidisciplinary scientific enterprise: the behavioral sciences.

With their success so deeply rooted in an empirical scientific approach, Western behavioral scientists saw little reason to suspect that they would find much of value in non-Western psychologies whose approaches are largely subjective and experiential. True, some of these psychologies had developed over thousands of years and made some extraordinary claims about mental processes, consciousness, and the potential for cultivating psychological well-being, but there seemed little reason to suspect that these were much more than primitive superstitions.

These suspicions appeared to be confirmed by preliminary investigations. In most cases, the major non-Western psychologies such as Buddhism, Hinduism, Taoism, and Sufism appeared to be linked to, or derived from, religious and spiritual systems and hence were immediately suspect. Then, too, many of their assumptions, goals, and practices seemed at first glance to be doubtful at best and nonsensical or pathological at worst. Who could make sense of claims that our usual state of consciousness is distorted, illusory, and dreamlike; that our minds are largely out of control and run us like conditioned automata, yet can be brought under control and elicit clearer states of awareness if we would be willing to spend long periods of time sitting and observing our breathing? Worse yet, who would believe such claims when they were accompanied by statements that we did not possess sufficient experiential background to fully assess these systems without engaging in their practices?

Not surprisingly, all but a few Western investigators confined their explorations of these traditions to reading a book or two or, less commonly, examining a few practitioners; perceived their suspicions as verified; and then dismissed these traditions as reminiscent of the superstitions from which, thankfully, Western psychology had been delivered. Very rarely indeed did anyone explore in depth, let alone undertake, the practices which the Easterners claimed were essential to understanding their disciplines. And who can really blame these behavioral scientists? Why undertake lengthy and demanding training in practices which at first glance appeared of dubious value at best?

Yet within recent years a rapidly growing number of Westerners, including behavioral scientists, have in fact begun such practices. For within both the behavioral sciences and the culture at large, Eastern philosophies, altered states of consciousness, voluntary control of psychophysiological processes, and searching within for a sense of existential meaning and satisfaction have begun to be more comprehensible.

In part this reflects some of the recent developments in the behavioral sciences which have made some of the claims of Eastern psychology seem less bizarre. For example, studies of altered states of consciousness have revealed a far broader spectrum of states than previously recognized; the phenomenon of state dependency makes the claim for the necessity of personal experience more plausible; meditation research has revealed a range of psychological, physiological, and biochemical shifts; and biofeedback has transformed the voluntary control of internal states from an unlikely hypothesis to an everyday practice. In addition, it has increasingly been recognized that beneath the surface differences of some Eastern systems can be found a surprising degree of underlying commonality. In this chapter those systems displaying these commonalities will be referred to specifically as the consciousness disciplines in view of their emphasis on the exploration and modification of consciousness.

In view of these facts, it is not surprising that there have been a growing number of evaluations of the consciousness disciplines by Western behavioral scientists. However, most of the assessments to date have been marred by a number of conceptual, paradigmatic, methodological, and experiential deficiencies, and have not taken into account many of the recent advances in relevant areas of Western science.

This chapter is intended to outline the principles and implications of adequate assessment. To do this, the nature of paradigms will be discussed; then the models of human psychology proposed by the consciousness disciplines and the behavioral sciences, which are both paradigms, will be outlined and compared. It will be seen that this comparison results in what Thomas Kuhn[2] called a "paradigm clash" and that unrecognized paradigmatic assumptions necessarily lead to erroneous conclusions. The methodological errors which most investigators have fallen into will then be discussed, and finally we will describe recent advances in areas of Western science which are relevant to an adequate investigation.

Since the aim of this chapter is primarily one of defining the criteria for adequate assessment, an exhaustive assessment and critique will not be presented here. This should not be seen as advocating a blanket acceptance of the consciousness disciplines, since like all psychologies they have their quota of inconsistencies. However the first step must be to determine the criteria and processes by which we are to assess them.

The term *consciousness disciplines* refers to a family of practices and philosophies of primarily Asian origin. Their central claim is that through intensive mental training, it is possible to attain states of consciousness and psychological well-being beyond those currently described by traditional Western psychologies, as well as profound insight into the nature of mental processes, consciousness, and reality. Some of these disciplines have been associated with the esoteric core of certain non-Western philosophies, psychologies, and religions (e.g., Buddhism and Hinduism). The term "consciousness disciplines" has thus sometimes been used more or less interchangeably with terms such as "Eastern traditions, psychologies, and philosophies," "mysticism," "spiritual disciplines," or the "perennial philosophy, psychology, or religion." However some of these terms have been so loosely used and misused that it is important to distinguish the consciousness disciplines from the religious dogma, beliefs, and cosmologies to which most religious devotees adhere, and from the occult popularisms of both East and West. Rather, the consciousness disciplines represent specific mental trainings designed to enhance perception and consciousness. If the individual desires, this enhancement may be used to deepen religious understanding, but it may also be employed and interpreted within a psychological framework.

PARADIGMS AND PARADIGM CLASH

Although the concepts of paradigm and paradigm clash have recently been criticized as being too loosely defined and overused they are still useful to our discussion and will be used here. We could simply speak of models or theories but since the theories we are describing are so large the term paradigm seems more useful and appropriate.

A paradigm is a kind of large theory, a theory or formulation about the nature of reality of such scope that it is capable of accounting for most of the known phenomena in its field.[2] Because of their success, paradigms tend eventually to be taken for granted and insinuate themselves into the researcher's psyche in such a way that they become implicit, unquestioned conceptual frameworks and filters which supply the "only natural and sensible" way of looking at things.[2,3] Like any model or belief, once a paradigm becomes implicit, it then acquires tremendous unrecognized controlling power over its adherents,[4] determining the investigation, perception, and interpretation of data in a self-fulfilling manner.[4-6] The introduction of a new paradigm at this stage becomes extraordinarily difficult and results in a paradigm clash.[2] In paradigm clashes, antagonism and poor communication between factions are common,[2,4,7] and even the greatest scientific innovations have frequently been discounted initially. Maruyana[7] describes the communication problems as follows:

> If the communicating parties remain unaware that they are using different structures of reasoning, but are aware of their communication difficulties only, each party tends to perceive the communication difficulties as resulting from the other party's illogicity, lack of intelligence, or even deceptiveness and insincerity. He may also fall into an illusion of understanding while being unaware of his misunderstandings.

We may now be confronting a paradigm clash between traditional Western psychological models and the models of the consciousness disciplines. If this is so, then to judge the validity of the consciousness disciplines paradigm we must also examine the presuppositions and logic of our own. Let us, therefore, begin by examining the assumptions and logic of each.

THE CONSCIOUSNESS DISCIPLINES PARADIGM

Most of the consciousness disciplines describe models of human nature which show a degree of consistency across cultures and ages, and which have been variously named "the perennial philosophy,"[8] "the perennial religion,"[9] or the "perennial psychology."[10] Obviously I cannot hope to do full justice to them here, but will attempt to delineate some of the dimensions which underlie such models and refer the interested reader elsewhere for more complete descriptions.[5,10-12,98,99]

Many traditions view consciousness as their central concern and make several claims that run counter to Western assumptions. The include statements that

1. our usual state of consciousness is severely suboptimal,
2. multiple states including true "higher states" exist,
3. these states are attainable through training, but
4. verbal communication about them is necessarily limited.

These tenets will now be examined in more detail.

Fully developed mystics state unequivocally that our usual state of consciousness is not only suboptimal, it is dreamlike and illusory. They assert that whether we know it or not, without mental training we are prisoners of our own minds, totally and unwittingly trapped by a continuous inner fantasy-dialogue which creates an all-consuming illusory distortion of perception and reality (maya or samsara). As Ram Dass remarked:

We are all prisoners of our minds. This realization is the first step on the journey to freedom.[13]

However this condition is said to go unrecognized until we begin to subject our perceptual-cognitive processes to rigorous scrutiny such as in meditation.

Thus, the "normal" person is seen as "asleep" or "dreaming." When the "dream" is especially painful or disruptive, it becomes a nightmare and is recognized as psychopathology, but since the vast majority of the population "dreams," the true state of affairs goes unrecognized. When the individual permanently disidentifies from or eradicates this dream he is said to have awakened and can now recognize the true nature of both his former state and that of the population. This awakening or enlightenment is the aim of the consciousness disciplines.[10,14-16,17]

To some extent this is an extension rather than a denial of the perspective of Western psychology and psychiatry, which have long recognized that careful experimental observation reveals a broad range of perceptual distortions unrecognized by naive subjects. The consciousness disciplines merely go further in asserting that we are all subject to distortions, that they affect all aspects of our perception, that without specific remedial mental training we remain unaware of them, and that the consensual reality we share is thus illusory. This has also been suggested by a number of Western investigators such as Erich Fromm[18] who suggested that

What is unconscious and what is conscious depends . . . on the structure of society and on the patterns of feelings and thoughts it produces. . . . The effect of society is not only to funnel fictions into our consciousness, but also to prevent awareness of reality. . . . Every society . . . determines the forms of awareness. This system works as it were, like a *socially conditioned* filter; experience cannot enter awareness unless it can penetrate the filter.[18]

The implications of this are awesome. Within the Western model we recognize and define psychosis as a suboptimal state of consciousness produced by a mind which is out of control and which views reality in a distorted way without recognizing that distortion. It is therefore significant to note that *from the mystical perspective our usual state fits all the criteria of psychosis,* being suboptimal, produced by a mind which is out of control, having a distorted view of reality, yet not recognizing that distortion. Indeed, from the ultimate mystical perspective, psychosis can be defined as being trapped in, or attached to, any *one* state of consciousness and its concomitant view of reality, each of which by itself is necessarily limited and only relatively real.[19,20]

To hold this as an interesting objective concept is one thing. To consider it as something directly applicable to our own experience is of course considerably more difficult. As Charles Tart,[21] one of the foremost researchers on the nature of consciousness and altered states, notes:

We have studied some aspects of samsara (illusion, maya) in far more detail than the Eastern traditions that orginated the concept of samsara. Yet almost no psychologists apply this idea to themselves. They assume . . . that their own states of consciousness are basically logical and clear. Western psychology now has a challenge to recognize this detailed evidence that our "normal state" is a state of samsara. (p. 286)

Of course it is very difficult, if not impossible, to recognize the limitations of the usual state of consciousness if that is all one has ever known. However, mystics repeatedly claim that anyone who is willing to undertake the strenuous but necessary training to extract awareness from the conditioned tyranny of the mind will be able to look back and see the formerly unrecognized limitations within which they lived. This process of reevaluating one state of consciousness from the perspective of another is called subrationing.[22] A common present-day analogy is that of people who live in a chronically smog ridden urban environment but only recognize the full extent of the pollution once they get out of it.

Most traditions acknowledge a wide spectrum of states of consciousness. In some disciplines, especially those emphasizing the importance of meditation (e.g., Buddhist psychology), this spectrum is described in considerable detail. Descriptions of the phenomenology of individual component states, and the techniques for attaining them, provide an articulate cartography of altered states.[10,16,17,23-25]

While knowledge of these many states is best obtained by direct experience, their existence has been recognized and acknowledged by some nonpractitioners. Perhaps the earliest and most eminent psychologist was William James[26] who around the turn of the century remarked:

> Our normal waking consciousness is but one special type of consciousness, while all about it parted from it by the filmiest of screens there lie potential forms of consciousness entirely different. We may go through life without suspecting their existence, but apply the requisite stimulus and at a touch they are there in all their completeness. . . .
>
> No account of the universe in its totality can be final which leaves these other forms of consciousness quite disregarded. How to regard them is the question. . . . At any rate, they forbid our premature closing of accounts with reality.

It is not just the existence of multiple states which is held to be important, but the fact that they may be associated with state specific properties, functions, and abilities. Perceptual sensitivity and clarity; attention, responsivity, sense of identity; affective, cognitive, and perceptual processes—all may vary with the state of consciousness in apparently precise and predictable ways.[17,24,27]

Some of these states are held to be functionally specific and a few to be true higher states. Functionally specific states are those in which specific functions can be performed better than in the usual state, though other functions may be less effective. True higher states are those which possess all the effective functions of the usual condition plus additional ones.[21,28]

Such states may be accompanied by perceptions, insights, and affects outside the realm of day-to-day untrained experience, some of which are held to be central to the growth of true higher wisdom.

Different traditions emphasize different techniques and combinations of techniques to obtain control over consciousness and perception, and the interested reader is referred elsewhere for a detailed classification of these practices.[10,12,17] In summary, it can be said that all involve training in controlling one or more aspects of perceptual sensitivity, concentration, affect, or cognition. The intensity and duration of training usually needed to attain mastery in these disciplines may be quite extraordinary by Western standards, and is usually reckoned in decades. In the words of Ramana Maharshi, perhaps the most respected Hindu teacher of the last century:

No one succeeds without effort. Mind control is not your birthright. Those who succeed owe their liberation to perseverance.[25]

The Swiss existential psychiatrist Medard Boss,[29] one of the first Westerners to examine both the Eastern and Western literature *and practice,* noted that compared with the extent of yogic self-exploration "even the best Western training analysis is not much more than an introductory course."

It may be, therefore, that we have underestimated the degree of dysfunction of our usual state, as well as the potential and the work required for observing and removing that dysfunction. As Jacob Needleman observes,

In our modern world it has always been assumed . . . that in order to observe oneself all that is required is for a person to "look within." No one ever imagines that self observation may be a highly disciplined skill which requires longer training than any other skill we know of. . . . In contrast to this one could very well say that the heart of the psychological disciplines in the East and the ancient Western world consists of training at self study.[100]

If one considers the different levels and aims of psychotherapeutic intervention, they may be broadly categorized as traditionally therapeutic (reducing pathology and enhancing adjustment), existential (confronting the questions and problems of existence and one's response to them), and soteriological (enlightenment, liberation, transcendence of the problems first confronted at the existential level).[101] Western psychologies and therapies focus on the first two levels[30] but have, as Gordon Allport noted, "on the psychology of liberation—nothing."[9]

Yet the human condition appears to include further possibilities: "what has been called 'salvation' by the Christians, 'liberation' and 'enlightenment' by the Buddhists, and love and union by the non-theistic humanist."[31] It is this latter level which is the primary goal of the consciousness disciplines.[24]

Interestingly enough, although these disciplines may start from different places and employ different approaches, they all aim for similar, though not necessarily identical,[12] soteriological states of consciousness, known by a variety of names such as enlightenment, samadhi, nirvana, liberation, etc.[9,13,15,17,19,32,33] This might be seen in general systems terms as "equifinality," in which a similar end stage is attained independent of the pathway by which it is reached.[34]

Although the instructions for attaining them may be quite explicit, the verbal descriptions of the states themselves are often considerably less so. This brings us to the last tenet of the consciousness disciplines which we will list in this section, namely the claim that language and even thought are inappropriate and inadequate modes with which to fully comprehend some of these phenomena.[10,102] For example, the Buddha, although clearly capable of the most sophisticated logical analysis[35] and "a thinker of unexcelled philosophic power,"[36] repeatedly stated that "the deepest secrets of the world and of man are inaccessible to abstract philosophical thinking."[37] Rather, students are told that they must experience these things directly for themselves if they are to have any true understanding.

THE BEHAVIORAL SCIENCES PARADIGM

There is nothing more difficult than to become critically aware of the presuppositions of one's own thought. . . . Every thought can be scrutinized directly except the thought by which we scrutinize.[38]

Perhaps the hardest part of assessing any paradigm or model is to examine the paradigm or model with which we are doing the assessing. The latter paradigm is so hard to look at because it is this with which we are doing the looking. Thus, we need to first become aware of our own (usually unrecognized) assumptions and beliefs in order to begin to recognize their possible distorting and biasing effects. The failure to take this difficult but essential step seems to have marred most previous assessments of the consciousness disciplines. Often what has not fitted within our own a priori system has automatically been assumed to be either false or pathological.[39]

What, then, are some of these relevant implicit assumptions of Western science? Concerning consciousness, the traditional behavioral sciences usually recognize only a limited number of normal states such as waking, dreaming, and nondreaming sleep. Very few others are recognized and are inevitably held to be pathological (e.g., delirium, psychosis). In addition the usual waking state is held to be optimal, predominantly rational, and under relatively good intellectual control.[4,40] Thus, no serious consideration is given to the possibility of the existence of either functionally specific or true higher states.

A similar situation exists for perception, for it is commonly assumed that ordinary perception is as close to optimum as is humanly possible. For example, concentration, the ability to consciously focus and fix perception, has been tacitly assumed to be trainable only slightly ever since William James at the turn of the century suggested an upper limit of three seconds for concentration on any one object.[26] This is very different from the statements of advanced yogis from a variety of cultures and disciplines who have frequently been observed to remain motionless for hours or days, and who claim that during that time they remained unshakably concentrated on their object of meditation.[17,24,41]

In the Western sciences, the intellect and objectivity reign supreme. All phenomena are held to be ultimately capable of examination by intellectual analysis, and such analysis is viewed as the optimal path to knowledge. A corollary of this is that all experiences are usually thought to be essentially verbally encodable and communicable. A final premise, which Western critics of mysticism have practiced, is that an intellectual, nonexperiential, nonpractical examination and appraisal of other traditions and practices represents an adequate approach for determining their worth.

COMPARING PARADIGMS

We can now examine each paradigm from the perspective of the other and observe how the two conceptual frameworks interact to produce a paradigm clash. Let us first view the claims and models of the consciousness disciplines from within the Western framework.

First, with respect to consciousness, since the Western model holds the usual state to be optimal, all claims for the existence of true higher states will automatically be dismissed. Not only will they be dismissed, but because these experiences are unknown to the usual state, they are necessarily viewed as pathological. For example, the experience of satori or shorter-lived transcendental experiences include a sense of unity or at-oneness with the universe.[10,42,43] However since unity experiences have been recognized by Western psychology and psychiatry only when associated with severe psychopathology, then reports of transcendental experiences have frequently been interpreted as evidence of severe regression such as to fetal stages or union with the primal breast.[44] This is a classic example of the pre-trans fallacy: the problem of confusing pre-egoic and transegoic stages of development.[12,45]

On the other hand, the yogi's claim that our usual state of consciousness is limited, fantasy filled, unclear and illusory, necessarily makes little sense to the Western scientist or mental health practitioner who has neither experienced clearer states nor rigorously examined his or her own consciousness. Fortunately, this is one claim where personal testing is relatively easy by any individual willing to undertake intensive practice of any of those meditative disciplines which aim specifically at examining the workings of mind. As a number of behavioral scientists have reported from personal experience, even within a few days of intensive investigation, the irrational, unclear, and uncontrollable nature of the untrained mind will rapidly become apparent, and the investigators will find themselves amazed that they had previously remained so unaware of these phenomena.[16,25,46-48,103,104]

The claim that the intellect is an inadequate and inappropriate epistemological tool for the comprehension of the reality revealed by the consciousness disciplines will meet with little understanding among traditional behavioral sciences. However, those who have examined the implications of recent advances in physics will be less surprised.[49,50]

Traditionally, three distinct modes of acquiring knowledge have been recognized in Western philosophy: Perception, cognition, and contemplation/meditation.[51,52] Each of these modes has its own unique properties and areas which are not fully overlapping and which cannot be fully reduced one to another, without producing what is called category error. Thus, in Western epistemological language the consciousness disciplines' claim for the inappropriateness of the intellect as the sole judge of yogic insights may be seen as a plea against category error.

When the yogi claims that physical empirical approaches are never appropriate or the scientist denies the validity of contemplation, then both are guilty of category error, meditation becomes pseudophilosophy, and science becomes scientism. It may be that these modes and types of knowledge are complementary, just as the wave and particle descriptions of subatomic particles are complementary. Thus, neither mode of knowing may encompass the totality, but rather each may see only that portion for which it is adequate, so that what is required for a fuller picture is a "dynamic epistemology."[53,54]

The claim that mystical experiences cannot be verbally communicated has traditionally met with little sympathy. However, this statement may be reasonable if we remember that language is conceptual and hence may result in category error when applied to nonconceptual material. Also, language may be excellent for communicating about experiences which people have in common, but otherwise surprisingly inefficient.[55] No overlapping experience means very little or no communication, e.g., the description of the color green for a blind person. This limitation is particularly evident in communication about altered states of consciousness and will be discussed in more detail subsequently.

However, mystics are not the only ones who claim that it is impossible to fully communicate the fundamental nature of reality with language. A number of scientists, working at the farther edges of their field, have reached the same conclusion and nowhere is this clearer than in the realms of quantum physics. Consider, for example, the words of the renowned physicist Walter Heisenberg:[56]

> In quantum theory . . . we have at first no simple guide for correlating the mathematical symbols with concepts of ordinary language; and the only thing we know from the start is the fact that our common concepts cannot be applied to the structure of atoms.

In addition, it seems that English is poorly equipped to deal with precise descriptions and analysis of consciousness, having a very limited descriptive vocabulary in this area compared to some other languages, e.g., Pali.[21] Since "we dissect nature along lines laid down by our native languages,"[57] which form the basis for our social construction of reality,[58] our linguistic limitations may limit our understanding and development in the areas of the consciousness disciplines.

Let us now shift perspectives and examine the Western model from the viewpoint of the consciousness disciplines. Since it involves a significantly wider range of states of consciousness and perceptual modes, the consciousness disciplines model is seen to be a broader one than that of the Western behavioral sciences. Indeed the Western model might be seen as a limiting case of the mystical model. The Western model, then, may have a position vis-à-vis the mystical model comparable to the Newtonian model vis-à-vis an Einsteinian model in physics. The Newtonian case applies to macroscopic objects moving at relatively low velocities compared to the speed of light. When applied to high-velocity objects, the Newtonian model no longer fits. The Einsteinian model, on the other hand, encompasses both low and high speeds, and from this broader perspective, the Newtonian model and its limitations are all perfectly logical and understandable (employing Einsteinian and not Newtonian logic, or course). However, the reverse is definitely untrue, for the Einsteinian logic is not comprehensible within a Newtonian framework. Furthermore, for a Newtonian physicist, reports of incongruous findings such as the constancy of the speed of light and objects increasing in mass at high speed are incomprehensible and suspect.

In terms of abstract set theory, the Newtonian model can be seen as a subset nested within the larger Einsteinian set. The properties of the subset are readily comprehensible from the perspective of the set, but the reverse is necessarily untrue. The general principle is that to try to examine the larger model or set from the perspective of the smaller is inappropriate and necessarily productive of false conclusions.

The implications of this for the comparison and assessment of the consciousness disciplines and Western behavioral sciences should now be clear. From a multiple states of consciousness model, the traditional Western approach is recognized as a relativistically useful model provided that, because of the limitations imposed by state dependency, it is not applied inappropriately to altered states outside its scope. From the Western perspective, however, the consciousness disciplines model must *necessarily* appear incomprehensible and nonsensical.

Once the possibilities of a multiple states model and the resultant paradigm clash are recognized, then it also becomes possible to obtain a different perspective on the relationships between different psychologies. Proponents of individual psychologies have usually argued for the superiority of their system and the incorrectness of others. However recently it has been suggested that various Western and non-Western psychologies and consciousness disciplines may, in part, address themselves to different states of consciousness and structures of the unconscious.[4,9,10,12,25,45,59] Therefore, different psychologies may not necessarily be oppositional. Rather they may to some extent be complementary, describing different perspectives, dimensions, states of consciousness, and layers of the unconscious, all of which may be relatively but incompletely correct.[5,10]

An interesting aside to this discussion concerns the implications of this spectrum of consciousness, or multiple states, model to the great religions. At their most esoteric and practical, certain aspects of the great religions are synonymous with the consciousness disciplines and can be considered as state specific technologies whose teaching and practices are designed to induce transcendental states. Thus, it may be possible to develop a state dependent psychology of religion and to recognize that the potential for achieving deeply transcendent and noetic states, which may be interpreted either religiously or psychologically as one chooses, may be inherent in all of us.[4,5,10,12,45]

METHODOLOGICAL PROBLEMS IN THE APPRAISAL OF THE CONSCIOUSNESS DISCIPLINES

In addition to the paradigmatic clash described above, a significant number of deficiencies of logic, knowledge, methodology, and experience mar most appraisals. Western investigators of the mystical literature almost invariably focus on the powerful, dramatic, and unusual experiences which yogis encounter. These span the whole range of human experience from unpatterned sensations, to muscular spasms, complex images, and intense effects. Such experiences are quite common for individuals commencing intensive practices and appear to reflect a deepening sensitivity to formerly subliminal mental processes as well as the appearance of formerly repressed material.[48,60] What investigators have not realized is that such experiences are not the goal of mystical traditions. Advanced practitioners view them merely as epiphenomena to be treated with detachment and benign neglect.[61]

Thus, a well-known Zen story tells of a student being taught to meditate on his breath who one day rushed to his master saying that he had seen images of a golden Buddha radiating light. "Ah yes," said the master, "But don't worry, if you keep your mind on the breath it'll go away." Western investigators have thus tended to base their assessment of mysticism on the very phenomena which the mystics themselves warn against taking seriously!

This assessment has also been founded on an intellectual analysis of the mystical literature, without examination or personal experience of mystical *practice*. However, mystics have explicitly warned against this, stating that deep conceptual understanding is dependent upon adequate personal experience.

> Without practice, without contemplation, a merely intellectual, theoretical, and philosophical approach to Buddhism is quite inadequate. . . . Mystical insights . . . cannot be judged by unenlightened people from the worm's eye view of book learning, and a little book knowledge does not really entitle anyone to pass judgement on mystical experiences.[62]

Several lines of evidence lend support to this claim. Several initially skeptical Western behavioral scientists with personal experience of these disciplines have remarked that only after they began practice, did some of the statements and claims which initially made little or no sense gradually become comprehensible.[46,47,61] The discussion earlier which noted the different modes and types of knowledge[51,52,56] is also supportive since it recognizes that to equate conceptual and contemplative knowledge may result in category error. Similarly, the recent recognition of state dependent phenomena such as state dependent learning and communication (to be discussed in more detail shortly) is consistent with the claim that this "is a learning in which a basic requirement is: First change your consciousness."[63]

Two philosophical principles are also relevant. the first is *adequatio* (adequateness) which states that the understanding of the knower must be adequate to the thing to be known.[38] Closely related is the concept of "grades of significance." The same phenomenon may hold entirely different grades of meaning and significance to different observers with different degrees of *adequatio*. Thus, for an animal a particular phenomenon may be merely a colored object (which it is), while to a savage it may represent marked paper (which it is). For the average educated adult it may be a book (which again it is) which makes patently ridiculous claims about the nature of the world, while for the physicist it is a brilliant treatise on relativity revealing new insights and depths to reality. In each case the phenomenon remained the same, but its level of meaning and significance was a function of the capacity and training (*adequatio*) of the observer. The facts themselves do not carry labels indicating the appropriate level at which they ought to be considered; nor does the choice of an inadequate level lead to factual error or logical contradiction. All levels of significance up to the highest are equally factual, equally logical, equally objective. The observer who is not adequate to the higher levels of significance will not know that they are being missed.[38] As Robert Laing[64] observed, "If I don't know I don't know, I think I know." This is precisely the claim of the consciousness disciplines: namely that only through personal mental training does a person become fully adequate to, and apprehend all grades of significance of, the knowledge which is the concern of these disciplines. This claim, then, is no different in principle from the claim that scientific research is best judged by those with appropriate scientific training, only the type of training is different.

Does this mean that *only* advanced practitioners can make assessments of the consciousness disciplines, or that Western scientists must all first become yogis? Obviously not! But it does mean that Western-trained scientists must recognize that without specific preparation there may be epistemological and paradigmatic limits to one's ability to comprehend and assess these disciplines, that scientific objectivity may need to be balanced (in at least some researchers) by personal experience and training, and that cautious open-mindedness to yogic claims may be a more skillful stance than automatic rejection of anything not immediately logical and comprehensible.

RELEVANT ADVANCES IN WESTERN SCIENCE

Any examination of the consciousness traditions should take into consideration certain recent advances in Western science. These areas include transpersonal psychology, state dependent learning, meditation research, clinical and sociological studies of peak and transcendental experiences, advanced psychedelic therapy, and the frontiers of modern physics.

Transpersonal psychology emerged in the sixties as the so-called Fourth Force of Western psychology (after behaviorism, psychoanalysis, and humanistic psychology) to study areas such as extreme psychological well-being and consciousness and to integrate Western and non-Western perspectives.[5,10,11,65] As such it has been especially concerned with topics such as states of consciousness, meditation, models of psychological health, peak experiences, mystical experiences, implications of modern physics, etc. It has thus already examined many of the issues raised anew by investigators of the consciousness disciplines, who should thus be familiar with this literature.

A second area concerns research and theorizing in the field of altered states of consciousness. Both animal and human studies have shown that learning, understanding, and recall may be dependent on, and limited by, the state of consciousness.[66] Thus, information acquired in one state by an individual may be neither recallable nor comprehensible by that same individual when in another state. Similarly another individual may be quite unable to understand the communication from someone else in an altered state (state dependent communication), but may be able to do so if he or she enters that same state also.[21,28] In some cases, information initially available in only one state may subsequently be retained or more easily learned in others (cross state retention).

Since the mystical traditions employ a range of altered states, the relevance of these recent findings is readily apparent. Mystics may enter altered states and acquire formerly inaccessible knowledge. However, because of the limits set by cross state communication, this information may make little sense to another individual with no experience of that state. The easiest but also most superficial judgment would then be that the mystic was speaking incomprehensible nonsense resulting from either psychopathology or an impaired state of consciousness. However, such a conclusion is premature because only by experiencing that same state will the observer be able to rule out the possibility that the mystic is expounding valid, though state dependent, knowledge.

It has not infrequently been suggested that mystical phenomena, even the supposedly highest and most illumined transcendental experiences, are essentially pathological, representing psychotic or near psychotic regressions towards an undifferentiated infantile state of consciousness.[67] Thus, for example, Freud[68] interpreted oceanic experiences as indicative of infantile helplessness, Alexander[69] regarded meditation training as self-induced catatonia and nirvana as regression to intrauterine stages, while the Group for the Advancement of Psychiatry[70] saw "forms of behavior intermediate between normality and psychosis." Such interpretations do not seem to consider the problem of paradigm clash or the now sizable body of experimental data on the psychology or sociology of transcendental experiences.

For the purposes of this discussion the term *transcendental experience* will be confined to an experience of an altered state of consciousness characterized by:

1. ineffability: the experience is of such power and so different from ordinary experience as to give the sense of defying description;

2. noesis: a heightened sense of clarity and understanding;
3. altered perception of space and time;
4. appreciation of the holistic, unitive, integrated nature of the universe and one's unity with it;
5. intense positive affect including a sense of the perfection of the universe.

Such experiences have been called by many names, including cosmic consciousness[71] and peak experiences.[72,73] Several lines of evidence suggest that such experiences tend to occur most often among those who are psychologically most healthy.[74] Clients working at advanced stages of psychotherapy may experience them[5,11,75] as may self-actualizers, those individuals identified by Maslow[73] as most healthy. Incipient experiences may occur in most people but may be repressed or misinterpreted because of fears of loss of control and intolerance of ambiguity. Indeed, those who report such experiences tend to score lower on intolerance of ambiguity scales.[72,76] Sociological surveys suggest that transcenders are likely to be better educated, more economically successful, less racist, and score substantially higher on scores of psychological well-being.[76-80]

Such experiences may apparently produce long-lasting beneficial changes in the individual.[72,73,81,82,105] Livingston lists 129 positive residual effects which may occur and concludes that positive residua may be a defining characteristic of transcendental phenomena.[82] This echoes the ideas of Carl Jung, who was the first Western therapist to affirm the importance of transcendental experience for mental health and wrote:[83]

The fact is that the approach to the numinous is the real therapy and inasmuch as you attain to the numinous experiences you are released from the curse of pathology.

Maslow[84] states that the transcendental, or as he called it "peak" experience, is "so profound and shaking ... that it can change the person's character ... forever after." Upon his return, the person "feels himself more than at other times to be the responsible, active, the creative center of his own activities and of his own perceptions, more self determined, more of a free agent, with more 'free will' than at other times." In his final formulation of the concept of the "hierarchy of needs," Maslow came to see the seeking of transcendence as the highest of all goals, even above self-actualization.[85]

It therefore seems inappropriate to equate transcendental experiences with psychopathology and psychosis. This is not to say that similar experiences cannot occur in the mentally ill or even that transcendental experiences might not be disturbing for some individuals. Only further research will tell. What is clear is that it is no longer tenable to view transcendental experiences as necessarily, or even usually, pathological or regressive. To do so is to commit the "pre-trans fallacy"[12,45]

Recent empirical research in two other areas also supports the idea of the existence of a spectrum of transcendental states of consciousness. Meditation research is still in an early stage, but most psychological and physiological data appear to be consistent with its claims to be able to induce a range of altered states and greater mental health.[41,48,86-88,103,104,106]

The second area, recent *advanced* research with psychedelics, appears to provide an independent line of evidence supporting the existence of multiple layers of the unconscious, states of consciousness similar to those described by the consciousness disciplines, as well as the phenomenon of state dependent learning.[5,59]

It is necessary to stress the word *advanced* because it is now clear that while the usual experiments employing either low doses, relatively few sessions, or subjects suffering from some form of psychopathology may provide extremely interesting information on perception and psychodynamics, this is far from being the whole story. Higher doses, more sessions, and healthy subjects inevitably seem to lead beyond these levels in an apparently predictable fashion through a stepwise series of experiences.[59,107,108]

According to Stanislav Grof, by far the most experienced clinical researcher of psychedelics, this progression seems to reflect the uncovering of deeper and deeper layers of the unconscious. It begins with traditional psychodynamic phenomena, progresses through Rankian birth trauma-like material and Jungian symbology, and ends in a variety of transcendental experiences. Grof advances considerable evidence to demonstrate that these effects represent an uncovering of layers of the psyche rather than a "pharmacological" or "organic brain syndrome" effect. Thus Grof[59,107] suggests, as have a number of others,[10,12] that various Western and non-Western psychologies and consciousness disciplines are not necessarily oppositional, but rather may address themselves to different structures of the human unconsciousness.

The last states of consciousness to emerge during psychedelic therapy, and hence assumed to correspond to the deepest levels of the unconscious, are the transcendental. There states and accompanying experiences not only closely resemble those described by advanced practitioners of the consciousness disciplines but, once experienced, allow significant insight and understanding of these traditions.

Everyone who experientially reached these levels developed convincing insights into the utmost relevance of spiritual and religious dimensions in the universal scheme of things. Even the most hard core materialists, positivistically oriented scientists, skeptics and cynics, uncompromising atheists and antireligious crusaders such as Marxist philosophers, became suddenly interested in spiritual search after they confronted these levels in themselves.[59]

Thus, this area of research appears to provide an independent line of evidence supporting the existence and availability of states of consciousness similar to those described by the consciousness disciplines, as well as the phenomenon of state dependent learning. In view of their significance, these studies should be replicated but in the current antipsychedelic research climate this appears unlikely. Indeed, it is distressing to recognize that there has existed in both the mass media and professional journals a bias towards publishing only negative reports on the effects of psychedelics.[112,113] Consequently it is little known that there is considerable evidence demonstrating their potential for clinical research and therapy.

Another supportive research area is, strangely enough, modern physics. In recent years, the physicists' picture of the world has undergone a shift which is so radical and far reaching in its implications as to shake the very foundations of science. For the reality revealed, especially that of the subatomic level, is so discordant with our usual picture of reality, so paradoxical, as to defy description in traditional terms and theories and to call into question some of the most fundamental assumptions of Western science and philosophy. The traditional descriptions of the universe, which were largely based on Greek philosophical concepts, as atomistic, divisible, isolated, static, and nonrelativistic, are being replaced by models which acknowledge a holistic, indivisible, interconnected, dynamic, relativistic reality, which is inseparable from, and a function of, the consciousness of the observer.[10,49,50,89,90]

These same findings, which do not fit at all with our usual pictures of reality, are strikingly reminiscent of those descriptions given repeatedly across centuries and cultures by advanced practitioners of the consciousness disciplines. Indeed, physicists themselves have suggested that some discoveries can be viewed as a rediscovery of ancient wisdom.

> The general notions about human understanding . . . which are illustrated by discoveries in atomic physics are not in the nature of being wholly unfamiliar, wholly unheard of, or new. Even in our culture they have a history, and in Buddhist and Hindu thought a more considerable and central place. What we shall find is an exemplification and encouragement, and a refinement of old wisdom.[1]

> For a parallel to the lesson of atomic theory . . . [we must turn] to those kinds of epistemological problems with which already thinkers like the

Buddha and Lao Tzu have been confronted, when trying to harmonize our position as spectators and actors in the great drama of existence.[91]

Indeed, it is sometimes difficult to decide whether descriptions of this reality are excerpted from a textbook of physics or of the consciousness disciplines. Compare, for example, the description of space-time by the Buddhist master Suzuki, with that first introduced into physics by Hermann Minkowski in 1908:

We look around and perceive that . . . . every object is related to every other object . . . . not only spatially but temporally. . . . As a fact of pure experience, there is not space without time, no time without space; they are interpenetrating. (Suzuki[92])

The views of space and time which I wish to lay before you have sprung from the soil of experimental physics, and therein lies their strength. They are radical. Henceforth space by itself, and time by itself, are doomed to fade away into mere shadows, and only a kind of union of the two will preserve an independent reality. (Minkowski[93])

At the most fundamental and sensitive levels of modern physics, the emerging picture of reality appears to parallel the most fundamental picture revealed by the consciousness disciplines. Thus it may be that whether perceptual sensitivity is enhanced by instrumentation or by direct perceptual training, the resultant view of the fundamental nature of reality may be similar, and may be radically different from our usual assumptions.[94,95]

ADEQUATE ASSESSMENT OF THE CONSCIOUSNESS DISCIPLINES

What then must Western behavioral scientists do if we are to conduct truly adequate investigations of the consciousness disciplines? First and foremost, they must recognize that the task is considerably more demanding than previously thought. Given the possibility of paradigm clash, the first essential step will require a thoroughgoing examination of the beliefs, models, and paradigms we ourselves bring to the investigation. Along with this goes the need for a willingness to be open to the possibility that these disciplines may represent systems and paradigms in many ways, although in different ways, as sophisticated as our own. Thus, initially unfamiliar or incomprehensible phenomena are not to be immediately assumed to be evidence of either inferior intelligence or psychopathology. Rather, the first response must be to inquire whether the investigation process is adequate to the task.

Thus, for example, it will be especially important to remember such factors as state dependent learning, the different modes of acquiring knowledge, and the different types of knowledge which they reveal. Investigators will therefore wish to examine both the literature *and practices* of these disciplines and will recognize the need for some investigators to have personal experience of these practices.

It may be necessary to adopt new research paradigms as suggested by Tart.[21,28] In one such design, the subject would be a participant experimenter or "yogi-scientist" trained in both the behavioral sciences and the consciousness disciplines. This is obviously an extremely exacting requirement but one which may be necessary for the fullest possible understanding of these practices.

It seems prudent to heed the warnings of the advanced practitioners of these traditions and, at least initially, to focus on those phenomena which they consider central. It will also be necessary to distinguish between the central consciousness disciplines and the degenerate popularisms with which they are so often confused.

One of the most subtle yet important tasks facing investigators may be the recognition that we may experience active resistances to some of the ideas and experiences presented by these disciplines, since our most fundamental beliefs and world views may be called into question.[10,12,45,61,63,96] These difficulties and resistances have been specifically noted by mystics who warn the investigator:

This is why it is so difficult to explain the path to one who has not tried: he will see only his point of view of today or rather the loss of his point of view. And yet if we only knew how each loss of one's viewpoint is a progress and how life changes when one passes from the stage of the closed truth to the stage of the open truth—a truth like life itself, too great to be trapped by points of view, because it embraces every point of view ... a truth great enough to deny itself and pass endlessly into a higher truth.[97]

This advice from the mystics is curiously similar to the solution suggested by William James.[109] He proposed that the key to the progression to broader perspectives for both the individual and for psychology as a whole lay in the recognition that

there is "always more," outgrowing the bonds of present self limitation for the apprehension of present reality, and the developing openness upon which the germinal—or not yet germinal—potentialities for new reals may come into existence ... not only with the real which can be independently shown to be real by ... now sober methods, but with the real which newly comes into existence as evolution goes on.

It is this openness to the "always more," this willingness to at least temporarily go beyond one's current viewpoint, which allows us to recognize that any viewpoint, theory, or paradigm is necessarily limited and selective in what it allows us to see and that there always exist undreamt of realms beyond its range.[110] It is this recognition and the willingness to explore both novel realms and novel viewpoints which, when combined with the best of the methodological rigor of the behavioral sciences and of the experiential training of the consiousness disciplines, may provide an optimal approach to exploring both paradigms.

REFERENCES

1. Oppenheimer, J.R. *Science and the Common Understanding*. New York: Simon and Schuster, 1954.
2. Kuhn, T.S. *The Structure of Scientific Revolution* (2nd ed.). Chicago: University of Chicago Press, 1970.
3. Wilson, T. Normative and interpretive paradigms in sociology. In *Understanding Everyday Life* (J. Douglas, Ed.) Chicago: Aldine, 1970.
4. Tart, C. (Ed.). *Transpersonal Psychologies*. New York: Harper & Row, 1975.
5. Walsh, R.N. and Vaughan, F. (Eds.). *Beyond Ego: Transpersonal Dimensions in Psychology*. Los Angeles: J. Tarcher Press, 1980.
6. Allport, G.W. *Personality: A Psychological Interpretation*. New York: Holt, 1937.
7. Maruyana, M. Paradigms and communication. *Technological Forecasting and Social Change*, 1974, *6*, 3–32.
8. Huxley, A. *The Perennial Philosophy*. New York: Harper & Row, 1944.
9. Smith, H. *Forgotten Truth*. New York: Harper & Row, 1976.
10. Wilber, K. *The Spectrum of Consciousness*. Wheaton, Ill.: Theosophical Publishing House, 1977.
11. Walsh, R. and Vaughan, F. Beyond the ego: toward transpersonal models of the person and psychotherapy. *Journal of Humanistic Psychology*, 1980, *20*, 5–31.
12. Wilber, K. *The Atman Project*. Wheaton, Ill.: Theosophical Publishing House, 1980.
13. Ram Dass. *Association of Transpersonal Psychology Newsletter*, 1975, *9* (winter).
14. Ram Dass. *The Only Dance There Is*. New York: Doubleday, 1975.
15. Ram Dass. Freeing the mind. *Journal of Transpersonal Psychology*, 1976, *8*, 133–140.
16. Goldstein, J. *The Experience of Insight*. Santa Cruz, Calif.: Unity Press, 1976.
17. Goleman, D. *The Varieties of the Meditative Experience*. New York: Dutton, 1977.
18. Fromm, E., Suzuki, D.T. and DeMartino, R. *Zen Buddhism and Psychoanalysis*. New York: Harper & Row, 1970.
19. Ram Dass. *Grist for the Mill*. Santa Cruz, California: Unity Press, 1977.
20. Ram Dass. *Journey of Awakening: A Meditator's Guidebook*. New York: Doubleday, 1978.
21. Tart, C. *States of Consciousness*. New York: Dutton, 1975.
22. Deutsch, E. *Advaita Vedanta: A Philosophical Reconstruction*. Honolulu: East West Center Press, 1969.
23. Buddhagosa. *The Path of Purity* (P.M. Tin, translator). Sri Lanka: Pali Text Society, 1923.
24. Brown, D. A model for the levels of concentrative meditation. *International Journal of Clinical and Experimental Hypnosis* 1977, *25*, 236–273.
25. Kornfield, J. *Living Buddhist Masters*. Santa Cruz, Calif.: University Press, 1977.
26. James, W. *The Principles of Psychology*. New York: Dover Publications, 1950.

27. Goleman, D. and Epstein, M. Meditation and well-being: An eastern model of psychological health. This book.
28. Tart, C. States of consciousness and state specific sciences. *Science*, 1972, *176*, 1203–1210.
29. Boss, M. *A Psychiatrist Discovers India*. New York: Basic Books, 1963.
30. Thetford, W., Schucman, H. and Walsh, R. Other psychological theories. In *Comprehensive Textbook of Psychiatry* (A. Freedman, H. Kaplan, and B. Sadock, Eds.; 3rd ed.) Baltimore: Williams and Wilkins, 1980, pp. 868–894.
31. Fromm, E. and Xirau, R. *The Nature of Man*. New York: Macmillan, 1968.
32. Wilber, K. The ultimate state of consciousness. *Journal of Altered States of Consciousness*, 1975, *2*, 231–242.
33. Johannson, R. *The Psychology of Nirvana*. London: George Allen and Unwin, 1969.
34. Bertalanffy, V. *General Systems Theory*. New York: Braziller, 1969.
35. Owens, D.M. Zen Buddhism. In *Transpersonal Psychologies* (C. Tart, Ed.). New York: Harper & Row, 1975.
36. Burtt, E. *The Teachings of the Compassionate Buddha*. New York: Mentor, 1955.
37. Govinda, L.A. *Psychological Attitude of Early Buddhist Philosophy*. New York: Viking Press, 1975.
38. Schumacher, E.F. *A Guide for the Perplexed*. New York: Harper & Row, 1977.
39. Elgin, D. *Voluntary Simplicity*. New York: Morrow, 1981.
40. Frank, J.D. Nature and function of belief systems: Humanism and transcendental religion. *American Psychologist*, 1977, *32*, 555–559.
41. White, J. (Ed.). *The Highest State of Consciousness*. New York: Doubleday, 1973.
42. James, W. *The Varieties of Religious Experience*. New York: Collier Books, 1961.
43. Kapleau, P. *The Three Pillars of Zen*. Boston: Beacon Press, 1967.
44. Lewin, B. *The Psychoanalysis of Elation*. New York: Psychoanalytic Quarterly, 1961.
45. Wilber, K. A developmental model of consciousness. In *Beyond Ego: Transpersonal Dimensions in Psychology* (R. Walsh and F. Vaughan, Eds.). Los Angeles: J. Tarcher Press, 1980, pp. 99–115.
46. Walsh, R. Initial meditative experiences: I. *Journal of Transpersonal Psychology*, 1977, *9*, 151–192.
47. Walsh, R. Initial meditative experiences: II. *Journal of Transpersonal Psychology*, 1978, *10*, 1–28.
48. Walsh, R. Meditation. In *A Handbook of Innovative Psychotherapies* (R. Corsini, Ed.). New York: Wiley, 1980.
49. Capra, F. *The Tao of Physics*. Berkeley: Shambhala, 1975.
50. Zukav, G. *The Dancing Wu Li Masters: An Overview of the New Physics*. New York: Morrow, 1979.
51. Wilber, K. Eye to eye: Transpersonal psychology and science. *ReVision*, 1979, *2*, 3–25.
52. Wilber, K. Eye to eye. In *Beyond Ego: Transpersonal Dimensions in Psychology* (R. Walsh and F. Vaughan, Eds.). Los Angeles: J. Tarcher Press, 1980, pp. 216–221.
53. Globus, G. Potential contributions of meditation to neurosciences. In *The Science of Meditation: Research, Theory, and Experience* (D. Shapiro and R. Walsh, Eds.). New York: Aldine (in press).
54. Vaughan, F. *Awakening Intuition*. New York: Doubleday, 1979.
55. Maslow, A.H. *The Psychology of Science*. Chicago: Gateway, 1966.
56. Heisenberg, W. *Physics and Philosophy*. New York: Harper Torchbooks, 1958.
57. Whorf, B.L. *Language, Thought, and Reality*. Cambridge: MIT Press, 1956.
58. Berger, P. and Luckman, T. *The Social Construction of Reality: A Treatise on the Sociology of Knowledge*. New York: Anchor, 1966.
59. Grof, S. *Realms of the Human Unconscious: Observations from LSD Research*. New York: Viking Press, 1975.
60. Kornfield, J. Intensive insight meditation: A phenomenological study. *Journal of Transpersonal Psychology*, 1979, *11*, 41–58.
61. Deikman, A. Comments on the GAP report on mysticism. *Journal of Nervous and Mental Disease*, 1977, *165*, 213–217.
62. Vimalo, B. Awakening to the truth. Thailand, Visaka Puja: *Annual Publication of the Buddhist Association*, 1974, 53–79.

63. Rajneesh, B.S. *Just Like That*. Poona, India: Rajneesh Foundation, 1975.
64. Laing, R.D. *Knots*. New York: Pantheon, 1970.
65. Wilber, K. *No Boundary*. Los Angeles: Center Press, 1979.
66. Overton, D.A. Discriminative control of behavior by drug states. In *Stimulus Properties of Drugs* (T. Thompson and R. Pickens, Eds.). New York: Appleton-Century-Crofts, 1971.
67. Ostow, M. Antinomianism, mysticism, and psychosis. *Psychedelic Drugs,* 1969, 177–185.
68. Freud, S. *Civilization and Its Discontents*. New York: W.W. Norton and Company, 1962.
69. Alexander, F. Buddhistic training as an artificial catatonia: The biological meaning of psychic occurrences. *Psychoanalytic Review,* 1931, *18*, 129–145.
70. Group for the Advancement of Psychiatry. *Mysticism: Spiritual Quest or Psychic Disorder?* New York: Group for the Advancement of Psychiatry, 1976.
71. Bucke, W. From self to cosmic consciousness. In *The Highest State of Consciousness* (J. White, Ed.). Garden City, N.Y.: Doubleday, 1972.
72. Maslow, A.H. *Religions, Values, and Peak Experience*. New York: Viking, 1964.
73. Maslow, A.H. *The Farther Reaches of Human Nature*. New York: Viking, 1971.
74. Wuthnow, R. *Peak experiences: Some empirical tests*. *Journal of Humanistic Psychology,* 1978, *18*, 59–75.
75. Bugental, J. *Psychotherapy and Process*. New York: Addison Wesley, 1978.
76. Thomas, L. and Cooper, P. Incidence and psychological correlates of intense spiritual experiences. *Journal of Transpersonal Psychology,* 1980, *12*, 75–85.
77. Greeley, A.M. *The Sociology of the Paranormal*. Beverly Hills, Calif.: Sage, 1975.
78. Allison, J. Adaptive regression and intense religious experience. *Journal of Nervous and Mental Disease,* 1967, *145*, 452–463.
79. Hood, R.W. Psychological strength and the report of intense religous experience. *Journal of Scientific Study of Religion,* 1974, *13*, 65–71.
80. Hood, R. Conceptual criticisms of regressive explanations of mysticism. *Review of Religious Research,* 1976, *17*, 179–188.
81. Chaudhuri, H. Psychology: Humanistic and transpersonal. *Journal of Humanistic Psychology,* 1975, *15*, 17–15.
82. Livingston, D. Transcendental states of consciousness and the healthy personality: An overview. Ph.D. thesis. University of Arizona, 1975.
83. Jung, C.G. Letters (G. Adler, Ed.). Princeton, N.J.: Princeton University Press, 1973.
84. Maslow, B.G. *Abraham H. Maslow: A Memorial Volume*. Monterey, Calif.: Brooks Cole, 1972.
85. Roberts, T. Beyond self actualization. *ReVision,* 1978, *1*, 42–46.
86. Shapiro, D. and Giber, D. Meditation: Self control strategy and altered states of consciousness. *Archives of General Psychiatry,* 1978, *35*, 294–302.
87. Shapiro, D. *Meditation: Self Regulation Strategy and Altered States of Consciousness*. New York: Aldine Press, 1980.
88. Walsh, R. Meditation research: An introduction and overview. *Journal of Transpersonal Psychology,* 1979, *11*, 161–174.
89. Bohm, D. Quantum theory as an indication of a new order in physics, B: Implicate and explicate order in physical law. *Foundations of Physics,* 1973, *2*, 139–168.
90. Beynam, L. The emergent paradigm in science. *ReVision,* 1978, *1*, 56–72.
91. Bohr, N. *Atomic Physics and Human Knowledge*. New York: Wiley, 1958.
92. Suzuki, D.T. Preface. In Suzuki, B.L. *Mahayana Buddhism*. London: Allen and Unwin, 1959.
93. Einstein, A. *The Principle of Relativity*. New York: Dover, 1923.
94. Walsh, R. Possible cross disciplinary parallels: Suggestions from the neurosciences. *Journal of Transpersonal Psychology,* 1979, *11*, 175–184.
95. Wilber, K. Physics, mysticism, and the new holographic paradigm. *Revision,* 1979, *2*, 43–55.
96. Goleman, D. Perspectives on psychology, reality, and the study of consciousness. *Journal of Transpersonal Psychology,* 1974, *6*, 73–85.
97. Satprem. *Sri Aurobindo or the Adventure of Consciousness*. New York: Harper & Row, 1968.

98. Hoffman, E. The Kabbalah: Its implications for humanistic psychology. *Journal of Humanistic Psychology,* 1980, *20,* 33–48.
99. Halevi, Z. *The Way of Kabbalah.* New York: Samuel Weiser, 1976.
100. Needleman, J. *A Sense of the Cosmos: The Encounter of Modern Science and Ancient Truth.* New York: Doubleday, 1976.
101. Vaughan, F. Transpersonal psychotherapy: Context, content, and process. In *Beyond Ego: Transpersonal Dimensions in Psychology* (R. Walsh and F. Vaughan, Eds.). Los Angeles: J. Tarcher Press, 1980, pp. 182–189.
102. Wilber, K. Two modes of knowing. In *Beyond Ego: Transpersonal Dimensions in Psychology* (R. Walsh and F. Vaughan, Eds.). Los Angeles: J. Tarcher Press, 1980, pp. 234–240.
103. Mahasi Sayadaw. *The Progress of Insight.* Kandy, Sri Lanka: Buddhist Publication Society, 1978.
104. Kornfield, J. Meditation: Aspects of theory and practice. In *Beyond Ego: Transpersonal Dimensions in Psychology* (R. Walsh and F. Vaughan, Eds.) Los Angeles: J. Tarcher Press, 1980, pp. 150–153.
105. Panzarella, R. The phenomenology of aesthetic peak experiences. *Journal of Humanistic Psychology,* 1980, *20,* 69–86.
106. Walsh, R. Meditation research: The evolution and state of the art. In *Beyond Ego: Transpersonal Dimensions in Psychology* (R. Walsh and F. Vaughan, Eds.). Los Angeles: J. Tarcher Press, 1980, pp. 154–160.
107. Grof, S. Realms of the human unconscious: Observations from LSD research. In *Beyond Ego: Transpersonal Dimensions in Psychology* (R. Walsh and F. Vaughan, Eds.). Los Angeles: J. Tarcher Press, 1980, pp. 87–99.
108. Pahnke, W. and Richards, W. Implications of LSD and experimental mysticism. *Journal of Religious Health,* 1966, *5,* 175–208.
109. James, W. *Psychology: Briefer Course.* New York: Hold and Company, 1910.
110. Erhard, W., Gioscia, V. and Anbender, K. Being well. This book.
111. Hixon, L. *Coming Home: The Experience of Enlightenment in the Sacred Traditions.* New York: Doubleday, 1978.
112. Grinspoon, L. and Bakalar, J. (Eds.). *Psychedelic Reflections.* New York, Human Sciences Press, 1982.
113. Walsh, R. Psychedelics and psychological well-being. *Journal of Humanistic Psychology,* 1982, (In press).

II
WESTERN PERSPECTIVES

Each being contains in itself the whole intelligible world.
Therefore, All is everywhere. . . .
Man as he is now has ceased to be the All.
But when he ceases to be a mere ego,
he raises himself again and penetrates the whole world.

Plotinus

What is the "I" which seeks or experiences well-being? This certainly seems a reasonable and relatively straightforward question from which to start our exploration of psychological health. Straightforward, that is, until we look below the level of our usual assumptions.

For what Ken Wilber suggests by integrating among an exceptionally broad range of psychologies is that what we assume to be our self or "I" and what we assume to be not-self or "It," as well as the boundaries between them, are extraordinarily plastic and arbitrary. Indeed the scope of our self-sense seems to parallel our degree of well-being, and may range from the drastically narrowed persona which we usually assume to be the norm and the limit of our identity, through successive mergings with what were formerly assumed to be various Its, to ultimately encompass the entire universe. At this point there are no Its, for all that was It has become I. Wilber suggests that various psychologies and psychotherapies have addressed different levels of this spectrum of identity and that the failure to recognize this fact accounts for much of the confusion and apparent contradiction which characterize the competing claims of different schools. The degree of integration and synthesis which this chapter suggests is quite extraordinary.

Ken Wilber is one of the most prolific and erudite writers in the fields of transpersonal psychology and consciousness. He is probably the major integrator and synthesizer of both psychologies and religions, both Western and non-Western, in the world today and draws on a prodigious range of knowledge from psychology, philosophy, religion, and science. His major books include The Spectrum of Consciousness *(Quest, 1977),* No Boundary *(Centre Press, 1979),* The Atman Project *(Quest, 1980),* Up From Eden *(Doubleday, 1981), and* A Sociable God *(MacMillan, 1982). He is the editor of the journal* ReVision *and a student of Zen.*

4

Where It Was, There I Shall Become: Human Potential and the Boundaries of the Soul

Ken Wilber

There is only the fight to recover what has been lost.

T. S. Eliot[1]

It is probably true that the organized search for expanded human potentials began in the modern West with the solitary figure of the "nerve doctor of Vienna": Herr Sigmund Freud. For Freud's discoveries—which we will presently examine in summary form—actually set the stage for the scientific, or at least the highly disciplined, Western search for hidden human potentials. With Freud's discoveries there began, for the first time in the modern Western world, the disciplined, organized, and incredible search and re-search for the lost potentials of the human mind, body, and soul. In the closing decades of the twentieth century, this search has apparently been destined to discover, or rather rediscover, in the depths of the human spirit, a potential that seems to many researchers so deep and vast and profound that it is no longer individual, but cosmic; no longer human, but divine; no longer only immanent, but transcendent as well. It is just this search for—and just this ultimate rediscovery of—the profoundest depths of human potential and the "farthest reaches of human nature" that I would like briefly to chronicle in this chapter, while, at the same time, setting forth some simple and general observations on the nature of human potential itself—its qualities and quantities, as it were—and the basic conditions necessary to elicit this potential. However, we begin at the beginning: with Freud himself.

In a now-famous passage from the *New Introductory Lectures,* Freud states that the therapeutic intent of psychoanalysis is "to strengthen the ego . . . , to widen its field of perception and enlarge its organization, so that it can appropriate fresh portions of the id. Where id was, there ego shall be."[1] Viewed in its simplest terms, this *reclamation* (which Freud likened to the Zuider Zee project) and integration of the lost or repressed aspects of the self—"*where id was, there ego shall be*"—remains to this day the major aim and goal of psychoanalysis. Thus in the widely circulated text on the *Technique and Practice of Psychoanalysis,* Greenson noted: "Resolving the neurotic conflicts means reuniting with the conscious ego those portions of the id, superego, and unconscious ego which had been excluded from the maturational processes of the healthy remainder of the total personality."[2] As Fenichel said, "The therapeutic task, then, is to reunite with the conscious ego the contents . . . which have been withheld from consciousness by countercathexis [repressing forces], that is, to abolish the effectiveness of the countercathexis."[3]

As succinct as these statements are, they nevertheless abound with technical jargon and complex conceptual ideas. Indeed, the whole theoretical framework of psychoanalysis is so vastly complex and intricate that literally years are required just to master the essential elements of the system. Yet the very complexity of the psychoanalytic framework—essential as it otherwise is—has actually served to obscure and mystify the essentially simple and straightforward message of Freud. Let us then, using Freud's own words, examine the essence and core of "reuniting ego and id." A brief examination of the psychoanalytic view—although it will be seen to be somewhat narrow—will nevertheless serve as an excellent introduction to the human potential in general. After all, it is important not only to discover new and vast and exciting potentials, but also to understand how we now prevent and resist the potentials we already have. What we want to examine in particular is how individuals surrender their own potentials, at *any* level. What occurs when any type of potential is alienated? What is the *form* of the lost potentials? How are they recovered? Why are they resisted? This overall resistance to aspects of our own selves is, traditionally, the domain of psychoanalytic ego psychologies.

Now I should say at the outset that this is not intended to be a simple summary of orthodox psychoanalysis or an absolutely faithful statement and explanation of purely Freudian principles. Rather, it is only a general and somewhat popular overview of the psychoanalytic orientation itself. In particular, I will be discussing the general nature of the "personal unconscious," and I will therefore be including some of the opinions of Jung, of Gestalt, of Transactional Analysis, and so on, in what may appear a rather eclectic or even indiscriminate fashion. The only reason I do this is that I want to discuss the personal unconscious in relation to some of the "deeper" or "more encompassing" structures of the psyche. And Jung's, Adler's, and Freud's views of the personal unconscious, however dissimilar they are in some aspects, are *by comparison* with these deeper structures, actually rather similar—if for no other reason than that they are *personal. In relation* to the deeper structures, these views of the personal unconscious are more similar than dissimilar, and it is in this atmosphere of general similarity that I will be proceeding. Finally, I should state that, in my opinion, Jung's view of the personal unconscious—which he called the shadow—is the more accurate one, and thus I will tend to discuss it from a Jungian perspective. To begin with, however, I will start with Freud himself.

Since this is a general and fairly popular discussion of the personal unconscious, I would like to present some tracts from Freud's only truly popular book, *The Problem of Lay-Analyses.*[4] What I find fascinating about this book is that it was the one place in which Freud really attempted to put his basic orientations into utterly simple and popular terms. For any great mind—whose owner usually tends to rather complex and formidable abstractions—this is always a revealing venture: for when the abstractions and technical jargon are set aside, and the individual tries to state in commonsense language just what he actually means, we tend to see the simple essence of the author's intellectual system emerge. At the same time, we might say that an author who cannot state the essence of his philosophic system in popular and simple terms, probably hasn't a true system to begin with, only abstractions about abstractions that, when translated into simple terms, leave not very much of substance. However, Freud passed on both counts, and in this book, *The Problem of Lay-Analyses,* we see his general and basic premises surfacing—his global "back of the head" intuitions that seem to guide all higher abstractions.

> This obscure soul apparatus, which serves as the agent for all processes of our soul, is conceived by us as an instrument consisting of several parts.[5]

He then begins to explain the two major "parts" of the soul apparatus:

> For argument's sake, let us accept the popular conception and assume that within us there is a psychical organization, recording sensations and perceptions of physical wants on the one hand, and releasing motoric actions on the other. This medium for establishing this definite cooperation we call the "I."[6]

Notice immediately that Freud uses the word "I"—not the word "ego"! In fact, in almost *all* of Freud's writings the term that his English translators rendered as "the ego" was actually *das Ich,* which is German for "the I." He used the pronoun "I," not the noun "ego." By looking to Freud's original terms, as Brandt[7] has pointed out, we recapture instantly a great portion of the basically simple and elegant message of Freud. "The ego" is an extremely difficult concept to define—no psychologist has yet perfectly done it—but all of us already know the meaning of "the I." We feel it.

So the I is one major portion of the soul apparatus as conceived by Freud: it is very simply your own immediate sensation of I-ness. You know it instantly by feeling, not remotely by definition. Freud now continues:

Aside from the "I," we perceive another region of the soul, much more extensive, much more impressive, and much more obscure than the "I," which we designate the "It."[8]

Again, how incredible! Freud does not use the word "id," which anyway is from Latin. He uses the impersonal pronoun "the It," or *das Es* in German. Thus at heart—on the immediate level of one's own experiental awareness—Freud was not concerned with the conflicts between the ego and the id, but the conflicts between the I and the It. Freud is very explicit on the use of the pronouns "I" and "It" to denote the two major regions of the soul:

Doubtless, you will raise an objection against our intention to refer to these two regions or stages of the soul with simple pronouns, instead of giving them beautiful euphonious Greek names. However, in psychoanalysis, we prefer to remain in contact with the popular way of thinking, and attach commonplace terms to our scientific conceptions, rather than look upon such nomenclature in contempt.[9]

Straightforwardly Freud then explains why he uses the term "the It"—what we of English tongue have learned to call the "id":

The impersonal pronoun "It" is most appropriate for our purposes, as is plainly proved by the fact that we frequently speak of something, averring that "'It' came to me quite suddenly"; "'It' gave me a shock"; "'It' was stronger than I." *"L'était plus fort que moi."*[10]

Here, then, are the two major aspects of the soul apparatus: the I and the It. Freud explains:

To all intents and purposes, the "I" is actually the front layer, the obvious, whereas the "It" is the inner layer, the hidden. To make it even more plain: the "I" is inserted between the reality of the outer world and the "It," the latter constituting the soul proper, the essence of the soul, as it were.[11]

In Freud's own popular words, then, the It is the hidden, the inner, the "essence of the soul"—and the I is the open, the obvious, the apparent. Now Freud in his technical works greatly qualified these generalizations: the It, in particular, was said to be the seat of libido, of sexual and aggressive energies, of primary processes or fantasy-dream thinking; and the I was subdivided into the I-proper or ego and superego. The It-proper and the I-proper were destined to forever remain at war. Only compromise, but never harmony, could be achieved between them.

Here, however, Freud is talking in popular and almost intuitive terms—the It is simply "aspects of the soul" which appear *it* or *other* to one's awareness, as when Freud uses the example, "It was stronger than I." In this special sense, Freud unequivocally states that "*there is no inherent opposition between the 'I' and the 'It,' both belonging together*" (my italics).[12] Every time I show that statement to a psychiatrist, he or she invariably states, "Freud never said that." Anyway, Freud continues and says that "in cases of normal health, it is practically impossible to distinguish between the two [the I and the It]."[13]

Now I am not suggesting that Freud ultimately and truly meant that the ego and the id could and should be one. Clearly, that was not his technical view. The real id, the deep It, could never even become conscious. Rather, the deep id sends up "derivatives," or "little its" if you will, and these derivative its can and must be integrated into the I, or they tend to show up in "substitute forms" as neurotic symptoms. When Freud technically says, "Where id was, there ego shall be," that seems to be what he means. He does not mean that the ego and the deep id are one and the same, but that the I and the little its must be brought together in a mutually satisfying *compromise*. As we will soon see, that appears to be essentially what Jung meant when he talked about integrating the persona and shadow—the narrowed I and the derivative its; but as for the "true" and "deep" It—there Freud and Jung absolutely parted ways.

At any rate, we return to Freud's popular exposition. Although "in cases of normal health it is practically impossible to distinguish between the two [the I and the It]," that is an ideal situation which is more the exception than the rule. For early on in the development of most individuals, some of the little its—which potentially could be integrated into the personality in a normal fashion—instead become dissociated or split off from the I. That is, the urges of the I are pitted against those of the It. Initiated by the I, this war has the object of banishing or throttling some of the desires of the It. Freud explains:

And now, I ask you to visualize what would happen in case this "I" is actuated by an urge arising from the "It"—an urge which the weak "I" would like to resist, because it feels that . . . this urge may involve danger, may result in a traumatic situation, a collision with the outer world.[14]

In this battle between the I and the It (if I may now follow Freud's popular version and not distinguish between little its and the It), something has to give—neither side will totally surrender its own wishes, and so one side simply has to be forcefully restricted:

The "I" makes an attempt at flight, deserting the specific part of the "It" and leaving it to its fate. It refuses all such assistance as it usually renders to urges arising from the "It." We refer to such a case as repression of urges by the "I" . . . . The repressed urge now goes its own way. . . . With its synthesis disturbed, a part of the "It" remains forbidden ground to the "I."[15]

Freud here does not distinguish between the superego and the I. He is still talking in popular, experiential terms—talking about the battle between I and It, I and my symptoms, I and my distresses, I and my desires. Experientially I never feel a battle between a superego and an id, whatever they are, but I do feel battles between my I and my desires, my I and my distresses, and I think Freud is being very true to his experiential intuitions at this point. Now I personally am not denying the existence of the superego; I am just pointing out Freud's simple intuitions on the nature of mental conflict: it takes the general form of I versus It, not ego versus id or superego versus ego.

Now this "repression of the It" might seem a fitting end to the whole war between I and It—the offending It is forcefully expelled from the field of consciousness, and the I is free to go its happy way. Alas, however, such is not the case: the It may be ordered off the field, but it doesn't leave the territory, nor does it rest quiet in its exile.

The isolated urge does not remain idle, however. Because normal gratification was denied it, it continues to compensate itself by engendering psychical derivatives which take its place and, connecting with other psychical activations, estrange them to the "I." Finally, in the form of an unrecognizable substitute, the isolated urge penetrates to the "I" and to consciousness, presenting itself as what is known as a "symptom."[16]

In other words, when the It is banished from consciousness, exiled from I-ness, it simply takes up an abode as a *symptom,* and thus *forces* its way into awareness in this disguised form. *The symptom becomes a new type of It,* and as a symptom, It continues its attack upon the unsuspecting I. "This revenge of the 'It' on the 'I,'" says Freud, "resulted in nothing less than a neurosis."[17]

Because the I has failed to come to terms with, and integrate, the It (the little its), the sphere of the I is somewhat reduced and restricted. Not only is the energy of the It "isolated" from the I, some of the I's energy has to be used to fight off the It. These are the countercathexes and defense mechanisms, some of which are necessary and normal in development, but which can become pathological if they are too severe. Modern psychoanalysis classifies defense mechanisms on a hierarchical scale from the most primitive (of the oral stage) to the more complex and structured (of the phallic stage). Introjection, projection, and denial are among the most primitive, and repression, rationalization, and displacement among the more sophisticated. In order to discuss the personal unconscious in general terms, however, I am going to follow Jung and Gestalt in emphasizing the central role of projection as a defense mechanism. "Everything unconscious is projected,"[18] say the Jungians, and while that is quite a generalization, it serves to point out in a simple way the relation between the I and the It. For in the Jungian (and Gestalt) system, what appears as an It first started out as part of the I, or as Jung put it, most of the personal unconscious was once conscious (or, secondarily, subliminal), but became dissociated and alienated and projected.[19] This is very similar to Freud's "popular" expressions given above, where I and It start out with "no inherent opposition." That, however, is not the technical Freudian view: although the ego grew out of the id, the two are fundamentally opposed in aims, in structure, and in organization. Again, I tend to side with the Jungian opinion: the personal unconscious, on the whole, was once conscious, the It was once part of the I, and so this discussion will reflect that opinion.

In this view, then, if certain personal tendencies, ideas, affects, or impulses are not integrated or assimilated they become It—they are defended against and warded off, and thus they are projected (bearing in mind that the only defense mechanism I am using here is projection). These denied and projected aspects cease to be a direct part of the I and appear instead as alien, foreign, outside, and other—they appear as It. They have been turned from I into It, from possible friend-in-here to enemy-out-there, from self to notself, from dynamic energy to painful symptom. I think Perls would here agree: something that should and could be I is *felt* and *perceived* as an It, as not-I. Further, since some part of the I is turned into an It, this constitutes nothing less than *the abandonment of one's own true potentials.* A radical boundary is forced upon the territory of the total ego, and the opposed forces of the I and the It begin their battle maneuvers.

To follow the Gestalt view (which is, in this respect, similar to Jung's), a simple example of the split between I and It might be this: suppose that as a result of some provocation or another, a hostile or angry impulse strongly wells up in a person. Now properly integrated with the total I (the whole ego), aggression can be a useful form of mobilization for overcoming obstacles and frustrations, but suppose that the individual in our example is one who has a great deal of difficulty effectively handling anger or aggression. Instead of using aggression in controlled forms, he condemns it altogether. He perceives that his angry impulses are absolutely dangerous, and thus he attempts to deny the existence of any angry urges that might arise in him. *So this anger is no longer I but It*—no longer a true part of himself but a banished and outcast and rejected "other."

Already he has abandoned some of his own potentials, for all angry impulses are now split off from the I and projected out of the ego—but that anger does not thereby simply vanish or evaporate. Rather, it continues to rise up again and again, and demand recognition from the I. Again and again the I refuses to accept It as a part of the I-system. There is now an intractable battle between the I and the split-off or It-anger.

We may suppose that in the back of his mind, this individual still continues to perceive or intuit these angry impulses. He knows *somebody* is angry, but since it can't be himself, it must be somebody else—*anybody* else—and so he must find a suitable candidate. He needs somebody to take over his projections—his Its. Instead of seeing the anger as *his,* he actually sees it in other people: he *projects* it out of his I and onto others, thereby "relieving" himself of the responsibility for his own energies.

Notice what results by projecting his aggressions: he no longer feels that *he* is angry at other people, but that other people are angry at him. He starts to feel that all sorts of people, for no apparent reasons, are angry at him, hostile towards him, "out to get him." His friends and associates will correctly deny this if he brings it up, but the feeling is insistent. It is so insistent because it's *his* anger—he keeps tossing this potential for action out of his I and it keeps boomeranging back to its true owner—and he can't figure out the source of the blows. Now even if certain people are actually angry with him, he simply compounds the problem by adding his projected anger to their actual anger; the threat then appears "double-strength."

Realize that this individual honestly feels that he totally lacks any hostile impulses and that others actually seem to abound with them. Under these circumstances, he understandably starts developing feelings of anxiety or fear, because "everybody's after him." He develops, that is, a *symptom,* a symptom of fear. His projected anger, as It, has returned to plague him with anxieties and fears, with thoughts of people hating or rejecting him, with feelings of inferiority, and so on. So projecting his anger—casting it out of his I as an It—doesn't leave a hole or empty space in his personality: it leaves a symptom. Thus (and I am now stating my own opinion, which is similar to Jung-Gestalt but not to Freud's technical view), to fail to recognize one's own potential is to turn that potential into a "dis-ease." When I become It, It becomes a symptom.

Now there is a fascinating twist to all this: when the It is a part of the I, then It is amenable to some sort of control. If a person is openly aware of his own angers (or wishes, hatreds, envies, positive virtues, or any of the egoic potentials that might be projected as Its), then he can more often than not exert a guiding influence over them: he can choose the aim and mode of the expression of the impulses. He is, in short, *responsible* for them, and they, in turn, *respond* to him.

On the other hand, when facets of the I are projected as Its, these Its are quite beyond conscious control. They seem to come and go as they please, without any reference to, or consideration of, the I. This "uncontrollability" is precisely why Freud, as we earlier saw, called these alienated aspects of the self "derivatives of the It." We say: "The symptom, It annoys me"; "It's an obsessive thought, I can't control It"; "My desire to eat, It's stronger than I am"; "This fear, It just happens to me"; and of each and every symptom: "I just wish It would go away."

Yet notice that all these little its are actually aspects of the total self, aspects of the total I. In other words, all these its—the symptoms, the tensions, the obsessions, the upsets, the neuroses, the dramas, the scares—are things an individual is doing to himself, with his own energies. He is clobbering himself and pretending that It is doing the clobbering, whereas It is merely an aspect of his own ego-self that he has ignored. His symptoms, then, are precisely as if he were pinching himself but didn't know it. Instead of saying, "I am hurting myself," he says, "It is hurting me." Therefore, in casting out the It from the I, we surrender our responsibility for It and thus our control over It. Then, in our projections onto other people and in our resultant symptoms, the It runs riot as it pleases.

You can probably see the general, overall effect of this casting out of the It from the total I: the true potential of the I is severely restricted and abridged. The very base and foundation of the I is narrowed, impoverished, and limited—the boundary of the I *shrinks,* as it were, by virtue of the exiling of the It. With the banishing, casting out, or projection of the unwanted aspects of the total I, the very *sense* of I-ness is narrowed. The potential of what the I is, and therefore what it can do, is narrowed. Both the substance and the function are curtailed. Since I am now siding with the Jungian view of the nature and generation of the personal unconscious, I will use Jungian terms: the sense of self shifts from the accurate I or total *ego* to an impoverished and inaccurate self, a "smaller I" or *persona,* and the alienated, cast-out, projected It remains "outside" of the self as the *shadow,* where, with sneak attacks and guerrilla raids, it torments the persona with symptoms. As I am generally discussing this matter, the battle between I and It is the same as the battle between the persona and the shadow.

Although it is not always a simple thing to do, the prescription for this battle can be simply put: the I must learn to drop its defenses against the It and to once again befriend, integrate, and take back the It. The I and the It—the persona and the shadow—must reconcile and reunite in some sort of a mutually satisfying integration. To take back the It is to regain the correspondingly lost potentials of the self.

To take back the It—this is usually a difficult and prolonged task. The task is further compounded by a peculiar situation: remember that the I doesn't really like the It—the I resists the It, defends against the It, suppresses the It. And this resistance to the It manifests itself in a loathing to take back, or even consciously touch, the It. In more medical terms, the I doesn't want to "get well"; the I doesn't want to release and let go of its symptoms, for not only do the symptoms provide a grim joy to the I ("substitute gratifications of neurotic pleasure"), but to actually renounce the symptom is to befriend the It which is hidden in the symptom. If the I were prepared to do that, the symptom would never have appeared in the first place. No, the I clings to its symptoms on the one hand while openly despising them on the other—and the I doesn't want to change. Because it resists the shadow, the persona secretly loves its "sickness," and in fact, the individual as persona will defend his suffering in the face of all comers. Perls and Adler both spoke often on that point. Perls used to say that neurotics enter therapy, not to get better, but to become better neurotics. Adler said that if you ask the client what he would do if he were completely better, what he tells you will be precisely what he is now trying to avoid (we may think of that in simple terms this way: his persona wants to do it, but his shadow doesn't, and he has to integrate the "I-don't-want-to" side first). Freud, too, spoke of this "fondness for illness." Of neurotics, he states: "They complain about their sickness, at the same time exploiting it to the limit. As a matter of fact, if an attempt is made to cure them of their ailment, they will protect this most cherished possession of theirs with the self-same fervor with which a lioness defends her offspring."[20]

If we now return to our simple example of projected anger or hostility, I think this will become more obvious. The individual in our example has an I (a persona) that will not tolerate and cannot bear an angry impulse (which thus becomes an It, a shadow component). Instead of honestly and innocently expressing his hostile feelings, he tries to deny them, but only ends up denying *ownership* of them by projecting them out of his I and onto others.

Thus, instead of feeling "I'm angry at the world," he feels, "The world is angry at me." In response, he develops *symptoms* of fearful anxiety.

For this simple example, let us suppose that the occasional and appropriate free flow of aggression is a highly satisfying experience. The *activity* of the impulse is gratifying, but when this impulse is suppressed and thrown out of the I as an It, the impulse is denied conscious satisfaction. Nevertheless, this It continues to operate and continues to seek release towards some type of object. Since the individual won't allow aggression to take an outlet in the environment, his aggression has only one place left to turn: onto himself. Further, the *source* of the aggression seems to be *from* others, from the environs.

Instead of attacking the environment, he attacks himself and *imagines* others are doing it. Instead of the satisfaction of attacking and working through obstacles in the environment, he is forced to settle for a *substitute* satisfaction: he attacks himself. He beats himself without knowing it, under the illusion that others are the culprits. Thus, what he directly *feels* is no longer hostility, but fear—fear of his own hostility which he now imagines to reside in others. His symptom of fear, then, gives him a type of substitute pleasure, because with this fear he is still exercising *his* hostile impulses—on himself, unfortunately, but that outlet is more satisfying than none at all.

That is one way of understanding why an individual will not let go of his symptoms: they are the only way he can extract satisfaction from the aspects of his I that he won't admit are his. In resisting the It, he is forced to embrace his symptoms with a mixture of love and contempt. Loathe his symptoms? Yes, that he does, but underneath he loves them as well and will, in fact, go out of his way to collect those feelings associated with his favorite symptoms: fears, depressions, guilts, scares, hysterias—all the different ways he can clobber himself with his own energies while pretending someone else is holding the club. TA calls this "collecting trading stamps"—actively (if unknowingly) seeking out one's favorite lousy feelings.[21]

The individual is, then, literally pinching himself, while pretending others are doing it: "I pinch the world" to "I pinch myself" to "The world pinches me." Notice how at each point of alienation, more of the I is turned into an It—in the person's feelings, thoughts, and language. This is especially evident in his language, as Fritz Perls constantly pointed out. The language of alienation and lost potential is an It-language. Perls states:

> Look at the difference between the words "I am tensing myself" and "There's a tenseness here." When you say "I feel tenseness," you're irresponsible, you are not responsible for this, you are impotent and you can't do anything about it. The world should do something—give you an

aspirin or whatever it is. But when you say "I am tensing" you take responsibility. . . .[22]

With alienation, a piece of the active I is shaved off and appears as a passive It—the "unwanted symptom." The responsible I is more and more converted into the irresponsible It, with a concomitant loss of potential: the potential of what one can be and thus the potential of what one can do. From this angle, a symptom is a sign of lost potential.

How to regain this lost potential? Let's go back to Freud's formula, which was quoted at the beginning of this article: "Where id was, there ego shall be." The original German is, "*Wo Es war, soll Ich werden,*" or "Where It was, I shall become." That, in one sentence, is the precise formula for the recovery of lost potentials: the passive It back into the active I; the irresponsible It back into the responsible I; the reactive It back into the active I. Where It was, I shall become.

Now that, of course, is my own interpretation of Freud's *popular* statement—"Where It was, I shall become." Freud's technical view was undoubtedly somewhat different, and I do not wish to appear to be citing Freud as a supporter of this interpretation. For Freud, the ego was almost always passive in relation to the true or deep id; the best the ego could hope for was to nudge the id a little in one direction or another. However, he does view therapy as a relative gain in the ego's control of the little its, the derivatives that could be brought under the purview of the I, with a resultant "strengthening of the ego." In Gestalt, however, the statement is much more forceful: the passive It back into the active I.

In a general fashion, then, the individual undergoing some sort of therapy on this level increasingly learns to convert all these little its back into this I. He learns to do this in his thoughts, his feelings, and his language. This is certainly true in Gestalt therapy, and can be seen in TA and the "reality" or "responsibility" therapies. However, it *seems* to be occurring in classical psychoanalysis as well. We already mentioned that Brandt was one of the first to emphasize that "where id was, there ego shall be" actually meant that "where It was, there I shall become." Loevinger gives another angle on Brandt's psychoanalytic view: "Brandt points out that patients sometimes use expressions where *it* stands for the id, but that more often derivatives appear in their speech *as the passive voice,* as something that happened to them without a sense of agency" (my italics),[23] that is, without a sense of responsibility. Further:

Brandt cites the case of a patient who described her feeling of being trapped by some part of herself over which she had no control by "I'm up here and *it's* down there." Brandt continues: "After repeatedly stating 'I am trapped,' then 'I am trapped by my emotions' and a little later, 'I am trapped by myself'—all passive voice statements which, transformed into the active voice say, 'It traps me'—this patient arrived at the insight 'I trap myself.' *The replacement of 'it' by 'I' as subject of the sentence corresponds to the process of 'it' becoming 'I' . . .".*[24] (my italics)

There is no question that Brandt, at least, thinks that *process* is the ultimate core of Freud's dictum ("where id was, there ego shall be"). Loevinger, in discussing this as a *psychoanalytic* (not Jungian-Gestaltian) issue, cites several support cases (such as Bruch,[25] Horowitz,[26] and Enright[27]), and concludes that "the clinical observations just quoted suggest a number of research projects. Is the change from speaking in terms of 'it' to 'I' discernable in all cases of successful psychoanalysis? Is there always a shift from passive to active voice in describing the self by patients treated successfully? Is successful therapy marked by transition from passive to active voice? Does 'it' literally become 'I'?"[28]

My own feeling is that It does literally become I, but I'm not sure that verbal behavior is the only measure of this transformation. At any rate, to return to the example of blocked aggression, we may follow—as a simple hypothetical example—this conversion of It-anger back into I. The individual might enter therapy complaining of fearful anxiety in the presence of others: he feels, somehow, that people seem to be zeroed in on him in a rejecting, negative, or openly hostile fashion. He himself feels no hostile intent towards anyone, but he is convinced that people seem covertly or even blatantly to hate him. He feels, in short, that certain people are "pinching" him, and he is but a passive victim.

There are many excellent and effective therapies that can help the individual with this particular type of problem, such as role playing, internal dialogue analysis, sub-personalities therapy, gestalt procedures, ego state analysis, and so on. For simplicity's sake, let us just take role playing in fantasy, and follow it through to its conclusion. The individual feels that some person or persons are constantly zeroed in on him in a peculiarly hostile fashion. He is asked, then, to imagine the threatening person and engage that person in dialogue.

At first, the image of the threatening person is an It—a frightening, uncontrollable, powerful other—and the individual will usually have a difficult time even playing the role of the persecutor. He has, that is, strong resistances to even contacting or touching this threatening agent, let alone playing the role of that agent. Much attention, and much work, might have to be given to this resistance.

The first turning point occurs when the individual can with relative ease assume the role of the hostile persecutor, for at this junction a certain transformation occurs: formerly, he felt another person was attacking and frightening him, but as he himself assumes the role of this attacking other, he realizes that *he* is attacking *himself*. No longer is there a battle between I and It, but between I and I; no longer, "It pinches me," but "I am pinching myself."

With amazement he discovers just how brutal he can be to himself. He finds the persecutor *within* himself, and begins to understand that by projecting his own hostile self-persecution, he populated the world with innumerable, external persecutors. However, by taking back his projection, he finds that the It is I. He starts to see and feel the form of his harsh superego: Controlling Parent, or torturing Top Dog.

At this point, the individual is halfway home. He has moved from "It pinches me" to "I pinch me." He now faces the decisive battle of transforming from "I pinch me" to "I am free to pinch the world" (and beyond this to "I don't need to pinch even the world"). He must learn, that is, to finally integrate the It (hostility) in its true form, namely, as energy mobilized *from* the self *to* the world. In dialogue work, this transformation first occurs at the point at which *he can address other individuals* (in fantasy, then fact) *while playing the role of the hostile persecutor.* Incidentally, this is the dramatic point in Gestalt therapy when the individual can address the group as the Top Dog; basically the same point at which the implosive layer ("I am pinching myself into suffocation") gives way to the explosive layer ("I pinch you!"). For at this point, he has finally turned the aggression back outward to its original form and, therefore, succeeded at last in truly integrating and absorbing this It into his I. He can approach others *as* the hostile persecutor, and thus the It-persecutor is correctly thrown back into his I—and here, we should note, it gradually resumes its original, less-than-violent form because it is integrated and balanced in the context of the total I.

In my own opinion, the individual has finally reversed the process of turning I into It: he has moved from "It attacks me" to "I attack me" to "I attack the world" (to "I don't need to attack the world"). He first had to see *that* he was pinching himself—and then *how* (and perhaps why) he was pinching himself, whereupon he was spontaneously free to pinch the world. At each point, the I drops more of its resistances to the It; more of the It is turned back into I; the I assumes more and more active responsibility for what previously was passive reactivity.

Perhaps the most decisive factor, in my view, is understanding just *how* he pinches himself, for once that is clearly perceived, growth seems to be almost spontaneous. If you clearly see that you are pinching yourself, you don't keep asking somebody else how to stop; and if you are asking someone how to stop pinching yourself, it only means that you haven't yet seen that *you* are doing the pinching! You don't ask how to lift your arm when you realize your arm is yours, and you don't ask how to control the It when It is seen as I. The control is almost spontaneous—the It flows with the I, not against it.

To take back the It, to reunite with the shadow, to reidentify with and integrate all those aspects of the ego that have been alienated—this is to actually broaden what one *is,* and thus expand what one can *do.* The enlargement of perceived essence brings an expansion of available function. Overall, this is nothing but the recovery of one's own potentials—potentials of being and of doing, of substance and of utility, of center and of activity. To put it all in a phrase: to recover the It is to recover lost potentials—potentials both of being and of doing.

Notice immediately, then, that this is not so much the sui generis creation of potentials previous lacking, but the recovery and reclamation of potentials once known but subsequently forgotten. *Forgotten:* the word is *amnesia,* and Freud himself found that behind every symptom, behind every alienation of an It, there lay a gap in memory, an amnesia pertaining to the It itself. The It was not really lost, just forgotten—forcefully forgotten, all too often, but forgotten nonetheless. We forget an It, and forget we have forgotten: that, in fact, is a definition of repression.

Thus, the aim is to *remember* something of ourselves that we had formerly forgotten. To remember: the word here is *anamnesia,* to remember or recollect, and we will very shortly see just how profound this notion really is. For now, the point is that *great potentials are not so much created as remembered.* To be sure, a remembered potential very often must be channelized, exercised, trained, extended in development, utilized. I do not wish to minimize that aspect of development. In my opinion, however, on the whole it is not the ground-up building of new and novel potentials, but the remembrance of buried and therefore untapped potentials. To remember lost Its is to remember or find again lost potentials—to make them conscious and therefore directly usable. Freud's own words, if not his technical view, can here be cited: "The aim of our efforts may be expressed in various formulas—making conscious the unconscious, removing the repressions, filling in the gaps in memory; they all amount to the same thing."[29]

Now I think we can capture the very essence of the secret power of anamnesis and remembrance: to remember is simply to re-member and re-collect, to *join together again* that which was dismembered and disjointed, to make whole that which was split and fragmented. For the I to remember the It is to re-member the I and the It, to join them together once again, "as it was in the beginning." To re-member that which was dismembered, and re-collect that which has been dispersed: there is the power of anamnesis, of "filling in the gaps in memory" and "making conscious the unconscious."

In my view, then, our true potentials are not so much created afresh as remembered again; they already exist, as it were, but in hidden or obscure forms. Our forgotten potentials lie with the forgotten It. But where, if we may put a rather loose question, does the forgotten It reside? The alienated and forgotten It, as we saw, is cast out of the I-ness and, in a special sense, continues to exist—but outside of the I. Thus, the It exists in and as our *projections* (remember I am only using projection in this chapter). That is, our hidden potentials, our lost Its, already exist but only as our own projections. The Its we perceive "out there"—there are our potentials! Fritz Perls was most explicit on this vital point: "Much material that is our own, that is part of ourselves, has been dissociated, alienated, disowned, thrown out [as shadow-It]. *But I believe most of it is available, but as projections"* (my italics).[30]

Thus, in a nutshell, the key to tapping lost potentials: *we recover our forgotten potentials by re-membering, or joining again with, our projections, our Its.* To underscore this point, let us, for the last time, draw again on our simple example of the individual who has persistently alienated and forgotten his own anger, and consequently suffers symptoms of fearful anxiety at the hands of innumerable "external" persecutors. Now this individual honestly feels that he absolutely lacks any trace of the potential for anger. He earnestly searches every corner of his I (his persona) and reports no hint of hostility. To him, his anger is absent, nonexistent. However, that is not absolutely correct: his anger exists, in its entirety, but in the projected form of the hostile figures of his "persecutors." There is his anger; there it already exists. He is, in fact, looking right at It! He sees his anger, he just doesn't see it as his. Likewise, he actually *feels* his anger, but in a disguised form—he feels it as *external* anger aimed at him, and this he calls "fear." Right there in his symptom, and right there in his projections, lie the forgotten potentials of his It. He does not have to manufacture his own anger; he does not have to invent it, he does not have to conjure it out of nothing. He has merely to remember it.

Now different schools of shadow therapy proceed in different ways to effect this anamnesis. Freud felt that the recovery of the actual and concrete memory of the event(s) that initiated the repression and alienation of anger (or sex, rage, envy, etc.) is necessary.[31] Others, such as Fritz Perls, felt that it is only necessary, here and now, to reunite with the projected anger, provided that one understands and assumes responsibility for the resistances to anger itself.[32] Nonetheless, both views come to essentially the same thing: to remember the traumatizing event is to remember the circumstances in which one first felt it necessary to repress or alienate anger because it was perceived as overwhelmingly dangerous. However, to remember when one first lost one's anger is to remember that it is one's *own* anger, and that is already the reuniting with the anger, the taking back of projections. Conversely, to absolutely befriend one's angers here and now is to make oneself available to traumatizing memories revolving around rage and anger, since the resistance itself is undermined. In any case, to remember is to re-member, and to recollect is to re-collect.

As the I ceases to resist the It, the projected It can be re-membered, taken back, re-owned. In my view, this brings both an expansion of the I's potentials for being and doing, as well as an expanded sense of the I's freedom. For when an individual is one with the It, he is free of the It. Being him, It no longer pushes him. Absorbing It, he is no longer restricted by It. Something that appeared not-self has become self; something that was thought to be other has become intimate; something which seemed to be out there has become in here: I have befriended the enemy, and It is I. And when the It is added to the I, *all the lost potentials of the It are thereby delivered to the I.* Very simply, one's potentials grow as Its become I's.

Thus the I, as persona, can be expanded, enlarged, and enriched by befriending and re-owning the shadow, the It. The inaccurate and impoverished persona can be transformed into the "accurate" and "strong" ego-self, a self-concept which harmonizes persona and shadow in one integrated self-sense. I believe that this exploration and "recovery" of the personal unconscious will be seen as Freud's lasting heritage to all those seeking their own hidden potentials—even though I disagree with the ultimate nature of Freud's It and even though he himself probably wouldn't call it "potential" (he had a very jaundiced view of the human core). For Freud at least—and this is what I have emphasized in this article—was the first great scientific discoverer and explorer *of an It-region:* "The obscured, the hidden, the essence of the soul," as he put it. He alerted us to the fact that there are depths to the soul unacknowledged by surface consciousness, that immense energies (and I will *add,* potentials) lie submerged in the psyche. With his initial breakthroughs, there began the great Western search for expanded human potentials.

To be sure, this search has taken on a hundred different forms. In particular, the shadow has been conceived in ways somewhat different from Freud's formulations. Jung viewed the shadow as *any* egoic potentials forgotten or repressed—positive and constructive potentials as well as negative, destructive, or "instinctual" ones.[33] Transactional Analysis sees the shadow as undifferentiated and therefore "unconscious" ego states that must be identified, brought into awareness, and then integrated.[34] Psychosynthesis, among others, tends to view the shadow as unconscious complexes of sub-personalities, both positive and negative in nature.[35] Nevertheless, the guiding insight has endured: get the It and the I together, move from persona to ego by befriending, re-owning, and integrating the shadow.

That has remained, then, the essential and core insight of ego, or ego-level, psychotherapy, and as far as it goes, I am certainly in perfect, if general, agreement. However, let us very quickly ask a striking question: we have seen that the I-boundary can expand, so to speak, from the persona to the ego. Does the I-boundary, therefore, necessarily have to stop at the ego? Freud already dramatically showed how incredibly plastic the I-boundaries are. As a matter of fact, they expand and shrink with what appears an alarming ease. And when we have enriched and expanded the I from persona to ego, why stop there? Are we justified in looking further? Is the isolated ego the greatest self to which my I can aspire? Are there no more potentials in the human organism than just the mental-ego? Are we unnecessarily restricting our potentials by restricting our conception of the self?

When we stand back and survey the richness of the total human organism on the one hand, and the ego-self on the other, simple subtraction gives us a huge It that has heretofore been ignored: the body itself. Truly, the body-global looms in the ego's awareness as an awesome It—the body-It seems somehow foreign, other, alien. While the body might be "mine," It is not I! The body is just downright—It-ish.

There are very good reasons for saying that just as to the persona the shadow is It, to the ego the body-global is It: an unbridgeable gap or hiatus seems to forever separate the mind and the body, the ego and the flesh, the psyche and the soma. Freud, by and large, simply accepted this mind-body split as irreducible. The persona and shadow could reunite in the total ego, but as for the ego itself and the body, no such loving embrace could be expected. Daniel Goleman explains:

> Freud believed in the "mysterious leap from mind to body," and based his early theory of anxiety on the transformation of physical into mental. But though he saw the brain and nervous system as "the bodily organ and scene of action" of mental life he saw no means of connecting acts of consciousness with their physiological substrata. He despaired of finding systematic connections between consciousness and the nervous system: "Everything that lies between these two terminal points is unknown to us and, so far as we are aware, there is no direct relation between them."

Thus, as Goleman points out, "From Freud on, mainline psychoanalytic practice if not thinking, has focused on the intra-psychic to the exclusion of the body."[36]

Now it seems odd to say that psychoanalysis has by and large ignored the body—we tend to think of psychoanalysis as operating exclusively with instincts, with sexuality, with erogenous zones, with organic energies. While that is true to some degree, psychoanalysis actually works with mental representations or symbols and mental displacements of energies that are presumed to arise in physiological tensions: the body as body rarely enters the psychoanalytic picture. Libido is *mental* energy; the pleasure principle is a *psychological* drive; sexuality is *psycho*sexuality. "Psychoanalysis recognizes the importance of body processes in psychological life, but it has traditionally been more concerned with mental experiences, especially those of a symbolic nature, than with body. . . ."[37] The importance of the body for psychoanalysis is that the body is a source of instincts—but, as we shall see, the body might also serve as the source of entirely different processes.

This acceptance by psychoanalysis of the mind-body dualism becomes all the more curious if we examine the origin of Freud's concept of the It. For Freud did not invent the id or *das Es* or the It-concept—rather, he borrowed the It-concept from Georg Groddeck, a renowned and brilliant physician operating a clinic at Baden-Baden. In fact, Freud's book *The Ego and the Id* ("The I and the It") was an acknowledged tribute to Groddeck's It-concept. Now as we saw, in practice the psychoanalytic It is a purely psychological item—a mental force with whose derivatives the ego must come to terms and integrate (the shadow-It). As we shall see, that view is all right—as far as it goes. However, for Groddeck, the It was not merely mental or egoic—it was psychosomatic, it was the functioning of the *total organism* which could express itself both egoically and bodily, or rather, *always* expressed itself both egoically and bodily. As Groddeck put the matter: "For the It there is no distinction between organic and mental. If I use the two terms body and mind, I understand by them phenomena of the It, or if you like, functions of the It. For me the two ideas are not mutually independent, and certainly are not antithetical. Let us drop this stale theme of an agelong muddle."[38]

"Yet one thing more," adds Groddeck. "Of the It, we know only so much as lies within our consciousness. Beyond that the greater part of its territory is unattainable, but by search and effort we can extend the limits of our consciousness, and press far into the realm of the unconscious . . . ."[39] *There, again, the formula:* where It was, I shall become; but here we see something novel—the glimmerings of a new and deeper It. The body-global can be directly re-owned in consciousness—in a special sense that I will later try to explain—to reveal the *total psychosomatic being*.

For what has slowly become obvious to us—as it was to Groddeck—is that the ego-mind and the body-global are not actually two different substances or two antithetical entities, but rather two different aspects of a single underlying process or reality: namely, the organism-as-a-whole, as Whitehead decisively pointed out. "The most satisfactory solution to the mind-body problem," states Hintz, "would seem . . . to be found along the lines thus indicated by Whitehead. It is to be found in the concept of organism which removes the 'problem' simply because it permits of no essential dichotomy in nature. . . . We cannot even legitimately refer to [mind and body] as separate entities . . . both of which may more likely be different aspects of the same fundamental natural reality and therefore not organically separable."[40] Or, as Feigl puts it, "Instead of conceiving of two realms or two concomitant types of events, we have only one reality which is represented in two different conceptual systems [physical and psychical]. . . . *This reality is known to us by acquaintance only in the case of direct experience*" (my italics).[41] This *direct experience* is a point we will soon focus on.

The situation is very much as if we were presented two pictures of Mt. Everest—one taken from the north slope, and one from the south. Not realizing that these are simply two different views of the same mountain, we have historically tried to develop a philosophy of the relationship between the north view (mind) and the south view (body). Some have held that only the north view is "really real", while others champion the south view only. Some tried to reduce the north to the south; others, vice versa. Some have maintained that the north *causes* the south; and others, again, vice versa. It has been most confusing.

The redeeming insight has been the simple recognition that these are but two different views of one reality. Mt. Everest, approached from one angle, gives us the north view; approached from the opposite angle, it gives us the south view. Notice, however, that we are not saying that the north view is the *same thing* as the south view: clearly they are not. They are quite different, as a matter of plain fact, and if you try to superimpose the two views, you get *not* a unitary view but a double exposure. North and south are not the same thing; they are different, to be sure, but different aspects of *one* reality, the mountain itself.

So it is with ego and flesh, self-concept and felt-body—they are different, but not alien—they are two different aspects of *one* underlying process, one reality. "We know," explains Benoit, "that the belief in the autonomy of these two parts [mind and body] is an illusion; there are not in man two distinct parts, but only two distinct aspects of a single being; man is in reality an *individual* artificially divided by an erroneous interpretation of his analytic observation. The error of our dualistic conception does not lie in the discrimination between two aspects in us—for there are indeed two aspects [north and south]—but in concluding that these two aspects are two different entities."[42]

"To tell the truth," Benoit continues, "our observation does not show us that there are two parts in us; it only shows us that everything happens in us as though there were two parts separated by a hiatus. It is our ignorant intellect that takes an illusory leap from the statement 'everything happens as though' to the erroneous affirmation that there are in us two parts separated by a hiatus."[43]

Benoit points out that, under the erroneous belief in this hiatus between ego and body, each individual misguidedly conceives himself as a horseman (ego) riding a horse (body)—the identical metaphor, by the way, that Freud evoked in *The Ego and the Id* to explain what he felt to be the correct view of the self: forever divided. Yet from a deeper view, Benoit reminds us, "We are not horseman and horse, with a hiatus between the two. The true symbolic representation . . . should be the centaur, single creature comprising two aspects separated by no hiatus. We are centaurs but everything happens in us as though we were horse and rider because we believe in the reality of a hiatus between our two aspects, or, more exactly, because we do not see the unity in which the two aspects are integrated."[44] This integrated unity, designated *bodymind*—the total psychophysical being—we will call, after Benoit, the "centaur."

Here, of course, we are running straight into the unsolvable philosophic problem of the mind/body relationship. After centuries of the most careful inquiry, Western philosophy has come to one fundamental and important conclusion: one may with complete intellectual respectability maintain any of four or five major different opinions on this relationship. Since each philosophical orientation seems to grab hold of an unshakable *aspect* of the truth, but none corners it fully, neither of the schools has finally been able to dislodge the others once for all. Further, since each school seems to have some merit, not only is it respectable to advocate a particular school, but it is acceptable to use the different schools in a type of *complementary fashion,* to utilize the tenets of each in the special situations that seem to reflect that viewpoint. One can only state one's viewpoint, cite the authorities, and move on from there.

Science doesn't—or has not yet— helped us with the matter. The Greens, for instance, who have worked extensively with biofeedback, proposed the "psychophysiological principle": "Every change in the physiological state is accompanied by an appropriate change in the mental-emotional state, and conversely, every change in the mental-emotional state, conscious or unconscious, is accompanied by an appropriate change in the physiological state."[45] Yet they have also championed the following statement: all of the brain is in the mind but not all of the mind is in the brain[46]—a view shared by some neurosurgeons turned philosophers, such as W. Penfield.[47]

Now my own view on this matter will not become finally clear until towards the end of this section—there are too many complementarities involved to present my position in a sentence. However, I would like to begin by pointing out that traditionally, when philosophers speak of the mind and the body, these words have carried several different meanings that have not always been specified, a fact that has compounded the problem immensely. For there have been at least three major but distinctly different issues involved, all of which have usually been subsumed under the same mind/body problem. (1) This problem has meant the relationship between my voluntary mental awareness and my material body. Since mind is ethereal (the argument goes), since no one has ever *seen* a mind, since even to myself the mind seems ghostlike, how then can it move my material body? All proper ghosts can walk through walls—they cannot easily move matter. How then does my ghost mind move my material body? (2) In other cases, mind has been used in the sense of the subject of awareness, and body has been used as *all* objects. Thus, the problem here is: What is the relationship between subject and object, inside and outside, organism and environment? (3) Recently, body has come to mean brain or nervous system, and the problem has now switched to, What is the relation between brain and mind?

Clearly, these problems are related, but they are also substantially different—and this seems to me quite important, because I believe there are three different answers to the above problems. For if by "mind" we restrict ourselves to "ego" or waking-state "self-concept," then I believe, as I have already suggested, that ego and body (as body, not brain) are two different aspects of the underlying centaur—and this "fact" allows the integration of the "total self," a bodymind autonomy, and a sense of existential I AMness not fragmented into segments (we will pursue that later). If by "mind" we mean "subject," and by body, "object," I believe that subject and object are ultimately one while conventionally separated (the Hindu and Buddhist doctrine of *maya*). If by body we mean brain and by mind we mean awareness, then I accept the suggestion that all of the brain is in the mind but not all of the mind is in the brain. That is, deeper aspects of mind (awareness) transcend the body, but the normal ego does not (and as normal ego cannot). The ego is implicated in the body and ideally integrated with it. In short, the deeper levels of awareness transcend *both* the normal ego and the body together.

What we are concerned with here is the first of the three versions: the psychological problem of the ego (self-concept) and the body-global (as felt-body, not brain), for I believe this relationship, or lack of it, is *representative* of a deeper mode of self, of awareness, and of experiencing—that the centaur is a deeper It that can become I, and that the body-global is the easiest (but not the only) way to center on this deeper or prior self. I will later connect this centauric self with one version of the mind/body solution called "neutral monism," a version espoused by both William James and Bertrand Russell. For the moment I ask the reader to accept the possibility that the self-concept (ego) and the body-global *both* exfoliate from a prior unity of experiencing, a unity called centaur by Benoit, sensibilia by Russell,[48] prehension by myself, experiencing by James,[49] and ongoing psychophysiological flow by Rogers.[50] Again, however, to say that ego and body issue forth, moment to moment, out of a prior unity, is not to say that they are identical. New York and Alabama are part of the Union, but they aren't identical. And one of the things we will be talking about is the secession of the south from the north—the disruption of that union, its meaning and its consequences.

We may begin our exploration of the centaur with Rollo May who, it seems to me, has absolutely nailed some of the important issues involved here. The whole thrust of May's work is that *prior* to anything that could be called the ego, the superego, the id, or the body, lies a sort of existential I AMness, a prehension of being-in-this-moment of which the body, the ego, and the superego are mere fragmentations. As I would state his case, a total sense of being precedes one's self-concepts about being and one's bodily orientations of feelings about being. In May's own words, "If it be countered that this picture of the multitude of egos [postulated by many schools of psychology] reflects the fragmentation of contemporary man, I would rejoin that any concept of fragmentation presupposes some unity *of which* it is a fragmentation. . . .*Logically as well as psychologically* we must go behind the ego-id-superego system and endeavor to understand the 'being' of whom these are expressions" (my italics).[51] Notice two things. (1) This is, for May, a logical or philosophical necessity *and also* a psychological *reality*— "being" is real and not just a philosophical suggestion or position. (2) He is not denying that, on a more superficial level, the ego-id-superego exist, just that they are expressions of, or follow after, beingness.

Further, for May this existential being *precedes both conscious and unconscious* tendencies. Speaking of existential intentionality, May says that "it is not to be identified with intentions but is the *dimension which underlies them* . . . , a dimension which cuts across and includes both conscious and unconscious, both cognition and conation" (my italics).[52] In the same way, this existential intentionality "is the missing link between mind and body,"[53] and this because it "goes below levels of immediate awareness, and includes spontaneous bodily elements and other dimensions which are usually called 'unconscious.' It refers to a state of being and involves, to a greater or lesser degree, the *totality* of the person's orientation. . . ."[54] (We will shortly examine the importance of these "spontaneous bodily elements" for the total being.)

In our terms, the existential centaur precedes not just the ego and the body, but the persona and the shadow as well. Further, according to May, it is not altogether incorrect to speak of this existential intentionality as being unconscious in a deeper sense than the id (or shadow or personal unconscious), for most individuals recoil against their own existence and identify instead with a particular fragment of their being (with the ego or persona, in our terms). In this sense, May is faithful to the general existential position: Sartre,[55] for example, maintains that the ego is a simple fiction conjured up to hide oneself from the contingencies of authentic and dynamic being.

In short, if I may state my opinions (based on the existentialists in general and May in particular), *before* an individual contracts as ego or self-concept *and* before he feels as an "objective body," he experiences his simple being-in-the-world, and *out* of that being, in the *present*, exfoliate specific mental impulses, bodily feelings, or general desires, any of which may (because of secondary reasons) be rendered unconscious (shadow). All of them, that is, exfoliate from sensibilia or prehension or neutral experiencing ("neutral monism"). That is the only reason, I believe, that Rollo May can time and again, in case after case, point up the existential dimension that *precedes* the ego or id or body or conscious or unconscious fragmentations. As I have elsewhere tried to argue, the centaur is microgenetically prior to the ego, body, persona, and shadow, and therefore is at least *potentially* capable of integrating them.[56] That seems to me a very important point, a point that lies behind the self-actualization and "full autonomy" movements—and makes them possible (as we will shortly suggest).

In my view, this existential centaur is a deeper level of awareness that many of the humanistic and existential psychologists are working with. A prime example is Carl Rogers, whose work also points up the importance of recontacting the body-global. Rogers has based much of his person-centered theory on "organismic experiencing," which means "to be aware how one attends, perceives, processes, and integrates information of one's internal, visceral world [the body-global] and one's external, interpersonal, and physical world. Openness to full organismic sensing comes when one experiences realness, caring, and sensitive, nonjudgmental understanding in relation with others."[57]

Rogers, in particular, is one of the humanistic researchers who have emphasized the importance of recontacting the body—for the body-global, of the many facets of the centaur, is the one most frequently alienated (we will examine possible reasons for this later). "One aspect of experiencing or organismic sensing can be conceptualized as heightened sensory awareness. Or, stated differently, the average person is dead to the body and needs to be awakened to the world inside his or her skin."[58] Now what we find here, which is quite novel and quite different from traditional psychoanalysis or even ego-level therapies in general, is an approach to the body not as an It, or as a mere source of instinctual or physiological needs, but as a *source of awareness per se*—a contributor to total organismic experiencing. The body-It can become the body-I, and this is instrumental, the theory goes, in awakening the total centaur or total psychophysical being.

"This concept of bodily felt sensing," write Holdstock and Rogers, "has become increasingly important, culminating in the Experiential Psychotherapy of Eugene Gendlin. . . . Experiencing emerged as a key concept in person-centered theory. It is variously referred to as organismic sensing, ongoing psychophysiological flow, or organismic experiencing. . . ."[59] Now when Rogers was first writing on the nature and importance of organismic experiencing, he tended, by his own account, to exclusively emphasize the sensory and bodily side, and somewhat ignore the cognitive side as well as the "external relationship" side. "Earlier, experiencing had been regarded largely in terms of awareness of the richness of subjective feelings. However, explaining experiencing in terms of inward references to feelings and bodily processes only represents at best a single aspect of the full human potential. Experiencing is more than just sensing visceral and feeling states. It involves being aware of the way one attends, perceives, processes, and integrates information of the internal visceral and external interpersonal and physical world."[60] Thus, if I may use my terms, centauric experiencing is not just bodily, or physical, but is a psychophysical or bodymind awareness.

Thus, organismic sensing or experiencing is more than heightened sensory awareness of internal bodily states and of limbic system activities. It is the integration of this awareness with awareness of those functions represented by the neocortex. It is also the integration of the activities of the left and right cortices.[61]

Now, according to Rogers, out of this ongoing psychophysiological flow, the person creates a self-concept (or what I am calling ego). The psychophysiological flow is both prior to the ego-concept and its ultimate ground and referent. Further, according to Rogers, *all* maladjustment comes about through an alienation of the self-concept from the prior psychophysiological flow—in my terms, the split between the ego and the centaur. "All maladjustment," he states, "of whatever degree, comes about through denial of experiences [or organismic sensing or ongoing psychophysiological flow] discrepant with the self-concept. . . . Thus the self-concept becomes increasingly inaccurate, unrealistic, and rigid over time [the persona]."[62]

Rogers acknowledges his close affinity to the whole existentialist position, and says, in effect, that this "rift between self-concept and ongoing psychophysiological flow" is tantamount to an existential alienation from I AMness. In his words, "Instead of 'I am,' the core identity of the person now becomes 'I am a teacher,' 'I am a student,' 'I am male,' 'I am female,' 'I am a Hell's Angel.'"[63] This leaves one open to second-person role relationships not based "on being, on 'I am.'" As the existentialists might put it, I simply AM before I am anything else: ego, body, role, id, or whatever. Pathology occurs when conditional regard switches from I AMness to I am this or that, for then one seeks to authenticate not his or her own being, but his or her being in the eyes of others.

We have seen that, while emphasizing contact with and actualization of the total psychophysical being or centaur, Rogers places much importance on the body-global aspect of being-in-the-world. In fact, he states that "each person is born with an *inherent bodily wisdom* which enables differentiation between experiences that actualize and those that do not actualize potential" (my italics).[64] I think Rogers would agree that the alienation of the body-global ("being dead to the body," in his terms), has far-reaching consequences—it is more than the loss of "just" the body, because this alienation acts to disrupt the prior psychophysiological flow. In this regard, Rogers has much in common with some other schools of the "human potentials movement," such as Gestalt therapy and Bioenergetic Analysis. All of these schools seek to contact the body as a *source of awareness* and prime contributor to a sense of bodymind union.

Thus, Perls et al. point out in *Gestalt Therapy* that most orthodox psychologists (ego level) would accept Federn's appraisal of an individual's ego sense: "The mental and the bodily ego are felt separately, but in the wake state always in such a way that the mental ego is experienced to be inside the body ego."[65] Now that is a very accurate phenomenological portrayal of the ego level, and I think it is an almost perfect description of the separate self as ego. Underlying the ego, however, is the centaur, the body-mind felt unity. Thus Perls et al. are very forceful in pointing out what they call the "underlying unity": "Fortunately, the *true underlying unity* can be demonstrated by a simple experiment: introspecting, try to include as objects of the acting 'I' more and more pieces of the larger passive body-self; gradually, then all at once, mind and body will coalesce, I and self will merge . . ." (my italics).[66] And the centaur will emerge.

Alexander Lowen believes that the dissociation (and not just the normal differentiation) between ego and body is a type of deeply seated blockage in the total self. "The block also operates to separate and isolate the psychic realm from the somatic realm. Our consciousness tells us that each acts upon the other, but because of the block it does not extend deep enough for us to sense the *underlying unity*" (my italics).[67]

In both of the above senses, one of the approaches to the centaur or existential self might be put in our formula this way: to take the body-It back into the I is to *re-member* the projected or alienated body and thus reawaken (anamnesis) the total centaur. That is not the only approach emphasized by the writers I have quoted, but it is a central feature of most. As Rollo May once said, "[Part of] what we are proposing is to take back the body." On the whole, however, the re-membrance of the body is simply one aspect of the move to reawaken and authenticate the total, organismic, or existential bodymind: the centaur.

In my opinion, the existential psychologists have done much to explain, explore, and "resurrect" the centaur. Beginning with Kierkegaard[68] and Nietzsche,[69] through Husserl,[70] Heidegger,[71] and Sartre,[72] to Binswanger,[73] Frankl,[74] Boss,[75] May, and Maddi, the potentials and crises of the total being were eloquently set forth in existential terms. Notions of authenticity, of concrete being-in-the-world, of Dasein, of intentionality and the will, autonomy, meaning, and the centered self—all of these were brought forth as potentials for and of *being,* and all of them were underscored by the central notion of the *total* being. Added to that were the organismic insights of Kurt Goldstein;[76] the Gestalt approach of Köhler,[77, 78] Wertheimer,[79] Koffka; the holistic view of Smuts[80] and unitas multiplex of Allport[81]—to mention a prominent few.

Now of course I am not implying that these authors—and the ones I have already quoted—are all in perfect agreement, or that they are all absolutely talking about the same "self," let alone about what I am calling the centaur. However, it does seem to me that they share a substantial and impressive number of common assumptions and conclusions (many of these writers acknowledge this fact by accepting in a general fashion the label "humanistic-existential"; see *Current Personality Theories,*[82] for instance, where the sections on Rogers, Adler, existentialism, holism, organismic theories, and personalism *all* acknowledge their general similarities to each other). It is my opinion, however, that the existential centaur is a real and prior level of awareness, and that the broad similarities of these writers result from the fact that they all either intuit, or are personally alive to, this prior level.

Now many of these existential-humanistic writers have gone to great lengths to explain, explore, and describe the *potentials* of the total bodymind or centaur. A prime concept in this regard is "self-actualization," a concept initiated by Goldstein and Karen Horney,[83] and made popular by Maslow[84] and Rogers and the whole human potentials movement. Rogers' whole theory, for instance, "focuses renewed attention on the importance of *actualizing the full potential* of each individual and on the meaning of concepts such as experiencing, organismic valuing, and organismic sensing which the theory holds to be of *crucial importance in fulfilling that unique potential"* (my italics).[85] The implication of this is that one's full potential springs from the total, ongoing psychophysiological flow, and not from any aspect or fragment of that flow—ego, body, superego, self-concept, and so on (and here I remind the reader that Rogers is no mere theoretician; he is known for his extensive experimental and clinical studies[86]). In our terms, self-actualization is, in general, intimately related to the centaur level, and is not directly available to the ego or persona levels.

Rollo May, for instance, states that "neither the ego nor the body nor the unconscious can be 'autonomous,' but can only exist as parts of a totality. *And it is in this totality* [or centaur] *that will and freedom must have their base"* (my italics).[87] *Presumably,* then, actual autonomy (and self-actualization) would result, and could only result by definition, with *the conscious resurrection of this totality*—a type of shift of identity from any of the fragments (ego, body, persona) to their prior source in I AMness. According to general existential thought, when an individual's self is felt or apprehended as the prior, total being, he assumes—*can* assume—responsibility for his entire being-in-the-world. He can, as Sartre puts it, choose himself. He can *choose* to accept his fate, and thus his choices or intentionalities, because they take into account his total orientation in the world, are meaningful in the deepest sense. Rollo May, for instance, links *meaning* (as in "my life has meaning") with intentionality, and quotes Husserl in support: "Meaning is an intention of the mind." From this prior, existential centaur, there is no reluctance to the present—no hidden corner of a self that balks at this existence. Although one cannot drastically change the nature of existence, one *can* learn how to face the situation and accept it. This does not change the nature of existence, but it greatly changes the person. He or she can start to move on the whole, as a whole—and that is what Leslie Farber called the "spontaneous will."[87a]

I particularly like the notion of the "spontaneous will," because—aside from its own intrinsic merits—it tends to point up the types of potentials available only to the centaur or total being, and not just the ego or persona. Rollo May explains Farber's conclusions: "Dr. Farber demarcates two realms of 'will,' the first consisting of an *experience of the self in its totality,* a relatively *spontaneous* movement in a certain direction. In this kind of willing, the *body* moves as a whole, and the experience is characterized by a relaxation and by an imaginative, open quality. This is an experience of *freedom* which is *anterior* to all talk about political or psychological freedom" (all italics mine).[88] We note here the significance of the body, the imaginative and open mental set, the emphasis on the total self, and the notion of its being *anterior* or *prior.*

"In contrast, the will of the second realm, as Dr. Farber sees it, is that in which some obtrusive element enters, some necessity for a decision with an element of an *against* something along with a *for* something. If one uses the Freudian terminology, the 'will of the super-ego' would be included in this realm."[89] The spontaneous will is of the total bodymind, whereas the second will is of the effortful and purposive ego (and superego). May equates the spontaneous will of the total self with the intentionality of the existentialists, which is why he says that intentionality "is the missing link between mind and body." As I see it, the connection is fairly simple and is pointed out by May himself: the body tends to be "involuntary" or "spontaneous," in the sense that we do not normally and consciously control its processes of circulation, growth, digestion, feeling, all the millions of spontaneous variables that add up to Rogers' "natural wisdom of the body." The ego, on the other hand, we generally assume to be the home of many voluntary, controlled, and purposive activities. The total self then, as the prior centaur or ego-body union, is a type of conjunction of both of these experiential realms: the voluntary and the involuntary. Thus, the "spontaneous will"—"the missing link between mind and body."

I cannot here elaborate on, or even adequately summarize, the analyses of May, Farber, Lynch,[90] and others on will, intentionality, and the total self or centaur. However, if we can accept the plausibility of their conclusions pertaining to these "two realms" (ego and centaur), and if we accept the existential equation of intentionality and meaning, then our inevitable conclusion would be something like this: the centaur has a spontaneous will, the ego has willpower; the centaur has meaning, the ego has purpose and goals.

James Broughton has recently completed an extensive phenomenological study on what individuals at different stages of development see as the relationship of mind, body, and self.[91] He divides his results into six stages of increasing development (influenced by Kohler, Piaget, and Baldwin[92]). At level 0, his lowest, the mind and body are not differentiated; self is "inside" and reality is "outside." At levels 1 and 2, mind and body are differentiated, and self tends to reside in the mind which "controls" the body (both mind and body seem to be "substantial"). At levels 3 and 4, the individual differentiates the social role or false appearance (our persona) from the "true" self-concept or "inner self." Going further, however, at level 5 (to use Loevinger's summary), "the self as observer is distinguished from the self-concept [our ego] as known. . . . *The physiological body is recognized as a conceptual construction just as mind is*" (my italics).[93] It appears to me that at level 5, the "self" is starting to shift to a center that is prior to both body and mind as separate entities, since both are recognized as mere *constructs*. At level 6, Broughton's highest level, this shift seems complete, because at that highest level *"mind and body are both experiences of an integrated self"* (my italics).[94] That, in my opinion, is the centaur, the integrated and total self, prior to body, mind, persona, and shadow, but embracing, as it were, all of them *as experiences* ("experiences of an integrated self," as Broughton's study showed). This highest level in Broughton's study does not, so far as I can tell, include any permanent or dominant states of transcendent awareness, unity, or "cosmic consciousness," and so on—that is, there are no strong transpersonal elements in it, no shift to a real transpersonal witness, etc. Rather, it is just what it appears to be, the "highest stage" of separate-self development, individual development, and humanistic integration. A type of "full self-potential," "self-actualization," or "self-integration."

In my own shorthand, I would generalize and summarize this entire integration in our simple formula: the boundaries of the soul have, as it were, "expanded" to the total self or centaur, so that, as far as the centaur goes, where It was, I have become.

With that, we are now faced with the same question we put to Freud at the end of the ego-level section: Can the boundaries of awareness, and therefore the potentials of the being, expand beyond the individual, beyond even the "total self" or centaur? Are there yet deeper and more encompassing I's? Perhaps more "obscured and veiled" Its? Is it all that fantastic to assume that there might be "further reaches of human nature"[95] and deeper "realms of the human unconscious"?[96] If these deeper realms do exist—if they are not just hallucinations or regressions—one thing is fairly obvious from the start: they would have to reach beyond the limits of individuality. They would have to be transpersonal.

Nevertheless, we should ask, how could there be a level of awareness "within" an individual which, in some sense, seems to transcend the individual—what could the meaning of "transpersonal" be? I do not mean to sound prosaic or maudlin about this, because it is a very difficult yet very important topic. Furthermore, since this whole idea initially sounds so puzzling, instead of jumping directly into the middle of a discussion of the possible existence of a "transpersonal self," I would like by way of introduction to briefly discuss the work of C. G. Jung, Freud's most brilliant and distinguished disciple. This will serve as some necessary background information—information that, in any other culture, would have been supplied in one form or another to a person from the time of his birth.

Jung began studying with Freud at the beginning of this century, and although Freud had designated Jung to be his sole "successor and crown prince," within a decade Jung had broken with Freud over doctrinal disagreements. After that celebrated parting of the ways, the two great men never again spoke to one another.

The ultimate basis of their mutual incompatibilities might be described as follows. We are already starting to see that consciousness might not be a one-dimensional affair, but might instead be composed of several levels or bands—a type of "spectrum of consciousness." We have thus far examined the persona, ego, and centaur levels, and we still have the possibilities of the transpersonal and the universal bands left, and these five levels—even if we admit their existence—probably are still only a prominent handful of the infinite levels and shades of the spectrum. At any rate, if we assume all that to be true, any researcher investigating a particular level of the spectrum might generally acknowledge as real all levels on and above his own, but he would probably deny reality to any level deeper than his own. He might proclaim these deeper levels to be either pathological, illusory, or nonexistent. Now he might be right—but he might not, and if we *assume* there are deeper levels of awareness, then we would also assume that this individual rejects these deeper levels simply because his mode of self-sense (his level of the spectrum) cannot by definition accommodate direct knowledge of the deeper levels. It is my opinion that something like this happened with Freud and Jung. For Freud ended up confining his truly remarkable and courageous investigations to the ego and persona levels. Jung, however, while fully acknowledging these upper levels, managed to push his explorations all the way down to the transpersonal bands, and this is to his greatest credit. Jung was the first major European psychologist to discover and explore significant aspects of the transpersonal realm of human awareness. This Freud could not comprehend, confined as he was to the upper levels, and thus the two great men had to travel their separate paths and answer to their own destinies.

What specifically was it that Jung stumbled onto? What was it that he discovered in the very depths of the human soul that pointed unmistakably to a transpersonal realm? What *in* a person could possibly be *beyond* a person?

To begin with, Jung had spent a great deal of time studying the primitive (and not so primitive) mythologies of the world—the whole pantheons of Chinese, Egyptian, Greek, etc., gods and goddesses, demons and divinities, totems and animisms, ancient symbols, images, and mythological motifs of all imaginable sorts. Yet what totally astounded Jung was that these primitive mythological images also appeared regularly and unmistakably *in the dreams and fantasies of modern, civilized Europeans,* the vast majority of whom had never and probably could have never been exposed to these myths at all. At least, they certainly did not possess the formidable and astonishingly accurate knowledge of mythology displayed in their dreams. Apparently, this information was not acquired during their lifetimes, and thus, Jung reasoned, in some sense or another these basic mythological motifs might be innate structures inherited by every member of the human race. These primordial images or archetypes, as Jung called them, would thus be common to all people—they belong to no single individual, but are instead trans-individual, collective, transcendent.

This is certainly a plausible hypothesis, especially if one carefully examines the reams of meticulously detailed data reported by Jung. Just as, for example, each person possesses one heart, two kidneys, ten fingers, four limbs, and so on, each person's deep structure might contain universal *symbolic forms* essentially identical to those of all other human structures. Jung himself felt these structures might be etched in the brain, for the brain is several million years old, and over that vast, vast expanse of time it necessarily evolved certain basic (and in this sense "mythological") ways of perceiving and grasping reality, just as our hands evolved in special ways to grasp physical objects. These basic imaginative, mythological ways of grasping reality are the archetypes, and because every person's brain structure is basically similar, every person houses deep within him the same basic mythological archetypes which slowly evolved over the millennia. Jung's theory is not, therefore, Lamarckian—a mistaken notion many psychologists seize upon to toss Jung's entire case out of scientific court. (I personally believe that the archetypes are metaphysical, or "psychoid" as Jung finally put it, which means they transcend the mind and body and are contained in neither.) Since these archetypes would be common to all people by virtue of a shared membership in the human race, Jung called this deep layer of the soul the "collective unconscious." It is, in other words, not individual or personal, but supra-individual, transpersonal, transcendent. Buried deep in every person's being, this theory would say, is the *mythology of transcendence,* a most powerful layer of the soul.

Jung felt that parts of the unconscious (corresponding with our persona, ego, and centaur levels) contain personal memories, wishes, ideas, experiences, and potentials. However, the deeper realm—the collective unconscious "within" you—contains nothing strictly personal whatsoever. Rather, Jung believed that it houses the collective memories, motifs, and potentials of the entire human race: all the gods and goddesses, divinities and demons, heroes, and symbols portrayed outwardly by the world's ancient mythologies are contained, in condensed and simple form, in the depths of each person's being. They live on, as it were, and continue to move us deeply in ways both creative and destructive. The collective unconscious contains not only demons which possess us, but also gods and heroes which inspire us. The demonic and heroic may be denied, but never robbed of their power or finally cheated of their due.

The basic aim of some types of transpersonal band therapies, such as Jung's, is therefore to help individuals consciously acknowledge and befriend and utilize these powerful transpersonal forces instead of being moved by them unconsciously and against their wills. "Such penetration and transformation," says Lama Govinda of some of the transpersonal aspects of Buddhist meditation, "is only possible through the compelling power of inner vision, whose primordial images or 'archetypes' are the formative principles of our mind. Like seeds they sink into the fertile soil of our subconscious in order to germinate, to grow and to unfold their potentialities."[97]

Let us, for the moment, simply assume there is some truth in Jung's conclusions, and let us draw out its possible implications. In the Jungian view, contacting this transpersonal realm would involve a special sense, relearning to live life *mythologically.* Now I realize instantly that this type of statement is apt to puzzle most people, for we moderns generally take an extremely dim view of anything that smacks of mythology. In our culture, for instance, if we say something is a "myth" we mean only one thing: it is an illusion, a primitive fantasy, wishful thinking, an untruth. We say, for example, that it is a myth that the sun circles the earth. Now that usage of the word "myth" is fine, but it is definitely not the way we are using it here. When Jung says we must learn to live life mythologically, I trust the reader realizes that he obviously doesn't mean we are to grasp some convenient illusion and build our lives around it.

To live life mythologically might mean, as one instance, to begin to grasp the transcendent, to see it alive in oneself, in one's life, in one's work, friends, and environment. And mythology at least shows us, opens us to, just such a world of transcendence. For the world of mythology is a world which temporarily suspends space and time—it is the world of "once upon a time," which, as Coomaraswamy points out, means the world *before* time and prior to time, a nonhistorical world that might open one to the nonhistorical aspects of one's own consciousness.[98] That, anyway, is the opinion of the great Mircea Eliade:

> Symbolic [or mythic] thinking is not the exclusive privilege of the child, of the poet or of the unbalanced mind: it is consubstantial with human existence, *it comes before* language and discursive reason. The symbol reveals certain aspects of reality—*the deepest aspects*—which defy any other means of knowledge. Images, symbols and myths are not irresponsible creations of the psyche; they respond to a need and fulfil a function, that of bringing to light the most hidden modalities of being. Consequently, the study of them enables us to reach a better understanding of man—of man "as he is," before he has come to terms with the conditions of History.[99] (my italics)

This aspect of one's being and awareness is before history and time. Eliade continues:

> Today we are beginning to see that the non-historical portion of every human being does not simply merge into the animal kingdom, as in the nineteenth century so many thought it did, nor ultimately into "Life"; but that, on the contrary, it bifurcates and rises right above Life. This non-historical part of the human being wears, like a medal, the imprinted memory of a richer, a more complete and almost beatific existence.[99]

Therefore,

> When a historically conditioned being—for instance, an Occidental of our own days—allows himself to be invaded by the non-historical part of himself (which happens to him much oftener and more completely than he

imagines), this is not necessarily a retrogression towards the animal stage of humanity or a redescent towards the deepest sources of organic life. Often he is re-entering, by means of the images and the symbols that then come into play, a paradisiac stage of primordial humanity . . . , a lost paradise.[99]

Now I realize that some of this might sound like completely unsubstantiated theorizing—nonetheless, I think there is a staggering amount of direct and indirect evidence accumulating in its behalf. In the physical sciences, for instance, the conclusion is starting to come down that this "mythological world prior to space and time" might end up being the ultimate substratum of the physical universe itself. Physicists are already saying as much themselves—for example, David Bohm (who, of anybody alive, deserves the title "dean of physicists") has joined forces with the neurosurgeon Karl Pribram in suggesting that the order of the universe is holographic.[99a] Thus, "ultimate reality" is said to be a timeless and spaceless realm, an "implicate order," wherein each part of the universe *is,* and *implies,* all the other parts as well. That is, it is holographic—*the part is the whole and the whole is the part.* Yet wasn't that what Cassirer pointed out decades ago as the single most defining characteristic of the mythological realm? In mythological thinking, Cassirer said, "the whole is the part, in the sense that it enters into it with its whole mythical-substantial essence, that it is somehow sensuously and materially 'in' it."[100] That the whole is in each part is not, according to some modern physicists, just a mythological thought—as if that meant "fantasy" or "pretend"—but it is really the physical nature of this world, the actual reality of this world.

Thus, when Eliade says that "the myth reveals the *deepest aspects* of reality," he might be very right. That is, the language and imagery of mythology might be much closer to the nature of reality than are linear logic and abstract thinking, for if the real world is indeed holographic, then only the multivalent nature of the mythic image would be capable of sustaining this vision and eliciting this understanding. The holographic-mythic image, wherein the whole is the part and the part is the whole, would be able to grasp states of affairs quite beyond the theory of logical types and the laws of contradiction and the excluded middle. This is why, I believe, that Coomaraswamy stated that "myth embodies the nearest approach to absolute truth that can be stated in words."[101] Mythological awareness is holographic because it begins to transcend conventional boundaries—boundaries of space and time, and opposites and selves—and for that very reason alone, mythological awareness might be one step closer to the real world, "the seamless coat of the universe," as Whitehead put it.[102]

Thus, from this angle, to live mythologically might mean to begin to open oneself to a "deeper" world of no-boundary and transcendence—*and the corresponding potentials therein.* This does not mean that we surrender altogether the conventional world of boundaries and fall into mythological fantasies (a dangerous state indeed). Rather, it would seem to mean that we open ourselves to mythological transcendence and bring that awareness down into our conventional world, thereby to enlighten, energize, and revitalize it by connecting it to a source much deeper than itself. We might even say this would be to *find the holographic and nonhistorical level of one's own awareness,* a level wherein the person is the Whole and the Whole is in the person, prior to space, time, and existence as a separate self—but perhaps I am getting ahead of the story.

Now—if I may quickly finish up this introduction to Jung's work on the mythological layer of the soul—Jung felt that these mythological images, these archetypes, are *already present* in each and every person, and they can be activated by any situation which corresponds to the particular archetype. The archetypal image then exerts an effect on behavior which ranges from mild influence to total possession—and no amount of upper-level therapies will suffice to assuage the assault. At the same time, the archetypal root might show up visibly in dreams, fantasies, daydreams, imaginations, or even hallucinations.

An individual, for example, might have a "key dream" where the central image is a sphinx, a gorgon, a medusa, a great serpent, a winged horse, or some other obviously mythological material. Through a little studying of ancient mythology, he might easily learn what these mythological images have meant to the human race on the whole, and thereby discover what these images *mean to his own collective unconscious.* According to Jung and his followers, by integrating this meaning—*by connecting this very deep type of It to his conscious I-awareness*—the individual is no longer forcibly controlled by It. The depth of his soul thus begins to loosen, the I begins to "grow down" into the depths of a transpersonal It, and the topsoil of normal egoic or centauric awareness begins to gently break apart to allow a growth of the transcendent—a growth, that is, of those processes which transcend his personal life but which nevertheless are aspects of "his" own deeper, transpersonal self.

Let me try to explain, in this context of mythological awareness, just how this shift to a deeper self, a transpersonal self, might occur. As the individual begins to reflect on his life *through* the eyes of the archetypes and mythological images common to mankind, his awareness necessarily begins to shift to a universal or global perspective, a transcendent, depersonal, supra-individual view. As Joseph Campbell so gracefully put it, the individual "may learn to see himself depersonalized in the mirror of the human spirit."[103] He is looking at himself not through his eyes, which are in some ways almost certainly prejudiced, but through the eyes of the collective human spirit—a different view indeed! As such, he is no longer exclusively preoccupied with his own personal disadvantage point. In fact, if this process quickens correctly, his very identity, his very self, would expand qualitatively to these more-or-less global dimensions, and his soul would become saturated with depth. He would no longer *exclusively* identify with just his ego or his centaur, and thus he would no longer be suffocated by his purely personal problems and dramas. (We will be examining this process in depth shortly—for the moment, I ask the reader to simply follow along.) In a sense the individual would be able to let go of his individual concerns and view them with a creative detachment and indifference, realizing that whatever problems his personal self faces, his deeper self would transcend to remain open. He would find, haltingly at first but then with an ever-increasing certainty, a profound center of awareness that persists unperturbed, like the depths of the ocean, even though the surface waves of consciousness be swept with ripples of pain, anxiety, or despair. He would find, in a word, his transpersonal self, the eye of humanity's spirit.

Now the discovery, in one form of another, or the transcendent self—assuming, for the moment, that it exists—is the major aim of transpersonal band therapies and disciplines. As one might imagine, however, the mythological approach which we have been exclusively discussing thus far is by no means the only path to the transcendent self. To every level of the spectrum of consciousness there seem to be numerous different but effective approaches, and an individual simply has to experiment a bit to determine which is the best for him. I have dwelt on the mythological as a convenient introduction to the realm of the transpersonal, but the strictly mythological route, as is probably very obvious, is a rather difficult one and usually demands a professional assistant to help guide an individual through the vast maze of the world's mythologies and his own archetypal layer.

However, there are simpler approaches to the transpersonal self—not necessarily shorter or easier, but definitely much less delicate and complicated. The "witnessing meditation" of Hindu jnana yoga, psychosynthesis, and preliminary zazen is a good example. Notice first of all the broad, distinguishing marks of the transpersonal self: it is a center and expanse of awareness which is creatively detached from one's personal mind, body, emotions, thoughts, and feelings. It is a center of awareness, in other words, which is not exclusively identified with one's mind or body or ego or centaur. Thus, the following "disidentification" exercise, adapted from psychosynthesis,[104] might be used to evoke and sustain this transpersonal center. One simply silently repeats the following several times, trying to realize as vividly as possible the import of the words:

I *have* a body, but I am *not* my body. I can see and feel my body, and what can be seen and felt is not the true seer. My body may be tired or excited, sick or healthy, heavy or light, but that has nothing to do with my inward I. I *have* a body, but I am *not* my body.

I *have* desires, but I am *not* my desires. I can know my desires, and what can be known is not the true knower. Desires come and go, floating through my awareness, but they do not affect my inward I. I *have* desires but I am *not* my desires.

I *have* emotions, but I am *not* my emotions. I can feel and sense my emotions, and what can be felt is not the true feeler. Emotions pass through me. but they do not affect my inward I. I *have* emotions, but I am *not* my emotions.

I *have* thoughts, but I am *not* my thoughts. I can know and follow my thoughts, and what can be known is not the true knower. Thoughts come to me and thoughts leave me, but they do not affect my inward I. I *have thoughts* but I am *not* my thoughts.

If an individual persists at such an exercise, the understanding condensed in it will quicken and he might begin to notice some fundamental changes in his sense of "self." For instance, he might begin intuiting a deeply inward sense of freedom, of lightness, of release, of stability. This source, this "center of the cyclone," would retain its pellucid stillness even amid the raging winds of anxiety and suffering that might swirl round its center. The discovery of this witnessing center—which Assagioli called the higher self and Maslow called the plateau experience (after Asrani)—is very much like diving from the calamitous waves on the surface of a stormy ocean to the calm and quiet depths of the bottom. At first the individual might not get more than a few feet beneath the agitated waves of the surface and down toward this quiet unknown It. With persistence, however, he might easily gain the ability to dive fathoms into the quiet depths of his soul, and as this ability matures and ripens, *this great transpersonal It is transmuted, converted, into an expansive transpersonal I.* Lying outstretched at the bottom, he gazes up in an alert but detached fashion at the turmoil that he once thought he was and that held him transfixed. In integrating this deeper and more pervasive It, he finds a deeper and more pervasive I.

To the extent that he actually realizes that he is not, for example, his anxieties, then his anxieties no longer *threaten* him. For even if anxiety is present, it no longer overwhelms him because he is no longer exclusively tied to it. He is no longer courting it, or fighting it, or resisting it, or running from it, or trying to "treat" it. In the most radical fashion, anxiety is thoroughly accepted as it is and is allowed to move as it will. He has nothing to lose, nothing to gain, by its presence or absence, for he is simply watching it pass by. Seen thus, anxiety is no more upsetting to him than a bird flying through the air, for he is not identified with either, but merely the witness of both.

These types of "plateau experiences," says Maslow, "represent a witnessing of reality. It involves seeing the symbolic, or the mythic, the poetic, the transcendent, the miraculous. . . . It's the transcending of space and time which becomes quite normal, so to speak."[105]

Thus, from this deeper, transpersonal level of the spectrum, any emotion, sensation, thought, memory, or experience that disturbs an individual is simply one with which he has *exclusively* identified his Self, and the *ultimate* resolution of the disturbance is simply to disidentify with it! Rajneesh always quotes Gurdjieff in this regard: "Identification is the only sin."

Slowly, gently, as the person pursues this disidentification "therapy," his entire *individual* self (persona, ego, centaur), which heretofore he had fought to defend and protect, begins to become transparent and drop away. Not that it literally falls off and he finds himself disembodied in space—rather, he simply begins to feel that what happens to his personal self (his wishes, his hopes, desires, hurts) is not a matter of life-or-death seriousness because there is within him a deeper and more basic self which is not touched by these peripheral fluctuations, these surface waves of grand commotion but feeble substance. The flight from the self to the Self is a flight from personal manipulation to transcendent witnessing.

Thus the individual's mind-and-body may be in pain, or humiliation, or fear, but as long as he consents to simply abide as the witness of these affairs, as if from on high, they no longer threaten *him*, and thus he need no longer manipulate them, wrestle with them, subdue them, or try to "understand" them. Because he is willing to witness them, to look at them impartially, he is thereby able to transcend them. As St. Thomas put it, "Whatever knows certain things cannot have any of them in its own nature." Thus, if the eye were colored red, it wouldn't be able to perceive red objects. It can see red because it is itself clear, or "red-less." Likewise, if we can but watch or truly witness our distresses, we prove ourselves thereby to be "distress-less," or free of the witnessed turmoil. That within which feels pain is itself pain-less; that which feels fear is fear-less; that which perceives tension is tension-less. To witness these states is to transcend them. They no longer seize us from behind because we look at them up front.

Thus, we might be able to understand why Patanjali, the codifier of yoga in India, said that ignorance is the identification of the seer with the instruments of seeing. Every time we become exclusively identified with or attached to the persona, ego, body, or centaur, then anything which threatens their existence or standards seems to threaten our very Self. Every attachment to thoughts, sensations, feelings, or experiences is merely another link in the chain of our own self-enslavement.

Heretofore I have been speaking of the release of human potentials as an "expanding" of identity, but now, rather abruptly, I am speaking of disidentifying. Isn't this contradictory? Actually, these are but two ways of speaking about a single process. Take, for example, the descent from the persona level to the ego level. Two things have happened in this particular descent: (1) the individual re-members or *identifies* with his shadow; but (2) he *disidentifies* with, or breaks his *exclusive* attachment to, his persona. His "new" identity, the ego, is thus a synergetic combination of both persona and shadow, and this can be described as either identification or disidentification, depending upon the referent point. Likewise, to descend to the centaur level, a person extends his identity to the body while disidentifying with the ego *alone*. In each case, not only do we expand to a new and broader identity, but also we break an old and narrowed one.

In just the same way, we "expand" to the broader identity of the transpersonal self by gently breaking or letting go of our narrower identity with the centaur alone. We disidentify with the centaur and all its aspects, but in the direction of depth and expanse.

Thus, as we begin to touch the transpersonal witness, we begin to let go of our purely personal problems, worries, and concerns. In fact—and this is the entire key to most transpersonal band therapies—we don't even try to solve our problems or distresses, as we surely would and should on the persona, ego, or centaur levels. For our *only* concern here is to *watch* our particular distresses, to simply and innocently be aware of them, without judging them, avoiding them, dramatizing them, working on them, analyzing them, or justifying them (Krishnamurti's "choiceless awareness"[106]). As a feeling or tendency arises, we witness it. If hatred of that feeling arises, we witness that. If hatred of the hatred arises, then we witness *that*. Nothing is to be done—but if a "doing" arises, we witness that. Abide as awareness. Let anything—any and all joys and distresses—come and go as they like, when they like, how they like.

This is possible *only when we understand that they do not constitute a real self*. As long as we are attached to them, there will be an effort, however subtle, to manipulate them. Understanding that they are neither the center nor the self, we don't resent them, try to move away from them or towards them. Every move we make to solve or work out a distress simply reinforces the illusion that we are that particular distress. Thus, ultimately (and viewed only from this level), to try to escape or solve a distress merely perpetuates that distress, or that distress in a disguised form. What is so upsetting to us is not the distress itself, but our *attachment* to that distress. We identify with it, and that alone is the real difficulty.

Instead of fighting a distress or in any way trying to remedy it (again, this is true only when we are approaching it from this transpersonal level), we simply assume the innocence of a detached impartiality towards it. The mystics and sages are fond of likening this state of witnessing to a mirror—for here we simply reflect any sensations or thoughts that arise, without clinging to them or pushing them away—just as a crystal mirror perfectly and impartially reflects whatever passes in front of it. Says Chuang-tzu, "The perfect man employs his mind as a mirror. It grasps nothing; it refuses nothing; it receives, but does not keep."[107]

Now if the individual is at all successful in developing and sustaining this type of detached witnessing—it takes time—he will be able to look upon the events occurring in his mind-body with the *very same impartiality* that he would look upon clouds floating through the sky, water rushing in a stream, rain cascading on a roof, or any other objects in his field of awareness. In other words, his *relationship* to his mind-body becomes the same as his relationship to *all other* objects.

In short, his mind-and-body totally become an *object* of his awareness, but in this sense: he starts to realize that because he can *see* them, they do not and cannot constitute a true seer. "May I remind you," said Zen Master Huang Po, "that the perceived cannot perceive?" Because he can perceive them, they cannot be the perceiver. Because he can know them, they cannot be the knower. Not one of them can be the conscious Self, because they are all, *all* objects. An object cannot see. Thus Ramana Maharshi called the higher self the "I-I" because it witnesses, as it were, the individual I.[108] When you watch the world, or think you do, the I-I watches you—as Shankara would put it, the I shines with the I-I's light.[109] The object of meditation is to eventually have the I "fall down abashed" into the prior I-I, which is, after all, only one's own true nature. Where It was, I-I shall become.

Prior to this, the individual had been using his mind-and-body as something with which to look at the world. Thus, he became intimately attached to them and bound to their limited perspectives, both conscious and unconscious. He became identified exclusively with them, and thus he was tied and bound to their problems, pains, and distresses. However, by consistently and persistently looking at them, giving them "bare attention,"[110] by emptying or exhausting them through witnessing, he realizes that they are—and always have been—merely *objects* of awareness, fleeting, ephemeral, empty: objects, in fact, of the transpersonal witness. "I *have* a mind and body and emotions, but I am *not* my mind and body and emotions." Up to that point, he had confused the seer with that which can be seen—a simple case of mistaken identity, but a mistake the East has called samsara, maya, avidya, adhyasa—bondage, limitation, constriction, death.

However, it is most important at this point to affirm that just because a person begins to contact, or even totally shift to, the transpersonal bands, he does not lose access to, contact with, or control over, any of the upper levels of the spectrum (except in cases of what we call "regressive involution," most notably schizophrenia). Remember that as an individual descends from an exclusive identity with the persona to a fuller and more accurate identity with his total ego, he does not thereby completely lose access to the persona—he is just no longer stuck to it! He can still don his persona if, for instance, he chooses to put on a "good show" or a temporary social facade for practical or decorous purposes, but he is no longer chronically anchored in that role. Formerly, he could not drop this facade, either for others or—and here is the pathological disaster—himself. Now, however, he can simply use it or not, depending upon circumstances and his own discretion. If he decides to put on his "good face," his persona (or one of them), then he consciously and temporarily checks his shadow; he holds back his negative aspects. He is still capable of being aware of them, however, and thus does not project them. So the persona itself isn't maladaptive or pathological—unless it's the only self you have. Thus, what is dissolved or destroyed when one descends from the persona level to the ego level is not the shadow or the persona, but the boundary and thus the battle between them—the boundary between I and It.

Likewise, when an individual descends to the centaur level from the ego level, he doesn't destroy the ego or body, but simply the boundary between them, the split between this I and this It. On the centaur level, an individual still has unobstructed access to the ego, the body-global, the persona, the shadow; but, because he is no longer *exclusively* identified with one as against the others, all of these elements tend to work in harmony—May's "autonomy"—or at least *concordia discors* (which we might translate as "lover's spats"). He has befriended them all and touched each with acceptance. There are no intractable boundaries between them (the Its have become I's) and so no major battles.

In the very same way, as an individual contacts the transpersonal self, he still has access to *all* the levels above it. No longer, however, will he be tied to those levels, bound to them, or limited by them. They become instrumental, not essential.

It should also be clearly stated that as a person begins this creative detachment from the exclusive and restrictive identification with the isolated organism, he in no way ceases caring for his centaur. He doesn't stop eating, refuse drink, abandon washing, drop all interest in those around him, or cease loving and living. Somewhat paradoxically, the reverse is actually the case. One becomes more caring and accepting of the mind-and-body. Since one is no longer bound by them, they no longer appear as a freedom-robbing prison, and thus the person's energies do not starve into a suppressed rage and hatred for his own organism. The moment we transcend the centaur, then and only then are we capable of truly accepting it. We saw that there are immense potentials in the centaur, and most of them can be developed by the centaur itself. Just the same—and only from the view of the transpersonal bands—only when we transcend the organism can the full potentials of the organism be realized, since only then is the full organism actually and wholly accepted. The organism as a whole thus becomes a perfectly accepted *expression* of the transpersonal self.

I also mentioned that, from the position of the transcendent witness, one begins to view the mind-and-body in the same way one would view any other object of awareness, be it a table, a tree, a car, a dog. Again, this might sound as if we would treat our personal organisms with the same disdain or disgust that on occasion we unleash on the environment, but once more, it actually works to the other side: we begin to treat all environmental objects as if they were our own Self.

In fact, this represents a preliminary intuition that the world is really one's body and is to be treated as such, and it is from this type of transpersonal intuition that begins to spring the universal compassion so emphasized by the mystics. For on the transpersonal bands, we begin to love others not because they love us, affirm us, reflect us, or secure us in our illusions, but because they *are* us. Christ's primary injunction does not mean, "Love thy neighbor as you love thyself," but "Love thy neighbor *as* thy Self." And not just your neighbor, but your whole environment! You begin to care for your surroundings just as you would your own arms and legs. At this transpersonal level, remember, your relationship to your environment is the *same* as the relationship to your very own organism. This is also why, in Zen, the true study of the moral precepts comes only *after* you have finished koan study, for only when you are one with all beings can you properly comprehend the deep significance of the moral precepts and the Bodhisattva's vows. Before that point, one's compassion is merely personic, egoic, or centauric: flattering, but corrupt.

At the level of the transpersonal witness, the archetypal self, an individual might also begin to regain a fundamental intuition, an intuition he certainly possessed as a child, an intuition that is said by the mystics and sages to be the one and only portal and op-*port*-unity leading from death to immortality. Namely, that since the Self fundamentally transcends the separate organism, then (1) it is single, and (2) it is immortal. If we grow down a bit and "become again as little children," this intuition is not so very hard to recapture. In fact, as a type of introduction, let me try to jar your memories of childhood.

Every child wonders (I did, anyway, and most people I mention this to seem to agree) at some time or another, "What would I be like if In had different parents?" I other words, it almost seems as if the child realizes, in his very innocent and inarticulate fashion, that consciousness itself—that inward I-ness or witness—is not really limited by the purely outer forms of mind and body that it animates. The child seems to realize that he would still be I even if he had different parents and a different personal organism. The child knows— and this is what prompts his question—that he would look and act differently, *but somehow he would still be an I,* because the inward witness of these outward forms is not bound by these forms! "I *have* a mind and body and emotions, but I am *not* the mind and body and emotions." The child asks this question—"What would I be like if I had different parents?"—because he wants the parents to explain, in a very nontechnical manner, *his transcendence,* the fact that he would still seem to be and feel the same I-ness even though he had different parents.

Further, the child might even realize that there is but *one* Self taking on these different outward forms, for every organism has the identical intuition of this *same* inner I-ness transcending the mind and body. Since these intuitions are formless, they could hardly be different. This single Self clearly transcends the mind and body, and thus is essentially one and the same in all conscious beings. The child knows—and the adult is asked to remember— that just as he can walk out of one room and into another without fundamentally changing his inward feeling of I-ness, so also he would not be fundamentally different if he possessed a different body, with different memories, and different sensations. He is the witness of these objects, but he is not tied to them. In other words, every child is very much in touch with the transcendent self, and only years of conditioning will convince him to surrender this intuition and identify exclusively with the particular mind and body he animates. "Well, Johnny, if you had different parents, I guess you'd be somebody *else.*"

What is forgotten can be recalled, and the recollection or collecting again of That alone which is worth remembering—this is the sole message of the great religious teachers, saints, and sages. From the Buddhist's *smrti* ("recollection") to the Islamic *dhikr* ("remembrance") to Christ's "Do this in *anamnesis* of me" (note anamnesis, "remembrance"), the call goes out to search one's heart and find the answer long forgotten. This answer is the remembrance of the great and ultimate It, the joining together *again* with the deepest Self—where that deepest It was, I shall become.

When I become that It, I am no longer just I. Because my sense of I-ness passes right out and beyond myself, the *potentials* that are opened to myself are no longer personal but transcendent, no longer secular but sacred, no longer limited but boundless. To the I are added the divine and cosmic potentials of that deepest It, and as a consequence the I is literally absorbed or dissolved in the prior fullness and limitless potential of that It. This is not a state of affairs that is manufactured or created, but an eternal state of affairs that is simply remembered. The word, again, is anamnesis—Plato knew all too well that ultimate truths are not learned but recollected. As Philosophia said to Boethius in his distress, "You have forgotten who you are."

If one had to summarize the final position and greatest contribution of Abraham Maslow, it would have to be the ultimate significance of, as he put it, "transcendence in the metapsychological sense of transcending one's own skin and body and bloodstream, as in identification with the B-values so they become intrinsic to the Self itself." There again: convert the transcendent It into a transcendent I. This "implies *identification* [re-membrance] with the B-values. . . . to become divine or godlike," for this is the ultimate "*potentiality of human nature*" (my italics), a state "in which one can *be* an end, a god, a perfection [a famous Zen koan asks, "How are you already absolutely perfect?"], an essence, a Being, sacred, divine," for this surely is "the very highest and most inclusive or holistic level of human consciousness."[111] There is Maslow's final view of human potentiality, and it is—as Tom Roberts puts it[112]—a potential "beyond self-actualization"—beyond, we would say, the centaur level. Self-actualization is, as we saw, a potential of the centaur: beyond the centaur is beyond self-actualization.

Now it should at least be mentioned—although we cannot pursue it at length—that just as the persona resisted the shadow, and the ego resisted the body-global, so also the centaur (and all levels above it) resists the transpersonal realm. The highest potentials—the transcendent ones—are basically threatening to the persona, ego, and centaur, for (as we will soon see) they threaten the death of the separate self. Maslow noticed this as the Jonah complex, and spoke of "defenses against metamotivation." Desoille called it "the repression of the sublime."[113] A true transpersonal therapy must handle this resistance as effectively as analysts handle shadow resistances. The same basic strategy must be used: help the individual see *that* he resists the sublime and *how* he resists It, so that, ultimately, It may become I. The truth is that, as a person loves his symptoms, so also he loves samsara. If not, he would already have effected enlightenment—and samsara is notorious for lasting a long, long time.

To continue: the insight that the transcendent self passes beyond the individual organism carries with it the intuition of immortality (strictly speaking, timelessness, but since immortality is a theological analogue of eternity, we will use it as a convenience). Even most adults harbor the inward feeling that they are immortal—they cannot imagine their nonexistence. I suppose nobody can; but the adult, because he exists *only* as the centaur, ego, or persona, falsely imagines—and deeply wishes—that his *individual* self will live forever: not that his true Self is already immortal, but that his ego should be! This is how he corrupts his intuition of eternity. Nonetheless, it is not true that the mind, body, or ego is immortal—as Buddha pointed out, they, like all composites, will die. They are dying now, and not one whit of any of them will survive eternally. Reincarnation does not mean that your ego moves through successive existences, but that the transcendent self is the "one and only transmigrant," as Shankara himself put it. That is to say, only the transpersonal self is immortal, timeless, or nonhistorical—not the individual ego.

Because the typical adult is identified exclusively with his separate self, the *otherwise correct* intuition that his transcendent self is immortal becomes deflected, and thus corrupted, into the wish that his ego be immortal—and he then views death as the end of all that he is. For this reason, he will not seriously entertain the idea that his ego will die. Says the *Mahabharata*:

> Of all the world's wonders, which is the most wonderful?
> That no man, though he sees others dying all around him,
> Believes that he himself will die.[114]

This whole confusion fires an explosive war between life and death, and drives man to ever more ersatz identifications, seeking to recapture that immortality which does lie at the base of awareness, but on the *other* side of egoic death.

In a certain sense, therefore, we have to "die" to our false, separate self (centaur-ego-persona) in order to awaken to our immortal and transcendent self. Thus the famous paradox, "If you die before you die, then when you die you won't die"; and the sayings of the mystics, "No one gets as much of God as the one who is thoroughly dead"; and Zen: "While alive, Be a dead man, Thoroughly dead; And act as you will, And all is good." For the greatest potential—perhaps the ultimate potential—lies only on the other side of death, not in any "afterlife" state, but here, now, in this lifetime, in this present moment. "You will know in due course," stated Ramana Maharshi, "that your true glory lies where you cease to exist." Your true glory, your greatest potential, lies just on the other side of *you*.

Perhaps we can approach this fundamental insight of the mystics and sages—that there is but *one* immortal Self common in and to us all—in yet another way. Perhaps you, like most people, feel that you are basically the same person you were yesterday. You probably also feel that you are *fundamentally* the same person you were a year ago. Indeed, you still seem to be the *same* you as far back as you can remember! Put it another way: *you* never remember a time when you weren't you. In other words, *something* in you seems to remain untouched by the passage of time. Yet surely your body is not the same as it was even a year ago. Surely also your sensations are different today than in the past. Surely, too, your memories are on the whole different today from those of a decade ago. Your mind, your body, your feelings—*all* have changed with time; but something has not changed, and you *know* that something has not changed. Something *feels* the same. What is that?

Even this time a year ago you had different concerns and basically different problems. Your immediate experiences were different, and so were your thoughts. *All* of these have vanished, but something in you remains. Now go one step further. What if you moved to a completely different country, with new friends, new surroundings, new experiences, new thoughts? You would still have that basic inner feeling of I-ness—you would still be you! Further yet, imagine that right now you forget everything that happened in the first five years of life. Leaving psychoanalysis aside for the moment, you would still feel that same inner I-ness, would you not? What if you even forgot the first 10 years or 15 years or 20 years of your life? Fundamentally, you would still feel the same *present* sense of I-ness. If right now you just temporarily forget *everything* that happened in your past and just feel that pure inner I-ness—has *anything* changed at all?

There is, in short, something within you—that deeply inward sense of I-ness—that is *not* memory, thoughts, mind, experience, surroundings, conflicts, sensations, or moods. For *all* of these have changed and can change and are changing now without substantially affecting that inner I-ness. *That* is what remains untouched by the flight of time—and that is the transpersonal witness and self.

Is it then so very difficult to realize that *every* conscious being has that *same* inner and nonhistorical I-ness? And that, therefore, the overall number of I's is but *one*? Did not the founder of quantum mechanics, Erwin Schrödinger, state that "consciousness is a *singular* of which the plural is unknown"?[115] Does not Zen speak of the One Mind?[116] Is not Brahman said to be "the One and Only Self, One without a Second"?[117] For my own part, I do not think they were all hallucinating, and I certainly do not think they were imposing mere "belief systems" on awareness. These people are not saying that all egos and all centaurs are the same—they are saying that there is only one ultimate and nonhistorical Self at the base of all historical egos and centaurs and, as William James might put it, for ought we know to the contrary, they might be right.

We have already surmised that if you had a different body you would still basically feel the same I-ness—but look around you: there *already* are all those other bodies with the same basic sense of I-ness. Isn't it just as easy to admit that there is ultimately but one, single I-ness taking on different views, different memories, different feelings and sensations?

This does not apply just to this time, but to all times—past and future. Since you undoubtedly feel—even though your memory, mind, and body are different—that you are the same I-ness you were 20 years ago, couldn't you also be the same I-ness you were 200 years ago? If I-ness isn't dependent upon memories and mind and body, what possible difference could it make? The answer, no doubt, is "none." In the words of the physicist Schrödinger:

What is it that has called you so suddenly out of nothingness to enjoy for a brief while a spectacle which remains quite indifferent to you? It is not possible that this unity of knowledge, feeling, and choice which you call *your own* should have sprung into being from nothingness at a given moment not so long ago; rather, this knowledge, feeling and choice are essentially eternal and unchangeable and numerically one in all men, nay in all sensitive beings. The conditions for your existence are almost as old as the rocks. For thousands of years men have striven and suffered and begotten and women have brought forth in pain. A hundred years ago, perhaps, another man sat on this spot; like you he gazed with awe and yearning in his heart at the dying light on the glaciers. Like you he was begotten of man and born of woman. He felt pain and brief joy as you do. *Was* he someone else? Was it not you yourself?[118]

Ah, we say, that couldn't have been me, because I can't remember what happened then. However, that is to make the mistake of identifying I-ness with memories—we just saw that I-ness is not memory but the witness of memory! Besides, you probably can't even remember what happened to you last month, but you are still I-ness. So what if you can't remember what happened to you last century? You are still that I-ness, and that I—there is only one in the whole cosmos—is the same I which awakens in every newborn being, the same I which looked out from our ancestors and will look out from our descendants—one and the same I. We feel they are different only because we make the error of identifying the inward I-ness with the outward memory, mind, and body, which indeed are different.

That there is only one highest Self has been obvious to the mystics, Eastern and Western alike—but how hard it seems for us moderns to grasp that fact. Even Maslow stumbled a little here, although he clearly saw the evidence. Speaking of *transcending* self-actualizers, he says that "the most highly valued part of such a person's self, then, is the *same* as the most highly valued part of the self of other self-actualizing people. Such selves overlap."[119] That is, at the deepest (or highest) point such selves overlap and are actually the same. Yet to say that all our deepest selves are really the same *is* to say that there is only one deepest self. There are lots of you's and me's in this world, but only one I.

As for that inward I—indeed, what is that? It was not born with your body, nor will it perish upon death. It does not recognize time or cater to its distresses. It is without color, without shape, without form, without size, and yet it beholds the entire majesty before your own eyes. It sees the sun, clouds, stars, and moon, but cannot itself be seen. It hears the birds, the crickets, the singing waterfall, but cannot itself be heard. It grasps the fallen leaf, the crusted rock, the knotted branch, but cannot itself be grasped.

You needn't try to see your transcendent self—which is not possible anyway. Can your eye see itself? Can your ear hear itself? Can your tongue taste itself? You cannot know that which is the knower. You need only begin by gently, consistently, and persistently dropping your false identifications with your memories, mind, body, emotions, and thoughts. Dogen Zenji said enlightenment was "mind and body dropped." Drop mind and body without losing them! This dropping entails nothing by way of superhuman effort or theoretical comprehension. All that is required, primarily, is but one understanding: *whatever you can see cannot be the seer. Everything* you know about yourself is precisely *not* your Self, the knower, the inner I-ness that can neither be perceived, defined, nor made an object of any sort. Whatever you think about yourself is precisely not your Self. Whatever you feel about yourself is precisely not your Self. Bondage is nothing but the misidentification of the seer with all these things which can be seen, and liberation begins with the simple reversal of this mistake. To abide as the Self is to step aside from limitations and thus finally to step out of them.

This, then, is the message of Jung; the message of Maslow, Assagioli, and the whole Fourth Force; and more, of the saints, sages, and mystics, whether Amerindian, Taoist, Hindu, Buddhist, or Christian: at the bottom of your soul is the soul of humanity itself, but a divine, uncreate soul, leading from time to eternity, from death to immortality, from bondage to liberation, from enchantment to awakening. To salvation in this life go those who comprehend the supreme identity. Listen to Kabir:

> O Friend, hope for Him whilst you live, know whilst you live,
>   understand whilst you live; for in life deliverance abides.
> If your bonds be not broken whilst living, what hope of deliverance
>   in death?
> It is but an empty dream that the soul shall have union with Him
>   because it has passed from the body;
> If he is found now, He is found then;
> If not, we do but go to dwell in the City of Death.[120]

At this point, we can hardly speak of potentials. What could one say, when the deepest potentials of *your* soul are already the very ones that move the planets and radiate as light from the stars; that explode as the thunderous crack of lightning and echo as the rain through the mists; that hurl the comets through the skies and suspend the moon in blackness of night? The little potentials of the persona, ego, and centaur which we nurture so carefully and of which we are so pleased, dare to stand up as candles in the sunlight. Dame Julian of Norwich cried out in her enlightenment: "See! I am God; see! I am all things; see! I do all thing; see! I never lift mine hands off my works, nor ever shall, without end; see! I lead all thing to the end I ordained it to from without beginning, by the same Might, Wisdom, and Love whereby I made it. How should anything be amiss?''

Nevertheless we have to be careful how we understand this ultimate potential, this divine and cosmic potential. It is not that the deepest I (or I-I) stands back from the cosmos and orders it around. It is not that this I has the potentials of the entire cosmos because this I can personally control the cosmos, but because this I *is* the cosmos. For as the very depths of the transpersonal self are pushed through, the transpersonal self gives way to the ultimate or universal self—the Self that *is* all realms of existence, manifest and unmanifest, in all directions and all dimensions.

For as the intuition of the transpersonal self begins to mature and deepen, it slowly—no, instantly!—dawns on you why you can't see the seer anywhere in the universe. You cannot see the seer anywhere in the universe because the seer *is all* of the universe. You cannot see the seer because it is everything which is seen, and thus could never be perceived as a separate entity apart from something else. Everything you are looking at is you who are looking at it. When this is understood, the seer and the seen collapse as each other; *all boundaries between all I's and all Its dissolve* in what has been called cosmic consciousness. Even the transpersonal witness crashes apart and falls into *everything* that is witnessed. No longer do you perceive objects or Its, because you *are* all objects and all Its. There is no separate subject standing apart from the entire field of awareness. As Zen puts it, everywhere you look you see only your own Original Face, "the face you had before your parents were born." (So, after all, it doesn't matter if you had different parents.) "The awakened one," explains Ramana Maharshi, "does not see the universe as different from himself."

Look at it this way: if you now close your eyes and attend very carefully to everything you hear, you will hear an extraordinary flux of sounds crashing around you: birds singing, cars honking, children playing, TV blaring, people chatting, crickets chirping; but notice that even now—just as you are—there is one thing that you cannot hear, no matter how hard you try, how long you try, how much you strain. Of all the sounds you can hear, you cannot hear—the hearer.

Now you cannot hear the hearer for a simple reason. As William James pointed out, you cannot hear the hearer because the hearer is nothing but the entire stream of sounds heard. You cannot hear the hearer because it is everything you hear! You do not hear the sound of thunder, you are the sound of thunder. Likewise, you cannot taste the taster—because what we have long thought of as a separate or subjective taster is really just the sum of present, "objective" tastes. There is no subject—the "taster"—that "tastes" special objects—the "tasted." There is just the present stream of tastes, with no split into subject and object. In just the same way, you cannot really see the seer because the seer is everything seen. What you are looking out of is what you are looking at. A famous Zen Master exclaimed upon his enlightenment, "When I heard the temple bell ring, suddenly there was no bell and no I, just the ringing."[121]

At that point, the whole realm of the transcendent collapses into the immanent. The supernatural world and the natural world turn out to be the same world. The extraordinary is finally only ordinary. Because there is no place that the Ultimate is not, the Ultimate is only present. Thus the ultimate potential is the very suchness of things as they exist now. The greatest human potential is not that you personally can make the sun move around in the sky, but that your own true Self is already the movement of the sun as it is now. All the activities of the cosmos now occurring are already activities of your own deepest I. That is why the absolutely ordinary is already the absolutely extraordinary. That is why the greatest potential of your cosmic self is already manifest all around you. It is already the case in every direction. And finally, that is why the Zen Masters say that Layman P'ang had the final word on the ultimate human potential:

How marvelous, how supernatural this!
I draw water, I carry fuel.

When your real self is the cosmos, then all the activities of the cosmos are already manifesting your greatest potentials: the birds sing in springtime; in fall the leaves turn yellow. To look elsewhere is to miss the point. Dogen hit it:

This slowly drifting cloud is pitiful!
What dreamwalkers we all are!
Awakened, the one great potential:
Black rain on the temple roof.

Yasutani Roshi used to explain enlightenment as—and these are his words—"the direct awareness that you are more than this puny body or limited mind. Stated negatively, it is the realization that the universe is not external to you. Positively, it is experiencing the universe as yourself."[122] As R. H. Blyth put it, "The experience by the universe of the universe." Says Dogen Zenji, quoting an old Zen Master:

I came to realize clearly that Mind
Is no other than mountains and rivers and the great wide earth,
The sun and the moon and the stars.

How incredible! For the entire universe has become the I. *The entire universe—that is the ultimate It.* Recall what the body and the shadow looked like before they were re-membered (or turned back into I). The shadow, for instance, really and truly appeared as an object-out-there; the persecutors (in our shadow example) appeared in every way to be *out there, not-self, alien.* Something that was really a part of the self was seen as not-self. Something that should have been I was felt and perceived as an It out there. Now, at the bottom of the soul, there lies around us the great and ultimate It: the universe appears as object-out-there; as really and truly not-self. *The cosmos is the ultimate It.*

Thus, the mystics have come with the great message, the message that unlocks the greatest and deepest potential of the human soul: *that ultimate It can become I.* That It can be *re-membered*—can indeed, like all the other Its we have studied, become I. *Tat tvam asi*—That art Thou: where It was, I shall become. Like all our projections, the cosmos itself is a part of I that is erroneously felt and perceived as an It. The trees, the stars, the cars and lakes, the tables, dogs, frogs, and rocks—these "environmental objects" or Its are just as much a part of our real self as the shadow is of our egoic self and the body is of our centauric self. And when that ultimate It, the universe, finally returns to I, then It is no longer It, and I am no longer I. A Zen text:

Without outer forms, without inner self, spring still arrives;
Unstopped, unhindered the moon traverses the sky.
Many born of the same branch, but
Few who die of the same branch.
The last word is, "just this;"
A wind-boat, having loaded the moon,
Bobs on autumn waters.

Could Freud have ever guessed? Could he even have suspected? "Aside from the 'I,' " we heard him say at the beginning of this paper, "we perceive another region of the soul, much more extensive, much more impressive, and much more obscure than the 'I,' which we designate the 'It.' " The It: Freud stumbled onto the very tip of the It, but an It that stretched down so much more deeply and profoundly than he ever surmised—an It that swirls down through the shadow to the ego, through the body to the centaur, through the cosmos to the true Self. Each of the levels of this incredible It can be *re-membered,* or joined again with, to disclose deeper I's. For *all* our projections can be re-membered and taken back. And every time an It is returned to I, then greater potentials are released, for the capacities and energies of the Its are given unto I. Then, at the very bottom of an individual's soul, the final anamnesis: looking at the cosmos, he sees his

Original Face; gazing into the firmament, he sees his own true nature; and of all the vast expanses of this marvelous universe, which he manifests with the clarity of a silver mirror, he truly and innocently knows within: where It was, I have become.

REFERENCES

1. Freud, S. New Introductory Lectures on Psychoanalysis: Standard Edition, Vol 22. London: Hogarth Press, 1964, p. 80.
2. Greenson, R. R. *The Technique and Practice of Psychoanalysis,* Vol 1. New York: International Universities Press, 1967, p. 26.
3. Fenichel, O. *The Psychoanalytic Theory of Neurosis.* New York: Norton, 1972, p. 570.
4. Freud, S. *The Problem of Lay-Analyses.* New York: Brentano's, 1927.
5. Ibid., p. 53.
6. Ibid., p. 55
7. Brandt, L. W. Process or structure? *Psychoanalytic Review,* 1966, *53,* 374–378.
8. Reference 4, p. 55.
9. Ibid., p. 55.
10. Ibid., p. 56.
11. Ibid., p. 57.
12. Ibid., p. 71.
13. Ibid., p. 71.
14. Ibid., pp. 73, 74.
15. Ibid., pp. 74, 75.
16. Ibid., p. 75.
17. Ibid., p. 76.
18. Jacobi, J. *The Psychology of C. G. Jung.* London: Routledge and Kegan Paul, 1968.
19. de Laszlo, V. S. (Ed.). *The Basic Writings of C. G. Jung.* New York: Modern Library, 1959.
20. Reference 4, p. 121.
21. Berne, E. *What Do You Say after You Say Hello?* New York: Bantam, 1974.
22. Perls, F. S. *Gestalt Therapy Verbatim.* California: Real People Press, 1969, p. 107.
23. Loevinger, J. *Ego Development.* San Francisco: Jossey-Bass, 1976, p. 369.
24. Ibid., p. 391.
25. Bruch, H. Transformation of oral impulses in eating disorders: A conceptual approach. *Psychiatric Quarterly,* 1961, *35,* 458–481.
26. Horowitz, M. J. Hysterical personality: Cognitive structure and the process of change. *International Journal of Psycho-analysis* (in press).
27. Enright, J. B. Thou art that: Projection and play in therapy and growth. *Psychotherapy: Theory, Research, and Practice,* 1972, *9,* 153–6.
28. Reference 23, pp. 393, 395.
29. Freud, S. *A General Introduction to Psychoanalysis.* New York: Pocket Books, 1971, p. 442.
30. Reference 22, pp. 66, 100.
31. Freud, S. *Analysis Terminable and Interminable: Standard Edition,* Vol. 23. London: Hogarth Press, 1951.
32. Perls, F. S., Hefferline, R. F. and Goodman, P. *Gestalt Therapy.* New York: Dell, 1951.
33. Frey-Rohn, L. *From Freud to Jung.* New York: Dell, 1974.
34. Harris, T. A. *I'm OK—You're OK.* New York: Avon, 1969.

35. Assagioli, R. *Psychosynthesis.* New York: Viking/Compass, 1965.
36. Goleman, D. Meditation as meta-therapy. *Journal of Transpersonal Psychology,* 1971, *3,* 1–25.
37. Shonta, F. C. Constitutional theories of personality. In *Current Personality Theories.* (R. J. Corsini, Ed.). Itasca: Peacock, 1977.
38. Groddeck, G. *The Book of the It.* New York: Vintage Books, 1961.
39. Ibid.
40. Hintz, H. H. Whitehead's concept of organism and the mind-body problem. In *Dimensions of Mind* (S. Hook, Ed.). New York: Collier, 1973.
41. Feigl, H. Mind-body, *not* a pseudoproblem. In *Dimensions of Mind.* (S. Hook, Ed.). New York: Collier, 1973.
42. Benoit, H. *The Supreme Doctrine.* New York: Viking, 1955.
43. Ibid.
44. Ibid.
45. Green, E. E., Green, A. M. and Walters, E. D. Voluntary control of internal states. *Journal of Transpersonal Psychology,* 1970, *2,*1–26.
46. Green, E. E. and Green, A. M. On the meaning of transpersonal. *Journal of Transpersonal Psychology,* 1971, *3,* 27–47.
47. Penfield, W. *The Mystery of the Mind.* Princeton: Princeton University Press, 1975.
48. Russell, B. *Analysis of Mind.* Humanities Press: Atlantic Highlands, N.J. 1978.
49. McDermott, J. J. (Ed.). *The Writings of William James.* New York: Random House (Modern Library), 1968.
50. Holdstock, T. L. and Rogers, C. R. Person-centered theory. In *Current Personality Theories* (R. J. Corsini, Ed.). Itasca: Peacock, 1977.
51. May, R. (Ed.). *Existential Psychology.* New York: Random House, 1969, p. 33–35.
52. May, R. *Love and Will.* New York: Norton, 1969, pp. 222, 224.
53. Ibid., p. 227.
54. Ibid., p. 234.
55. Sartre, J. P. *Existential Psychoanalysis.* Chicago: Gateway, 1966.
56. Wilber, K. Microgeny. *ReVision,* 1978, *1,* No. 3/4, p. 52–84.
57. Reference 50, p. 125.
58. Ibid., p. 144.
59. Ibid., p. 127.
60. Ibid., p. 129.
61. Ibid., p. 145.
62. Ibid., p. 134, 135.
63. Ibid., p. 136.
64. Ibid., p. 132.
65. Reference 32, p. 389.
66. Ibid.
67. Lowen, A. *Depression and the Body.* Maryland: Penguin Books, 1973.
68. Kierkegaard, S. *Fear and Trembling and the Sickness unto Death.* New York: Anchor, 1954.
69. Nietzsche, F. W. *The Philosophy of Nietzsche.* New York: Modern Library, 1927.
70. Husserl, E. *Ideas: General Introduction to Pure Phenomenology.* New York: Macmillan, 1931.
71. Heidegger, M. *Being and Time.* New York: Harper & Row, 1962.
72 Reference 55.
73. Binswanger, L. *Being-in-the-World.* New York: Basic Books, 1963.
74. Frankl, V. E. *Man's Search for Meaning.* New York: Washington Square Press, 1963.

75. Boss, M. *Psychoanalysis and Daseinanalysis*. New York: Basic Books, 1963.
76. Goldstein, K. *The Organism*. New York: American Book, 1939.
77. Köhler, W. The mind-body problem. In *Dimensions of Mind*. (S. Hook, Ed.). New York: Collier, 1973.
78. Köhler, W. *Gestalt Psychology*. New York: New American Library, 1959.
79. Wertheimer, M. *Productive Thinking*. New York: Harper, 1959.
80. Smuts, J. *Holism and Evolution*. New York: Macmillan, 1926.
81. Allport, G. *Pattern and Growth in Personality*. New York: Holt, 1961.
82. Corsini, R. J. (Ed.) *Current Personality Theories*. Itasca: Peacock, 1977.
83. Horney, K. *Neurosis and Human Growth*. New York: Norton, 1950.
84. Maslow, A. H. *Toward a Psychology of Being*. New York: Van Nostrand Reinhold, 1968.
85. Reference 50, p. 129.
86. Rogers, C. *On Becoming a Person*. Boston: Houghton Mifflin, 1961.
87. Reference 52, p. 199.
87a. Farber, L. *The Ways of the Will*. New York: Basic Books, 1966, pp. 1–25.
88. Reference 52, p. 217.
89. Ibid.
90. Reference 52.
91. Broughton, J. M. The development of natural epistemology in adolescence and early adulthood. Unpublished doctoral dissertation. Harvard University, 1975.
92. Baldwin, J. M. *Thought and Things*. New York: Arno Press, 1975.
93. Reference 23.
94. Ibid.
95. Maslow, A. H. *The Farther Reaches of Human Nature*. New York: Viking/Compass, 1971.
96. Grof, S. *Realms of the Human Unconscious*. New York: Viking Press, 1975.
97. Govinda, L. *Foundations of Tibetan Mysticism*. New York: Samuel Weiser, 1973.
98. Coomaraswamy, A. K. *Time and Eternity*. Switzerland: Ascona, 1947.
99. Eliade, M. *Images and Symbols*. New York: Sheed and Ward, 1969, p. 13.
98a. Bohm, D. J. and Hiley, B. J. On the intuitive understanding of nonlocality as implied by quantum theory. *Found. Phys,* 1975, *5*(1), 93–104.
100. Cassirer, E. *The Philosophy of Symbolic Forms,* Vol 2. New Haven: Yale University Press, 1955.
101. Coomaraswamy, A. K. *Hinduism and Buddhism*. New York: Philosophical Library, 1943.
102. Whitehead, A. N. *Process and Reality*. New York: Macmillan, 1969.
103. Campbell, J. (Ed.). *The Portable Jung*. New York: Viking, 1972.
104. See reference 35.
105. Kripner, S. (Ed.). The plateau experience: A. H. Maslow and others. *Journal of Transpersonal Psychology,* 1972, *4*.
106. Krishnamurti, J. *The First and Last Freedom*. Wheaton: Quest, 1954.
107. Giles, H. A. *Chuang Tzu*. Shanghai: Kelly and Walch, 1926.
108. Ramana Maharshi, *The Collected Works of Ramana Maharshi* (A. Osborne, Ed.). London: Rider, 1959.
109. Prabhavananda. *Shankara's Crest Jewel of Discrimination* (C. Isherwood, translator). New York: Mentor, 1970.
110. Thera, N. *The Heart of Buddhist Meditation*. London: Rider, 1972.
111. Reference 95.
112. Roberts, T. Beyond self-actualization. *ReVision,* 1978, *1*, 42–47.
113. See *Synthesis* 1.

114. Quoted in Smith, H. *Forgotten Truth*. New York, Harper, 1976.
115. Schrödinger, E. *What Is Life? and Mind and Matter*. London: Cambridge University Press, 1969, p. 95.
116. Blofeld, J. *The Zen Teaching of Huang Po*. New York: Grove Press, 1958.
117. Hume, R. E., translator. *The Thirteen Principal Upanishads*. London: Oxford, 1974.
118. Schrödinger, E. *My View of the World*. London: Cambridge University Press, 1964, p. 20.
119. See reference 95.
120. Quoted in Huxley, A. *The Perennial Philosophy*. New York: Harper, 1970.
121. In Kapleau, P. *The Three Pillars of Zen*. Boston: Beacon Press, 1965.
122. Ibid.

One of the problems that we get into with the issue of paradigms is that each paradigm argues for itself. The Eastern paradigm says that holism, altered states, and higher consciousness are the truth and the way. The Western paradigm says that segmental precision and piecemeal approaches are the truth and the way. In this article, Werner Erhard, Victor Gioscia, and Ken Anbender argue eloquently (a) that what is needed is not another paradigm, but an understanding of how paradigms shift, and (b) that we can be the ones who shift the paradigm. In so doing, they point out the limits of both the Eastern and the Western paradigms. They suggest the critical importance of taking responsibility for this, and also note that the individual, by the very nature of the ability to create nondichotomous awareness—the awareness "I am" and "I am able to cause"—is healthy at the most fundamental and core level. By developing a paradigm of paradigms, the human species is empowered to experience mastery in the matter of its own further evolution. This article discusses clearly and cogently the shift that is necessary in order for individuals to have the ability to choose among paradigms.

Werner Erhard has been researching the nature of individual and social transformation since 1963. As a product of that research, he has developed specific technologies which enhance people's ability to transform the quality of their own lives and to contribute to the lives of others. In 1971, he created the est Training, a transformational experience in which over a third of a million people in the United States, Canada, Europe, and India have participated. He is a principal founder of the Hunger Project, a multinational organization of over two million members who have undertaken to produce a grass-roots commitment to end death by starvation within two decades. Mr. Erhard has lectured widely in academic and professional institutions in Europe and America.

Victor Gioscia, Ph.D. (Philosophy, Fordham, 1963), is a research consultant at Werner Erhard and Associates, and one of the people who leads the est Standard Training and the Communication Workshop. He is the former Executive Director of the Center for the Study of Social Change, Senior Sociologist in the Department of Psychiatry at Roosevelt Hospital in New York, and Director of Research at Jewish Family Services in New York. Dr. Gioscia has preferred several disciplines at several universities including The City University of New York and is an experienced clinical theoretician. He is currently working on a transcendental sociology.

Kenneth Anbender, Ph.D. (Clinical Psychology, Adelphi University, 1975), is the Director of Research for Werner Erhard and Associates, and is one of the people who leads the est Standard Training and the est Com-

munication Workshop. Dr. Anbender has taught classes in the areas of psychology, extreme health, and communication at the University of Michigan, Adelphi University of Advanced Psychological Studies, and the California Institute of Asian Studies. His studies in altered states of consciousness, mystical experience, creativity, and health have led to a deep commitment to a shift in the quality of life on the planet through individual and social transformation. His participation with Werner Erhard and Associates, in the field of psychology, and in writing this chapter is an expression of that commitment.

5
Being Well

Werner Erhard
Victor Gioscia
Ken Anbender

All observation is selection.   A. N. Whitehead

The way is the way.   Lao-tzu

Good Luck.   Anonymous

INTRODUCTION

Our intention in the following essay is to offer the reader an opportunity to reflect on an issue which is central in our time—the search for a new paradigm—a profound new definition of human well being.

Since we regard the reader's reflection as a sufficient resource to arrive at a satisfying conclusion, we shall not ourselves attempt to define—or redefine—human illness or wellness; nor shall we present a new paradigm from which an intelligent definition of well being might reasonably be deduced.

We will elucidate paradigms in general and paradigms of well being in particular. Also, since the issue of paradigms old and new, as well as the transitions between them, is curently receiving much careful attention, we shall focus on the issue of paradigm shifts and some of the problems that arise during times of paradigm shifts.

The reader is asked to suspend defining well being until after we have more completely examined the nature of paradigms, paradigm shifts, and their relation to the issue of human freedom.

We shall not add conceptual complexity to the issues at hand. In fact, our purpose will be to move the reader toward that dimension of knowing in which such complexities resolves themselves naturally and spontaneously, not by conceptual clarification or even by experiential exercise, but by a knowing of the most fundamental kind.

We shall present the thesis that each of us has access to a dimension of knowing that most of us have only accidentally used. It is present and unseen, powerful, seldom employed, ordinary, and rare.

We intend to provide access to this dimension of knowing so that the reader can select confidently from among the available options those (s)he finds most satisfying.

Our method will be to pass in review:
1. aspects of the Western paradigm which until recently defined all wellness as not-illness;
2. aspects of the Eastern paradigm of well being which are currently evoking interest;
3. the nature of paradigm shifts in general. We shall thus raise the issue of paradigm mastery—the power to select paradigms freely, after careful consideration.

Finally, we shall present a paradigm of paradigms as the basis of paradigm mastery.

I. THE SEARCH FOR PARADIGMS

We live in interesting times. Each day brings us fresh news of breakthroughs, innovations, and discoveries, along with bold new models and paradigms for their comprehension. Humanity seems intent on articulating a new paradigm of human nature which will at long last render health and well being universally possible.

So earnest is this search for new paradigms of human well being that there are an abundance of them, whose very number how now become problematic. We seek not only new ways to be well, but new ways to seek new ways to be well.

Currently, for example, there is much interest in the paradigms of the East. These, it is hoped, when somehow combined with those of the West, will more deeply heal us. Many hope that a shift away from the Western paradigm, toward the Eastern paradigm, will at last put us on *the* road to lasting well-being.

There is, in addition, a growing enthusiasm that our current explorations will not merely combine new knowledge with old, but will occasion a *paradigm shift* in the definition of human health and well being.

The search is on for a profoundly new *kind* of inquiry, which will enable us this time to see not only where we have been, where we are, and where we are going, but more essentially, will empower us from now on to *be* who we are *while* we journey onward.

The authors gladly acknowledge their fraternity with those who seek to articulate a paradigm which no longer locates well being beyond our human reach. Precisely what is wanted is a paradigm which locates well being *within* our nature. Not only is a shift toward such a paradigm currently underway: what the shift reveals is clearly sound and fundamentally important.

Yet, paradigms have shifted before. In fact, it is their nature to shift, each eventually giving way to its successor as inevitably as the waves of the sea. So the issue in our time is not *whether* a paradigm shift is underway, but whether we can discover the principles underlying *any* paradigm shift which will enable us from now on to experience our full humanity *during* the shift not, as ever before, in the hope that true well being will come *after* the next shift has been accomplished.

What is wanted and needed during an era of multiple paradigm shifts is not yet another paradigm shift, but the *ability* to shift paradigms confidently, ably, powerfully, i.e., paradigm mastery. The purpose of this essay is precisely to articulate the principles by which such mastery is occasioned.

We will ourselves neither promote a new paradigm, nor defend those useful in the past, nor justify or rationalize current paradigm shifts. Our aim is to assist, enable, and empower all those participating in the shift of fundamental notions of human well being, so that their work may draw on a mastery of paradigm shifts.

Our purpose then is the articulation of the principles by which paradigms are generated—what might be called the "paradigm of paradigms": that set of principles, access to which serves as the *source* of the power and the ability to *cause* a shift from one paradigm to another.

Our search for the principles of paradigm mastery is occasioned by two central observations:

1. There are now so many new paradigms, models, theories, philosophies and practices which address themselves to redefining the nature of human health and well being, that selection from among them has become increasingly problematic in the absence of independently established bases of selection.

2. We have historically accumulated no principles or markers which might serve as guides *during* a time of paradigm shift. We don't know, really, what is required to shift from a Ptolemaic to a Copernican model of the cosmos, or from a Newtonian to an Einsteinian paradigm.

Currently the sheer number of old and new models offered as paradigms of health and well being makes it difficult for us to shift masterfully from one paradigm to another. It no longer suffices to shift unknowingly from one paradigm to the next. What is required now is the know-how, the ability to shift masterfully. What is needed is a paradigm of paradigms.

Happily, contemporary logicians are now aware that it is unworkable to construct endless ladders of knowing about knowing about knowing in an infinite regression. So, as we present the principal outlines of the paradigm of paradigms in the following pages, we shall at the same time demonstrate that the search for a paradigm of paradigm *of paradigms* is *not* only unnecessary, it is an absurdity—for the first qualifying characteristic of the paradigm of paradigms is that it may *not* locate mastery beyond our logical reach, in an endless infinity of logical steps. Minimally, to qualify, the paradigm of paradigms must reveal that paradigm mastery is possible.

II. PARADIGM OF PARADIGMS

Initially the problem of locating the paradigm of paradigms seems simple enough: first, describe the currently dominant paradigm by which we have sought, until very recently, to define health and well being. Next, describe the principal features of the paradigm we seek to develop. It then remains only to specify the bridging operations from one to the other—listing the essential steps we took from where we were to where we want to go.

This strategy presents two alternatives:

1. Describe the new paradigm from within the old.
2. Describe the new paradigm from within itself.

In the first alternative, one must fail, because the new paradigm cannot be held *in* the old paradigm. If it could, it would be *within* the old paradigm (or, at best, be an extension of it) and therefore *not* a *new* paradigm at all.

Using the second alternative, one must again fail because, when one is seeking a new paradigm (i.e., when one is shifting paradigms), one obviously does not yet have the new paradigm with which to describe the new paradigm.

Furthermore, in the second alternative, even when one attains the new paradigm, one must fail because in the current paradigm of description, self-referential statements, while true, lack content and thus have no "information". Such statements therefore provide no basis of description.

Even if both paradigms—the old *and* the new—were clearly described, the question would still remain: What is required to shift from the old to the new? What are the guidelines through the labyrinth of assumptions and postulates which currently obscure the path toward paradigm mastery?

The first step is to recognize that the path *is* labyrinthine.

The second step is then at least metaphorically clear—to see *into* the labyrinth, one must see from beyond it.

What is required, then, is not just another paradigm—another vision of health and well being—another point of view. It is not even sufficient to classify and search among *kinds* of paradigms. This approach only postpones the inevitable problem of the criterion of selection by adding to the already long list of selectable approaches we already have.

What *is* required is an investigation into the nature of paradigms—into the ontology which sustains them, the epistemology which reveals them, and the integrity which guides their right employment. What is wanted is nothing less than the discovery of those principles which can release us from our dependency on an endless sequence of models and paradigms, with no fore-seeable end in view.

What is called for is mastery in the matter of paradigms, a transformed rela-tionship with paradigms, which enables us to shift confidently and power-fully *from* paradigms which continue to locate health and well-being forever beyond us—always in the next paradigm—*to* a paradigm of paradigms, which enables and empowers us to:

1. locate health and well being here and now, where we are, within our selves
2. use any paradigm masterfully, to the full extent of its usefulness
3. mix the principles and techniques of various paradigms precisely, potently, and usefully
4. shift paradigms ably, confidently, masterfully

What is called for, therefore, is not simply another paradigm, but that set of principles which will enable us to use and shift paradigms confidently, so that we experience ourselves as masters of paradigms and of paradigm shifts.

This will transform us from considering ourselves a helpless species *confined* by its paradigms, to experiencing ourselves as a species *able* to celebrate its mastery of paradigms and paradigm shifts.

Only a paradigm of paradigms—or, more exactly, an awareness of the principles by which mastery in the matter of paradigms and paradigm shifts is had—can elevate us above the labyrinth of assumptions which presently confine us.

Clearly, even the emerging consensus that we should look carefully into the wisdom of the East, or that we should now see wholes where we saw only ag-gregates of parts, while obviously sensible, cannot suffice. Surely these views too will eventually be superseded, and we shall be asked to shift again through another labyrinth of assumptions left over from what today appears to be tomorrow's paradigm.

It has now become clear that an endless series of shifts from one paradigm to another no longer suffices. Not a few writers now announce that we must begin to abandon our current positions and examine in earnest *really* new paradigms, as revolutionary and different *in kind* from our contemporary visions as, let us say, the theory of evolution was from the theory of special creation.

However, before congratulating ourselves that the search for a paradigm of paradigms is already well under way, let us examine *as a case in point,* a current paradigm shift—the shift from a Western to an Eastern paradigm of well being—so that we can begin to assemble observations on the nature of paradigm shifts.

III. THE WESTERN PARADIGM

It is an old story. We cannot see our eyes—we see with them.

So it is with any point of view. In our search for a way of searching, we are able to avoid the more obvious pitfalls only when we are willing to hold up a mirror to our favorite strategies.

Let us inquire then into the major structural characteristics of the Western paradigm we have used until very recently to define health and well being for ourselves. Among its principal characteristics are the following:

1. *Positivism:* Since its historical inception, contemporary science has clung steadfastly to a sense-amenable test of its hypotheses, wishing never again to return to the time when truth came by edict from those in power. This initial democracy of the sensorium is now increasingly regarded as a set of unwelcome blinders, limiting our knowledge to the narrow spectrum of the senses of "comparably trained" observers, augmented to be sure by technological instrumentation.

2. *Reductionism:* Reductionism asks of anything that it examines, "What is it made of?" One answer holds that all things are made of "stuff"— essentially matter and/or energy, deployed in space and/or time. This view, currently known as materialism, is usually contrasted with another view which holds that some things are *not* material. One of the corollaries of reductionism holds that wholes are made of parts, and so, restoring broken parts (e.g., John's liver) restores health to the whole (John). Variations include healing John's feelings (parts) so that John (the whole) will feel "better."

3. *Change:* The Western paradigm posits change as fundamental. Thus, members of the clinical professions routinely assume that some thing must be changed if the "ill patient" is to be restored to health. Things, it is said, need to be put back in order. This view generates a corollary that only *action* brings about *reaction.* The thought that nothing need be done frustrates advocates of the current Western paradigm.

4. *Dichotomy:* The dichotomous nature of the contemporary Western paradigm is essential to it. One either is, or is not, sick. Healthy is not-sick. A corollary is: one hopes to change that which is *not* (sickness, or not-health) into that which *is* (health, or not-sickness) by *doing* some thing.

5. *Cause–Effect:* In the West, causes generate effects, and effects result from causes. Hence, there is a curious blend of voluntarism and victimology in the dominant paradigm of health, which hold both that we can cause (i.e., "do something" about) an illness, *and* that most illness in life happens *to* us (i.e., is an effect) hence not our doing. Thus, we may cause our health to get better only after our health has been made worse. Thus, hope.

6. *Emergence:* Perhaps the most fundamental postulate in the Western paradigm is what we shall term a "bottom-up" view. In its larger aspect, this postulate envisions evolution as having started with the big bang, gradually building up clouds of gas, then stars, then planets, eventually plants, animals, and finally, us. "Higher" life forms are said to have "emerged" from "lower" ones. Our own "lower" functions are said to be animal, and our "higher" functions, human.

Notice that the summary of the Western paradigm reads very like a naive restatement of Cartesian-Newtonian cosmology.

There is a material universe. It is composed of things and forces—e.g., atoms and gravity. It is a huge machine. Somehow—a long time ago—it got started, and now it includes biological, psychological, and sociological *parts,* which, though *apparently* very different, consist, like everything else in this universe, of constellations of things and forces.

Note also that mastery in this mechanical paradigm accrues to the mechanic, whose essential clinical task *can only be* putting things back where they normally belong, with the least possible force.

It is interesting to observe how the Western paradigm structures each of its subsidiary fields of inquiry. Just as "cause" is that which occasions an effect, and "effect" is that which results from a cause, so order is the absence of disorder and, correlatively, health is not-sick. We are biologically healthy if we have no disease. We are psychologically healthy if we have no anxiety. We are sociologically healthy if we have no alienation.

Note that each of these disciplines embodies each of the structural characteristics of the Western paradigm. Each in its turn is positivist, reductionist, change oriented, dichotomous, mechanical, and emergent. Note also that *within* this paradigm, disciplines may come and go, as they have in great variety in our own time, yet the central principles of the paradigm have remained unchanged for centuries.

By reason of their very generality, paradigms sustain the coming(s) and going(s) of literally hundreds of specifications, without themselves changing an iota. In this way, schools come and go, each no more satisfactory than its predecessor, each generating no more *ability* than before. Indeed, the apparency of constant change guarantees the unexamined persistence of the paradigm. The contents change—the contexts remain.

IV. THE EASTERN PARADIGM

"Granted," says an advocate of the Eastern paradigm, "there is no true mastery in the old Western paradigm. But our *current* explorations take place well beyond these limitations. We no longer assume things are mechanical. Today we know that things are holographic—each "part" containing the whole. Today we are holists, no longer trying to obtain health by attempting to put back together parts we took apart by our overspecializations. Today we regard materialism, reductionism, positivism, and all of their associated corollaries, as an obsolete paradigm precisely because that mechanical paradigm precludes the experience of true human mastery. This is in fact the driving energy behind our search for an Eastern paradigm, which cannot be said to suffer from the sort of naive materialism whose central features you have delineated in your foregoing paragraphs."

"We are fully aware," our Eastern protagonist continues, "that most of what we now know to be our true human potential was buried under the West's obsessions with exterior technology and material progress. We will not repeat these mistakes. We seek to release humankind from the grip of the Newtonian paradigm and restore to humanity the right and the ability to actualize its full potential. The Eastern paradigm encourages us to bring forward what the West counseled us to leave behind—the higher reaches of human nature, unitary consciousness, mysticism, the Experience of Being."

"Furthermore," our advocate continues, "we shall not again make the mistake of throwing out the baby with the bath water. We will retain those findings of the Western paradigm which foster actualization, without subscribing to the limiting premises from which they were derived. We seek a true synthesis, the best of East and West, in a new leap forward. We want to be full humans, not emergent machines.''

These remarks are unexceptionable. They witness a shift toward a paradigm which, in our opinion, has room for everything that our protagonist wants to put in it, including some Western hardware. The vision is noble. Clearly, the Western exclusive preoccupation with matter, energy, time, and place rules out interest in the inmost reaches of ''inner space'' and in the spectrum of neglected human abilities which will soon be discovered to reside there *''in potentia.''*

The question remains, by what criterion shall we *shift* from one paradigm to another, without locating mastery *in* one *or* the other? Even granting that the Eastern paradigm looks wonderful from where our protagonist sits, has (s)he not already made the very same mistake (s)he sought to avoid? Has (s)he not looked with Western eyes enviously to the East—to find there what was lacking in the West? Let us put the question in its least flattering aspect: Is our Eastern advocate not simply attempting to repair the holes in the Western paradigm with Eastern patches? Or vice versa?

Furthermore, what response can be made to the advocate who *combines* pieces from both the Eastern and the Western paradigms, in what appears to be a useful meta-assembly? Is not at least some small measure of mastery gained thereby? Do not those who refuse to prefer either the right brain *or* the left, who insist on the whole, have something which advocates of either half lack?

Unfortunately, the attempt to gain mastery by resort to an additive strategy can confer no additional mastery, for precisely what is wanted is the power to know *which* elements to combine and the power to employ the resultant combination masterfully.

Thus, the additive strategy only postpones the search for mastery. For it leaves unanswered the very question it sought to resolve: What is the *source* of paradigm mastery?

It may be useful at this point to begin to distinguish further between contents and contexts. We are neither for nor against the *contents* of the Eastern model, or the Western for that matter, for it may well be that the combination of Eastern and Western elements that our protagonist champions will turn out in the end to be useful. Indeed, this is very probably the case.

The point continues to be: Is this *shift* of paradigms—this *way* of changing—undertaken *from* or *toward* mastery? That is, must we wait again, and hope that we shall experience our true wellness *after* we shift to the new Eastern paradigm? Does it matter whether we hope Eastern or Western style? Can a paradigm tell us whether we are well or ill if we are its authors? Or must we stand paradoxically outside our paradigms for them to be expressions of our mastery?

V. MATRIX OF PARADIGMS

To formulate the matter more rigorously, we might construct the following matrix, in which:

WP = Western Paradigm
EP = Eastern Paradigm
PS = Paradigm Shift
PP = Paradigm of Paradigms

	WP	EP	PS	PP
WP	1	2	3	4
EP	5	6	7	8
PS	9	10	11	12
PP	13	14	15	16

We read the contents of these cells as follows:

1. The Western paradigm argues for itself. (All paradigms do.)
2. The Western paradigm is looking more and more fondly at the Eastern paradigm.
3. The Western paradigm prefigures what a shift beyond itself would look like.
4. According to the Western paradigm, there is no paradigm of paradigms, only a *next* paradigm.
5. The Eastern paradigm regards the Western paradigm as reductive and insufficient.
6. The Eastern paradigm argues for itself. (All paradigms do.)
7. The Eastern paradigm prefigures what a shift beyond itself would look like.
8. The Eastern paradigm regards itself *as* the paradigm of paradigms.
9. There is a shift away from the Western paradigm under way.
10. There is a shift toward the Eastern paradigm under way.

11. The issue of shifting how we shift paradigms is a central concern of our time.
12. Only paradigm shifts which are shifted from the paradigm of paradigms reflect mastery.
13. The paradigm of paradigms must transcend the Western paradigm.
14. The paradigm of paradigms must transcend the Eastern paradigm.
15. The paradigm of paradigms supplies criteria by which to shift paradigms.
16. The paradigm of paradigms cannot itself be simply another paradigm.

(We will develop cells 13–16 later in this essay.)

What is meant by statement 12: "Only paradigm shifts which are shifted *from* the paradigm of paradigms reflect mastery"?

This: We are wholly free only if we may accept or reject *any* paradigm.

The problem is, since every paradigm argues in its own favor, every paradigm defines what is outside itself as false. Each paradigm argues for itself by setting its own standards for the definition of paradigms. Another way to state this matter is as follows: In any set *called* "This set," there must be an element called "not this set." It is a symbol *in* this set of what is *outside* the set. Except "not in this set" is not *really* "not in this set"—it is an item *in* this set *called* "not in this set." It represents (symbolizes) what is *outside* this set as if it were *inside* this set.

Paradigms, similarly, contain *representations* or *symbols* of what lie beyond themselves—including all other paradigms. But the mere manipulation of the symbol of what lies outside a set can bring with it no true mastery, since what remains beyond the set remains beyond the set untouched, even though the *symbol* in the set of what is beyond the set may indeed have undergone all sorts of (only) symbolic manipulations. What is *in-here* is precisely *not-out-there* and vice versa.

This is the reason why Eastern masters sound "funny" to Westerners. Eastern masters often say something about what they say it is impossible to say something about. Zen masters say, "Not this . . . not that . . . not not . . ." until there remain no symbols of what is outside the novice's symbol system. Such masters are very clear that symbolic statements about what is beyond symbolization are worthless and, in fact, deceive, since they foster the illusion that one is outside one's symbol system if one is talking *as if* one were.

True mastery is not merely symbolic. So, in the matter of paradigms, we might paraphrase the Zen master who says, "You may not decide, and you may not not-decide," by saying, "You may not elect the Eastern paradigm from the Western paradigm, and you may not elect the Eastern paradigm from the Eastern paradigm. Nor may you elect a Western paradigm from an Eastern paradigm, nor a Western paradigm from a Western, *or from any combination*. Now, elect a paradigm."

Since mastery is, above all, the ability to cause, mastery cannot be caused by *any* paradigm. Only a "paradigm" which is not itself a paradigm can confer paradigm mastery, i.e., be a cause of paradigms.

Statements of this sort when approached from within a paradigm of causes and effects are tautological and hence without descriptive power. But what of a cause which does not cause effects? What of a cause which causes itself? What are the qualities of such a cause? Before moving to a discussion of this issue, it may be useful to summarize the main points we have made so far:

1. There is a Western paradigm. It stamps its subsidiary models and theories of health and well being in its own image.
2. There is an Eastern paradigm. It promises to empower processes of health and well being not currently available in the West.
3. We define mastery as the ability to cause paradigm shifts.
4. Mastery of paradigms cannot be conferred by any paradigm.
5. The paradigm of paradigms cannot itself be just another paradigm. If it were, it wouldn't be the paradigm *of* paradigms.
6. The principles *by* which we shift paradigms cannot be found *within* the paradigms being shifted.

We consider next that realm in which paradigm shifts take place—that context, the contents of which are paradigms. Interimly, we shall say that paradigm shifts prompted by the precepts of other paradigms are not wholly free, and we shall call those shifts of paradigms which are wholly free "Transformations."

IV. WIDENING THE FRAME OF INQUIRY

It is time to widen the frame of our inquiry and to bring into focus the fact that the current shift in paradigms of health and well being participates in a much larger paradigmatic shift, encompassing not only Eastern and Western paradigms of health and well being, but a shift in our experience of the nature of human evolution.

Observation reveals that fundamental redefinitions are underway, not only in matters of health and well being, but far more widely. Cosmologists report that "singularities" and so-called black holes require entirely new *kinds* of theory. Nuclear physicists report that quarks and "gluons" simply do not fit into prior theories of subatomic "particles." Half the nations of Africa are not yet half a century old. We have walked on the moon and sent rockets to the stars.

Scientists and philosophers across the spectrum of inquiry are currently redefining the spectrum of inquiry. The philosophy of science thrives as does the theory of information. We have an ecology of ideas which prompts us to look deeply at learning, at learning to learn, and at learning to learn to learn. Human experience has been redefined. So has human nature. We require far more of ourselves than ever before. We now expect whole societies and cultures to engage in transformation—to generate whole domains in which to evolve, and thence to evolve responsibly, i.e., the evolution of evolution.

This is one of the reasons why the phrase "human potential" is not wholly satisfactory, since it tends to imply the fixed existence of predetermined potentialities and possibilities, which we ought thus to fulfull. It may be that we ourselves are now required to generate and manage our own evolutionary options and opportunities. The discovery that this in fact is the case was not entirely a welcome one, since it came with the recognition that we have now accumulated the wherewithal either to wreck our evolution (via nuclear holocaust) and/or to redesign it (via genetic "engineering").

We have entered into an era in which we *are* responsible for the evolution of our own further evolution. The opportunity exists. The criteria do not. Those are up to us. And there are no precedents.

In our prior discussion of the matrix of paradigms, we postponed detailed discussion of the "paradigm" of paradigms. The place for that discussion is here. For the paradigm of paradigms *is* the source of those criteria.

We may begin our discussion by recalling what we have said so far about the "paradigm" of paradigms. First, it must demonstrate unequivocally that it does not lead to a topless ladder of logical steps. Thus, it is required to be the *dimension* of paradigms—an abstract space *in* which paradigms are *contents.*

Within this abstract space, or dimension, the number of paradigms may be large or small. The dimension of paradigms—"paradigmness"—is itself not numbered. It is not *a* paradigm.

Further, it was required of the paradigm of paradigms that it provide opportunity for the experience of mastery—which is the ability to come *to* any paradigm, and hence the ability to shift *from any* one *to* any other, in freedom.

A master of paradigm shifts could as easily shift from an Eastern to a Western paradigm, or the reverse, or for that matter, from an Einsteinian to an Newtonian one.

It begins to be apparent that the paradigm of paradigms must itself be without content—or, to use another metaphor—it must be dimensionless. It is no one paradigm. It is neither Eastern nor Western, nor some of each, thus not even planetary. It is paradigmness itself—the abstract possibility or "space" in which paradigms themselves are contents.

VII. CONTEXT, CONSTRUCT, CONTENT

Before spelling out the further characteristics of the paradigm of paradigms (to the extent that this is possible), it may be useful to formalize the principles we have been implying in our discussion so far. To do so, we shall construct a table in which three characteristics of the paradigm of paradigms are compared with, and contrasted to, the characteristics of the Western paradigm, the Eastern paradigm, and aspects of a paradigm shift. We shall then discuss some additional characteristics of the paradigm of paradigms itself, which we have said to be the source of paradigm mastery.

The three characteristics we shall discuss are:

1. *Context:* the principles which generate paradigms—the abstraction, space, or idea out of which particular paradigms arise.
2. *Construct:* the organizing principles which unite the concepts of a paradigm in a coherent, logical whole.
3. *Content:* the concepts which constitute a paradigm—what the paradigm states.

Schematically, the table reads:

	CONTEXT	CONSTRUCT	CONTENT
Western Paradigm	1 Survival	2 Change	3 Parts
Eastern Paradigm	4 Transcendence	5 Enlightenment	6 Full Nature
Paradigm Shift	7 Becoming	8 Change of Change	9 Planetary Well being
Paradigm of Paradigms	10 Paradigmness	11 Transformation	12 Mastery

The cells may be summarized as follows:

1. The Western paradigm of emergent evolution is based on the premise of survival.
2. The Western paradigm calls for change, i.e., *doing* something.
3. The Western paradigm defines the whole as well if the parts are in order, i.e., not sick.
4. The Eastern paradigm is based on the transcendence of ego.
5. The Eastern paradigm calls for enlightenment.
6. The Eastern paradigm calls for attainment of one's Full Nature.
7. The paradigm shift currently under way entails a shift from a Western-oriented *becoming* (trying to get there then) *to* an Eastern-oriented *being* (here now).
8. The paradigm shift currently under way reflects an awareness of "second-order" change, or change of change.
9. The paradigm shift currently under way embraces responsibility for the whole (i.e., planetary evolution.)
10. The paradigm of paradigms is the dimension of paradigmness, that realm in which paradigms are contents.
11. The paradigm of paradigms calls for transformation, i.e., a shift from paradigm-generated options to generating paradigms as options. (We will expand our discussion of this point below.)
12. The *paradigm of paradigms* empowers the human species to know mastery in the matter of its own further evolution. That is, it states that humanity can responsibly generate the paradigms with which to guide its own further evolution. It is humanity's coming *to* para-

digms, from beyond paradigms, as the *source* of paradigms, i.e., as the cause of paradigm mastery.

VIII. ENLIGHTENMENT AND TRANSFORMATION

How shall we describe this space—this dimension of source—this ability to *cause* paradigms, and thus to experience mastery?

The traditional Eastern answer to the search for mastery has been, "Find an enlightened master, apprentice yourself, and, *if* you work diligently, you will one day transcend your ego and be enlightened. When you are enlightened you will know what source is. A source is one who enables others to transcend ego. In short, source is *the* distinguishing quality of a master."

This traditional answer was a useful beginning, which, like all beginnings, left much unsaid.

First, we confront here, in another of its ubiquitous forms, the problem that enlightenment/transformation—the ability to transcend paradigms—cannot be captured in conceptual terms, since enlightenment/transformation is *by definition* the transcendence of definition. Any attempt to describe it conceptually must by definition fail. Thus, enlightenment/transformation cannot be held by the conceptual mind. It does not fit into the faculty of symbols and concepts of experience. Nor can those aspects of ourselves constructed by the assembly of symbols and concepts of experience—our personalities, our egos, our identities—hold or contain enlightenment/transformation.

Many Westerners therefore conclude that those enlightened/transformed must eliminate their conceptual minds, their personalities, their identities, and/or their egos. And, since the Western paradigm defines this as impossible, many Westerners believe enlightenment/transformation to be impossible.

In fact, real enlightenment/transformation does not require *eliminating* one's identity. This *is* impossible. Enlightenment/transformation is transcendence of ego: *having* an ego, not *being* one. Trying to have no ego *is* ego.

Enlightenment/transformation—the ability to come to *any* paradigm with equal ease—is not describable within the Western paradigm precisely because enlightenment/transformation is *not:*

1. positivist, i.e., sense-amenable
2. reducible to configurations of matter-energy in space-time
3. change-oriented
4. dichotomous
5. the effect of any cause
6. an emergent property of matter

It is worth noting that Westerners and/or those who prefer the Western paradigm will hear descriptions of enlightenment as violations of intelligibility itself—as making no *sense*—since it *is* the principal function of the Western paradigm to render the "material" universe intelligible. (It is also worth noting that Easterners also develop symbols of enlightenment.)

The problem of communicating enlightenment and/or transformation to adherents of the Western paradigm is even more difficult than noted above, since, it will be recalled, from *within* any paradigm, only a *symbol* of what is outside the paradigm exists *or can exist*. So Westerners who reject enlightenment or transformation, or regard it as impossible, are not in fact rejecting the reality of enlightenment but only its *symbol*. Eastern masters who have acquainted themselves with the Western paradigm have thus come to see why some Westerners refuse to take even the *possibility* of enlightenment seriously. Conversely, Westerners who have acquainted themselves with the Eastern paradigm have begun to appreciate Easterners' compassionate concern that Westerners unacquainted with the Eastern paradigm are allowing the possibility of enlightened mastery to escape through their paradigmatic fingers.

In truth, one must both give up (i.e., transcend) one's ego *and* retain it (have it as an ego) to experience transformation. To any enlightened being—Eastern or Western—this is obvious.

Transformation/enlightenment is not, in itself, a content. Nor is it, in itself, another paradigm. It is, in a manner of speaking, a quality of being.

A further difficulty in describing transformation/enlightenment is what has been called the "Horseless carriage" problem. When automobiles were first invented, they were called horseless carriages. Similarly, radio was called "wireless." Just so, the domain specified by the paradigm of paradigms is often referred to as "mindlessness" or "egolessness." Such terms can communicate little if anything to minds or to egos, and must be particularly irritating to those who hold that the conceptual mind is par excellence *the* faculty of knowing, or to those who hold that what is not conceptually knowable is not knowable at all. Hence the principal barrier to humanity's ability to experience mastery in the matter of its own further evolution is the paradigm which defines mastery as impossible because mastery is not conceptually intelligible.

For it lies in the very nature of the conceptual mind to define what is by what has been, to compare and contrast the unfamiliar with the familiar, the unknown with the once known—in short, to define the present by what was once known in the past. It is precisely the function of paradigms to define what is knowable and what is not knowable by counseling the comparison of the unknown with the known, by suggesting this is *like* that.

In the West, mind makes metaphor; and in the West, "mind" has been par excellence *the* faculty on which we have relied to steer our historical course. In the East, transcendence of the ego has been attempted. Unfortunately, elimination of the ego has often been substituted—in both East and West—for its transcendence.

Most Westerners, therefore, until very recently, have ruled out even the possibility of transformation/enlightenment, and remained steadfastly within the confines of the Western rational paradigm, which defines transformation/enlightenment and any mastery that might be associated with it, either as impossible, and hence unattainable, or as attainable only by the mindless, and hence, the deluded. Correlatively, most Easterners, until recently, have actively avoided the transcendental *inclusion* of ego in their steadfast wish not to be trapped in conceptuality and mere symbolic mastery.

Clearly, no simple mixture of bits and pieces of Eastern and Western wisdom will add one whit to humanity's ability to stear its evolutionary course, for even if there were some valuable insights in both East and West—as there surely must be—there seem to be no independent criteria by which to select them.

Surely it is no longer sufficient merely to adapt to each successive paradigm as it appears. It is one of the distinguishing characteristics of our age that we seek to transcend this endless sequence of the models and paradigms which pretend to tell us who we are and how at last to attain well-being.

What is required now is not just another shift in paradigms.

What is wanted is mastery in the matter of paradigms.

We examine next the relations of mastery and transcendence.

IX. THE TRANSCENDENCE OF EXPERIENCE

The crucial distinction is the difference between a genuine and a merely symbolic transcendence, between an ability and a conceptual explanation of ability, between mastery and mere symbols of mastery.

Ancient and modern masters are agreed that release from our symbolic prisons is possible, and comes from time to time to those whom we thereafter call enlightened or transformed beings.

Somehow, these human beings attain to a luminosity of experience and selfhood which escapes our daily power to explain it, and yet awakens within us a spark of recognition. These beings seem to have a freshness of experience unburdened by preconceptions and symbolic comparisons. They seem, in other words, to have a vitality unconfined, uncompared, and uncontrasted. Their *ability* to experience seems equally unbounded and incomparable. Each experience for them seems to be whole, entire, and complete unto itself—being exactly what it is and exactly what it is not—without reference to what it may have been and what it might become.

This quality of completeness, of wholeness, of *entirety in each moment* is the quality which lifts experience beyond dichotomy: not dichotomous, not not-dichotomous, and not both. It is "non-dual," as Zen masters say.

It is virtually impossible for most people to experience without comparison and without distinction. Most of us find it impossible to see *this* as just *this,* and not *not-that*. Actually, enlightened experience calls for, "This is. It *is* this. It is not that. *And* it is not-this. And it is not not-that."

This cumbersome language conceals a quality of enlightened "experience" which is brutally and unbearably simple. Enlightened Experience is—to make matters even more difficult—not actually an experience at all. It is the *ability* to come *to* experience *freshly,* unfreighted by memories of how one experienced before, by expectations of how one is going to experience now, or by hopes of how one will experience in the future.

Here is an example:

    Pupil: I wish I didn't have this terrible headache.
    Master: What is terrible about it?
    Pupil: It hurts.
    Master: Yes. Now what is *terrible* about it?
    Pupil: Well, it's in my way—I can't concentrate.

> Master: Why not have a headache when you have a headache and concentrate when you concentrate?
> Pupil: You know, it's not really so terrible.
> Master: Good. Now, have your headache.
> Pupil: But it's gone!
> Master: Good. Now, concentrate.

Anecdotes of this sort abound in the literature of the East. It has a both-and/neither-nor quality which infuriates uninitiated Westerners. Things are said to be simply what they are!

Note that "things," the defined contents of the Western paradigm, are dichotomized spatially (this is here—not there) and/or temporally (this is now—not then). Indeed, what "things" are, *are* designated halves of such dichotomies.

It is interesting to observe, parenthetically, that contemporary physical speculation is moving rapidly beyond these spatiotemporal dichotomies, even while psychological theorists are examining theories which go beyond locating awareness "in" time and space. Many now speak of particles without mass and experiences without content.

We observe the following:

At the center of human experience lies a quality of being simply what one is and not being what one is not. This quality is concealed from moment to moment by our insistence on comparing now to then and here to there.

Were we simply willing to be fully here, fully now, not not-there and not not-then (or not-*yet*-here and not-*yet*-now), we would uncover what is eternally and quietly now—the origin and source of all experience—the awareness-without-content, "I am."

Awareness is without content. It is the awakened context of conscious experience, which it precedes, not chronologically, but ontologically.

It is complete—whole—entire—
Neither divided nor undivided
Neither here nor not-here
Neither now nor not-now
And here now
And only here now
And not here now.

Lacking parts it is whole and indestructible.
Lacking location it cannot be lost.
Lacking time it is immortal.
Lacking form it is substance.
Lacking substance it is form.
Lacking form and substance it is nothing.
Lacking nothing it is everything.

Being everything it is complete.
Being complete it is satisfied.

Itself no thing it excludes no thing.
Itself no thing it enables everything.

It is the truth, "There is being!"
It is the awareness, "I am cause."
It is the awakening, "I experience."

Thus undefined by anything exterior or prior to itself, our deepest awareness *is* mastery. In our most fundamental being, we *are* well.

Each of us comes *to* experience whole, entire, and complete, well able to master experience.

Mastery *is* being well.

Nothing is more laughingly obvious than this truth while we are aware of it. Nothing is more elusive when we are not.

Awareness of this domain may take those who have it by delicious and untoward surprise—arising suddenly, often hilariously—often leaving just as quickly, without a trace. Eastern *and Western* mystical literature abound with these astonishing moments.

There is a kind of knowing characteristic of this realm which is epistemologically prior to ordinary experience, for it is itself without content. It is the awareness of experiencing what we experience.

It is experiencing experience—like waking again after waking from ordinary sleep.

It is the awareness of consciousness' constructs and contents as the source of that awareness.

As source of our consciousness, we create the laws of form, and, as their creators, know—in their creation—that we are that which is their source. We are—in this domain—cause of that which is caused—our conscious experience.

Indeed, *in* this domain (truly speaking it is not *a* domain at all), we do not actually experience. We generate and intend experience. In this domain, we are aware of generating and intending *what* we are consciously experiencing, and *that* we are consciously experiencing. We are aware that we *are,* and that we *are* experiencing.

In "awareness," things are exactly what they are *and* exactly what they are not. In "experience," we either experience the things we experience *or* we do not.

Consciousness divides. Here from not here, and now from not now. Either/or. Thus we are conscious of this content *or* that.
Awareness is beyond division. It is both/and.
Awareness is consciousness' context; consciousness, its content.
Awareness is the possibility of consciousness, its cause, its source, its genesis, its space, its origination, its creation.
Concepts are the contents of experience.
Consciousness is the *construct* of experience.
Awareness is the context, "I am."

X. BEING WELL

Context

Awareness of being well, experiencing well being, and a concept of health are thus *not* synonymous. They are in fact reflections in three entirely different domains of ourselves.

Awareness of being well is the fundamental knowing of who we are by who we are. Who we are comes *to* consciousness and *to* the realm of things from beyond consciousness and from beyond the realm of things. We *are* not our daily consciousness, we have it. When we are aware we come *to* consciousness. When we are aware that we come *to* consciousness from who we quintessentially are, then we are whole, entire, and complete, *and* we are conscious of things.

That we are, and that we are aware that we are, is context to consciousness' content.

Being well *is* the awareness of the miracle that we are, and that we are aware, and that we come *to* experience, wholly, entirely, and completely able to be.

Who we are—each of us—*is* being who we are able to be: being who we *are*.
This awareness is simple, first, and fundamental.
Somehow, we have become unaware of it.
Yet it is available. And once gained, is known never not to have been.
We are. And we are aware of being able to be who we are.

This aspect of ourselves—our fundamental being—examines the paradigms presented to us, to see whether we are there fully or only partly enabled.

It is this aspect of ourselves which responds with gladness when a paradigm truly reflects us and promises to add to our lives by expanding our opportunity to be and to express who we truly are.

Our ability to recognize in paradigms, images of our true selves by which we can expand our participation in life *is* the paradigm of paradigms—the freedom to participate in life masterfully.

Construct

Since we enact our intentions in time, it may be said that contexts generate constructs. Consciousness construes. It divides the universe into things that (apparently) serve us, and things that (apparently) do not. This tree of knowledge is simultaneously a garden of opportunity and the site of paradise lost, for we often confuse who we *are* with our ability to divide the world into things.

Who we are *is* who we are, *and* we are conscious of things.

One of the most blinding of all errors in our search for our true nature and for paradigms which enhance our participation in life is the confusion of who we are with our consciousness of things. We confuse being with being conscious.
We *are* not our consciousness.
We *are,* consciously.
And we live, consciously.
Consciousness is our constuct, our process, our way, our path, our manner of living.
It is *not* our self, our "essence," our source, but only *a* style of being in the world.
In consciousness, *we* divide this from that, now from then, here from there.

This same consciousness judges wellness or illness, employing criteria normally drawn from the world of things, not from the realm of who we most fundamentally are.

We often confuse criteria of well-being drawn from our *consciousness* with criteria drawn from our essential selfhood, and thus confuse *being* well—which we *are*—with consciousness of experience, in which we distinguish sickness or wellness. No error is more misleading than this confusion of selfhood with the constructs of consciousness.

This fundamental consideration—that we consider ourselves to be our consciousness—leads us to seek the source of our well being in consciousness, and in the predicaments of consciousness, rather than in the apartments of our fundamental selfhood.

In this way *we* define ourselves as being defined by what we are conscious of, rather than being aware that it is we who are, conscious of whatever we are conscious of,—whether it be illness or health. In this way we seek in paradigms of consciousness for paradigms of selfhood, and in this way selfhood is lost.

Content

We are aware of being aware.
We are aware of being conscious.
We are aware of being conscious of things.
Each has its logic.
Each has its paradigm.
The logic of awareness does not apply to consciousness.
The logic of consciousness does not apply to awareness.
Neither logic applies to things.
Nor does the logic of things apply to awareness or consciousness.

Similarly:

Paradigms of awareness do not apply to consciousness.
Paradigms of consciousness do not apply to awareness.
Neither paradigm—whether of awareness or of consciousness—applies to things.

It remains to demonstrate that the logics and paradigms of things do not apply to our awareness of being or to our awareness of being conscious.

We have seen that the Western paradigm regards things as the source of our being, thus confusing substance with form, reality with appearance, selfhood with manifestation. Small wonder that we no longer find true reflection of ourselves in a paradigm designed to define what is less than what we are.

This much has long been known.

What has only recently become clear is that many have been attempting to define the essential wellness of our being—which transcends the dichotomies of consciousness—by employing a logic derived from the dichotomous operations of consciousness.

That we are is neither well nor ill. We are.
That we are conscious is neither well nor ill. We are conscious.
What then may we say of health and sickness?
In what paradigm shall we locate these?
To which aspects of ourselves do these notions pertain?

We have come now to the heart of the matter.

Note that it is we ourselves who mistakenly consider ourselves to be things and thus ruled by the laws of things.

From which it follows that healthy and sick are only adjectives which describe those aspects of ourselves which *are* things—our materiality, our here–not–thereness—in short, those aspects of our lives which are "governed" by the laws of things.

Note also that it is we ourselves who mistakenly consider ourselves to be defined by the constructs and processes of our own consciousness and thus ruled by the laws of consciousnesses.

It follows that healthy and sick are adjectives which describe our *process*—our being-in-time, our now–not–thenness—in short, those aspects of ourselves which are ruled by the laws of construction: process, flow, and eventuation.

We may now pose our central question: What if we no longer consider these to be complete, sufficient, or satisfying paradigms by which to define ourselves and our essential well being? What then?

We have already implicitly answered this question. As contemporaries, many have examined carefully the precepts of the Western paradigm and found them insufficient for mastery. Many are no longer satisfied by a paradigm which reduces our essential natures to configurations of matter.

As contemporaries, many examined carefully the precepts of the Eastern paradigm and found them, too, insufficient for mastery—to the extent that it identifies our essential selfhood with configurations of consciousness.

We consider either, or both, of these paradigms to be insufficient—not simply to define our fundamental wellness, but to foster it, generate it, and enable it to be a ubiquitous human quality.

We have defined ourselves by paradigms inappropriate to our task, and thus have allowed ourselves to be defined inappropriately.

By confusing context with construct and construct with content, we have confused principles of generation with principles of construction with principles of content.

And in so doing, we have confused (1) being well with (2) consciousness of well being, with (3) the presence (or absence) of illness.

Conclusion

We *are* well.
Being well is the awareness of the miracle that we are able to be.
We are the ones who come to consciousness, able to be, ill or healthy.
We *are* the paradigm of paradigms—able to come to *any* paradigm—to discern whether we are there truthfully portrayed.

It is time to shift to a paradigm which accords us more of our full and entire dignity.

This time—as our species welcomes greater and greater responsibility for its own further evolution—let us not allow ourselves to be defined *by* the next paradigm, no matter how wondrously and magnificently it portrays us.

For true mastery lies not in things or in paradigms,
but in our ability to cause life to *be*
serenely, magnificently, completely,
what is.

To oversimplify the matter somewhat, it is as if Freud supplied to us the sick half of psychology and we must now fill it out with the healthy part.

Abraham Maslow

One of the major themes of this book, and one of the reasons for writing it, is the dearth of information and research on well-being in Western psychology. One of the most notable exceptions to this theme has been Douglas Heath whose research and scholarship have made major contributions to our fund of objective data.

In "The Maturing Person," he summarizes much of his research and thinking. He first delineates the difficulties and then the necessary theoretical assumptions and methodological guidelines involved in this type of research. Then he presents his multidimensional model and shows how maturing can be traced across various personality factors. There are many strengths to his approach including the use of both longitudinal and cross-cultural studies, a methodological approach which allows an increasing refinement and precision of concepts and criteria, and the breadth and vision of his scholarship which includes both psychological and religious perspectives.

Dr. Heath is Professor of Psychology at Haverford College in Pennsylvania. He is one of the most respected researchers of psychological well-being and one of the very few people who has amassed a large body of empirical findings. He has published extensively, and his most recent books include Humanizing Schools: New Directions, New Decisions *(Hayden Book Co., 1971) and* Maturity and Competence: A Transcultural View *(Gardner Press, 1977). Since Dr. Heath was one of the earliest contributors to* Beyond Health and Normality, *which had a long gestation period, some of the most recent research in the field may not be cited. Readers wanting a more detailed discussion of his work may wish to consult one of his books.*

6

The Maturing Person

Douglas Heath*

What a paradox! Our Western languages are replete with terms like self-realization, self-actualization, self-fulfillment, psychologically healthy and sound, positive mental health, maturity, emotional stability, becoming, sane, fulfilling our potential, well-integrated, wholeness, the good life, virtue. Our Western philosophical heritage is rooted in symbols of growth and fulfillment: the Hellenistic ideal of arete, *humanitas,* paideia, or the self-realization of the autonomous person in harmony with his community; the model of Socrates enabling a youth's intrinsic virtue to develop and blossom; the Christian assumption that we have the capacity to grow and approach the ideal of Christ; the European existentialist call to become more authentic "as the Dasein undergoes the *arduous process* of choosing itself and growing into maturity" (Binswanger, 1963, p. 346); the American philosophical emphasis on continued growth, as seen in Whitehead's goal of "developing the self," Dewey's "growing healthily," and Van Doren's cultivating the "skills of being."

Such is the vision of our Western heritage, but what is the reality of our scientific knowledge about how to respond to such a call? The paradox is that in spite of the preeminent advance in knowledge and insight that our Western scientific methods have gathered about our physical world and our selves, we still must turn to both Western and Eastern humanistic and

*The research referred to in this chapter was supported by the Spencer Foundation, W. Clement and Jessie Stone Foundation, and the National Institute of Mental Health, Grant No. 11227.

religious traditions for wisdom about what "growing into maturity" and becoming "authentic" mean in fact.

Why has our Western scientific tradition provided us with so little wisdom about how to live "the good life," to "grow more healthily"? Why do our helping scientifically based professions, like psychiatry, define their goals as furthering mental health but talk almost exclusively about mental illness? Why do we channel millions of dollars annually into the study of diseased and deficient people, and only thousands into the study of healthy and mature persons? And why do we use the rhetoric of nurturing the "whole child" but hold teachers accountable only in terms of technically impeccable achievement tests measuring factual information that is only temporarily retained in any case?

At least six reasons account for the marginal contribution that Western science has made to our understanding of psychological maturity. The first is that the current psychological sciences cannot deal very well with the level of analysis that is most appropriate for concepts like "self-realization" and "maturity." "Healthiness" is a holistic concept that refers to the characteristics of a complex system functioning harmoniously as a whole over time. It is the clinician-scientist, like a Freud or a Rogers, who, keeping the whole person in view, has contributed more to our understanding of healthy systemic growth than the research scientist who, ignoring the person as a person, has focused on a highly specific aspect of development, such as changes in depth perception with age. Although current personality research has its roots in the holistic views of persons like Henry Murray and Robert White during the early post-World War II era, contemporary scientific research has fled from its early molar, systemic, and contextual assumptions to embrace more molecular, fragmented, and reductionistic topics and modes of analyses that have little or no relation to the functioning of the person as a system. The prospects are not favorable that the analytic, reductionistic bias of American personality researchers, in particular, will be moderated in the future. The type of graduate training, the publication policies of journals, the criteria for research funding, and the contemporary scientific ethos that one should work with objectively and precisely manageable topics conspire to lock most researchers into a highly reductionistic way of defining what is a significant issue to explore. Scientism is crowding out spirit, substance, and significance.

A second reason for the scientific neglect of concepts like psychological health and maturity may be rooted in our Western assumption that objective, valid knowledge can only come from active, manipulative control of the antecedents that affect a dependent variable. The research that is valued, therefore, is that which takes place in a laboratory where the influences that affect a person's response can be controlled. Such research, of course, at least with humans, is essentially time-bound. Concepts like maturing, becoming, growing, on the other hand, refer to changes occurring over long periods of time in complicated, uncontrollable settings. Although researchers somewhat plaintively write that we will never have an adequate understanding of development until we observe persons throughout their lives (Wohlwill, 1973), extraordinarily few have committed themselves to just such longitudinal studies (Block, 1971; Cox, 1970; Grinker, 1962, 1974; Heath, C. W., 1945; Jones et al., 1971; Kagan and Moss, 1962; Vaillant, 1971, 1972, 1974, 1975, 1976, 1977, among others).

A third reason for the paucity of valid empirical knowledge about the mentally healthy person has been the preference to induce generalizations about healthy persons from studies of the unhealthy rather than of healthy persons themselves. This rather strange and circuitous approach is defended by the claim that we can only know what is healthy and mature by observing their opposites. However, the unexamined assumption that mental health is the converse of mental illness has not been compellingly demonstrated (Jahoda, 1958). Besides, the assumption is a very complex one. The issue will probably not yield to any simple resolution because it involves more fundamental problems, like the probable discontinuity of pathological behavior as a result of biochemical alterations.

Certainly, another formidable barrier to the direct study of maturing persons is the timorous attitude of researchers about involvement with issues and concepts whose definitional criteria may involve value judgments. The professional loses status if he cannot purify his criteria of subjective bias. What is diseased and dysfunctional is palpable, immediate, objectively determinable, if not measurable. What is healthy and mature is an idiosyncratic, amorphous value judgment—at least so the argument goes. If we are to study healthily growing persons we must rely on judges to identify them for us. Judges have their own biases and subjective criteria. Therefore, when we study such selected persons, we will only rediscover the values of the judges who selected the persons to be studied in the first place. I will return to this argument shortly.

A fifth barrier that has handicapped our understanding of healthy growth has been the relativistic bias that has dominated Western social science for the past 40 years. The argument has been that each society defines who is mentally healthy in somewhat different terms; therefore, no scientific model of healthy growth that applies to all persons irrespective of cultural background is possible. Szasz pursues the argument even further when he claims that each society's definition of what is mentally ill only disguises its own value judgment of what is a preferred way to live (1961, 1970). It is a myth that there are universal transcultural mental health insights to be discovered. By implication, any mental health term is only an ethical-legal fiction, not a scientifically based fact. Yet, a review of the substantive cross-cultural findings of the past decade reveals an increasing number of researchers who believe that they have objectively demonstrated that there are recurring behavioral similarities among diverse cultures (Ashton, 1975; Cantril, 1965; Dohrenwend and Dohrenwend, 1974; Gutmann, 1975; Harmon, Masuda, and Holmes, 1970; Kohlberg, 1968, 1970, 1973; Osgood, May, and Miron, 1975). The psychiatric nihilism and relativistic bias implied in Szasz's argument may be slowly yielding to an emerging zeitgeist within the behavioral sciences, a changing paradigm that is more receptive to the possibility of establishing such transcultural universals (Osgood et al., 1975).

There is one final and more down-to-earth reason for our limited progress in reaching an empirically based understanding of healthy growth. An early intriguing allegedly empirical model of studying self-actualized, mature persons, while provocative and highly influential, was so methodologically inadequate that it discouraged others from pursuing subsequent empirical studies. I refer to Maslow's well-publicized, allegedly empirical, but extraordinarily subjective study of self-actualized persons (Maslow, 1950). Recall that he alone selected persons from our historical past (e.g., Lincoln, Eleanor Roosevelt) and induced from their lives qualities that he claimed represented self-actualized persons. The sheer complexity and abstractness of the qualities identified made many refractory to more objective measurement. The subjectivity of the methodology provided no acceptable scientific model to others about how one might empirically explore self-actualization (M. B. Smith, 1973). The delayed evolution of the Personal Orientation Inventory, designed to assess some attributes of self-actualization (Knapp and Comrey, 1973; Shostrom, 1964; Shostrom and Knapp, 1966), its associated research, and some research on peak experiences have been the only significant scientific consequences of the rich intuitive legacy that Maslow left behind.

What pathways for the future study of positive mental health does this brief analysis suggest? The concept of healthy growth or maturing is a theoretical nodal point at which many disciplines meet. Not only philosophers, theologians, and the great religious traditions of the planet but also behavioral scientists and psychiatrists, as well as educators and humanists, have concerned themselves with the qualities of the good life, the meaning of healthy development, the goals of liberal education, and the portrayal of the fulfilled person. It is a nodal point at which the issues of what is fact and what is value become fused, as Maslow asserted (1963). An empirical approach to the issue of healthy growth or maturing must faithfully represent its complexity as sketched by the humanist; it must be deeply systemic. To grapple with the complexity of a developing person means our approach must be multifaceted, must examine different "levels" of the personality, must be developmental in assumption and probably longitudinal in design, must not become paralyzed by fears about evaluative issues and, if it is to establish universal developmental principles, must not flinch from seeking transcultural confirmation. Finally, we need more persuasive methodological models of how to proceed, models that are as empirically objective, reliable, and valid as adherence to the integrity of the phenomenon permits us to create.

Even a cursory review of our Western tradition's view of healthy growth and maturing immediately reveals a confusing babble of tongues. No two philosophers, educators, clinicians, psychologists, or social scientists identify the same number of traits or even the same trait to be a core defining quality of the maturing person. However, a closer analysis of the writings and findings of those who empirically, whether as clinicians, observers, or researchers, have worked with actual persons who are changing, reveals considerable agreement about the qualities of healthily functioning persons. Several recurring themes weave through the claims and findings of clinicians like Freud (1923), Jung (1939), and Rogers (1961); developmental psychologists like Piaget (1947), Erikson (1963), Murphy (1962), Kohlberg (1964), and Werner (1948); social psychologists or sociologists like Cantril (1965) and Inkeles (1974); biologists like Sinnott (1959); and researchers like Barron (1963), Warren and Heist (1960), Loevinger (1976), and Vaillant (1977) who are directly studying sound, mature persons. For example, most agree with Socrates that accuracy of self-insight is a central quality of a mature person. Self-confidence is another such quality. Although large chunks of empirical research have been done on self-esteem and other qualities that I will shortly induce from the research literature, I cannot systematically review such research here. Much of it has been gathered bit by bit, piece by piece, without any organized effort to relate it to some systemic view of the maturing person. Its empirical linkages to the organismic concept of psychological health are thin and fragile.

The editors have charged me, instead, to provide an overview of a model of healthy growth, identify assumptions that a scientific understanding of maturing must make, and then use such a model to integrate where possible the available evidence. After the tentative effort to order comprehensively the theoretical and empirical findings about maturity, I will turn to some key theoretical issues, like the relation of maturing to adult effectiveness, adaptation, and modernism, and then discuss the implications of the model of maturing for understanding healthy development throughout the life span, for educating youth, and for the formation of religious values. I will conclude by identifying the edges of the frontier which researchers might profitably risk exploring. In a short chapter, I can only be schematic; more detailed theoretical analyses, discussion of new methods of assessment, and the presentation of supporting evidence have been reported elsewhere (Heath, 1965, 1968, 1977c).

NECESSARY THEORETICAL ASSUMPTIONS OF A SCIENTIFIC MODEL OF MATURING

Systemic

Since, as we have said, concepts like self-actualization and maturing concern a person, not just a sector of his personality, a holistic and systemic model is required. Any viable psychobiological system must have equilibrating properties that allow it to remain flexibly open to new information at the same time that it retains its essential structural stability. A healthy system is one that has the requisites for adapting without so distorting its own structural needs that subsequent growth is interfered with. At the outset, we must distinguish between adjustment, self-fulfillment, and adaptation. Adjustment is accommodation of oneself to fit the expectations or demands of some external source or role. Self-fulfillment is the alteration of the external requirements to fit or satisfy one's own needs and talents. Adaptation, on the other hand, is the creation of an optimal equilibrium between fulfilling the demands to adjust and fulfilling the demands of one's own needs. Too severe demands to adjust, as in response to too high expectations, or too intense needs for self-fulfillment, as seen in wish-dominated thinking, may distort the system's subsequent healthy growth. We can state the equilibrating principle governing healthy systems this way: too extended development in one dimensional sector of a personality may induce resistance to further growth in that sector until compensatory development occurs in the neglected sectors. We sometimes clinically find, for example, this systemic principle operating in intellectually gifted persons whose cognitive maturation far outpaces their emotional and interpersonal maturation. At some point, if they are not to snap and break, like the proverbial rubber band, they may overcompensate by suddenly abandoning their intellectual talents and self-discipline to pursue drugs, orgiastic, or other deinhibiting experiences that help them to recover a sense of equilibrium. Such an equilibrium may seem, and may be in fact, regressive on some dimensions but such a regression may, as Jung suggested, be necessary before *systemic* growth can resume.

As every perceptive diagnostician knows, we cannot evaluate the "healthiness" of most specific behaviors. Their meaning depends upon the "healthiness" of the system of which they are only partial manifestations. For this reason, diagnoses based on specific behaviors, e.g., reporting "hearing voices" as in Rosenhan's study (1973), are likely to be very unreliable. This is why I cannot identify homosexual behavior in and of itself to be unhealthy, immature, or pathological. It may or may not be, depending upon the maturity or healthiness of the person manifesting such behavior. I prefer to talk of pathological systems, not of pathological behavior.

Universality

While persons as systems differ in certain relatively irreversible ways (i.e., ethnic stock, gender, cultural background, and social class), every person is similar by virtue of being a human system that must ceaselessly adapt. Therefore, any model of maturing, becoming, or actualizing the self should seek to identify those universal qualities that describe an adapting system. I make the powerful claim that it is possible to construct a perfectly general model of the maturing process that applies to all persons, regardless of their race, religiocultural background, or sex. It then becomes an empirical question, not an ideologically based argument, to discover if, for example, mature Nigerian males and females differ as predicted from less mature Nigerian males and females; or if mature females differ from less mature females in ways that are similar to how mature males differ from less mature males. Sex, social class, and cultural background then serve as moderator variables, altering the timing, extent, and patterning of maturing effects on the system's given structural dimensions.

Abstract

The assumption of universality requires a model of health that is sufficiently abstract to not be dependent upon any specific behavioral trait, like "hearing voices" or participating in homosexual activities. It needs to identify more general genotypic, so to speak, rather than phenotypic, qualities—for it is in the area of the latter that cultures are likely to have their most diverse effects. For example, if we examine cultures in terms of the content of their pubertal initiation ceremonies for clues about maturing, we probably will fail to find transcultural similarities. However, if we examine the way cultures stabilize an adolescent's sexual identity, of which a pubertal rite is only one of numerous phenotypic possibilities, we are more likely to identify a transculturally universal proposition, e.g., clarity of the timing of a rite facilitates the early stabilization of sexual identity.

Developmental

Increasingly, researchers are recognizing that a process rather than a state model is necessary when talking about psychological health. True, we may be able to specify eventually what degree of psychological health a person has at a particular moment in time, but the more significant fact about that temporary state is its potential degree of adaptability to changing internal and external demands in the future. That requires not only an assessment over time but a conception of health that is developmental, that consists of qualities that enable a system to change and adapt to varying situations. For this reason, I technically talk of a "maturing person." I talk of "mature" or "maturity" only for reasons of style or convenience. To say a 21 or 32 year old is now "mature" is to make a normative judgment, the bases of which may vary from one judge or society to another. Furthermore, it implies a static ideal point that violates the assumption of continued growth. We can, however, by taking a developmental or dimensional view, say that this person is more mature than he was last year or than this other person.

The theoretical issue becomes clouded when we talk about psychological "health" as a developmental concept. Because our ideas about development are frequently chained to chronological age, it makes no sense to us to say that the typical nine year old is more psychologically healthy than the typical five year old. However, if we define the psychological health of a system as its ability to adapt over time, then we would have to admit that a typical nine year old is more able to adapt to a wider range of demands than a typical two year old. In fact, the two year old is so psychologically unhealthy we must protect him from himself by putting him behind bars—of his playpen. What rescues us from this awkward terminological position is that we cannot talk about adaptation independently of the maturational level of the structure of a system and the types of adjustments it must make. So it is not reasonable to compare the psychological health of children of different ages for they must adapt to different kinds of demands. It is reasonable to compare the psychological health of one infant with that of another infant and of a prepubertal child with that of another prepubertal child. Theorists like Sanford (1962) and Loevinger (1976) quarrel with this equation of psychological health with maturing. Sanford believes that a term like *development* refers to increasing complexity, and a term like *health*, to the potential for maintaining stability. Loevinger does not believe that there is any necessary relation between her personality typology and psychological health. Only studies of the relation of psychological healthiness to her developmental typology will clarify the issue.

We confront another cloudy issue when we propose a developmental model of maturing that concerns the upper age range. Does it make any sense to talk about psychological health improving or maturing continuing with 80- and 90-year-old persons? My answer is yes, though plateaus and even regressions may occur more frequently. Persons of any age still must adapt to changing external as well as internal physiological events. The elderly must confront both types of changes. Some evidence suggests that the more psychologically healthy a person has been when younger, the more likely will he be to adapt more effectively when older to the crises that face him. We have remarkably little information about the course of psychological health over long periods of time, but my studies of maturing from 17 to 32 clearly demonstrate that maturing can continue, i.e., the adult men studied improved at high levels of statistical significance on six of seven diverse measures of their mental health during the intervening years (Heath, 1977d).

Dimensional

I suggest that any system is characterized by certain genotypic, independent, structural qualities or dimensions on which it may be developed to different degrees. The systemic assumption suggests that the health of a person may be adversely affected by too great differential development on some dimensions at the expense of development on others. For example, most theorists agree that a system becomes more differentiated and complex over time, thus becoming more integratively flexible and so more adaptable. Another dimension of a growing system about which there is widespread agreement is that it becomes progressively more stable, but excessive stability relative to growth in integration may result in rigidity which reduces the capacity of the system to assimilate and differentiate new information, thus limiting its eventual adaptability.

A system does not necessarily become more dimensionally mature in some continuous, linear way. Development is marked by differing rates of growth throughout the life span as well as by the emergence of differently timed physiological and/or socially defined "crises" which disturb a system's equilibrium. We normally call such periods "stages" and identify them by the kinds of dimensional growth that are demanded at that period. Erikson, for example, has identified late adolescence as a time when one must integrate and stabilize one's identity (1963). Increasing evidence suggests that another period during which physiological and/or social factors disrupt an achieved equilibrium is at mid-life, when one must again, at a different and more complex level of maturity, reintegrate and restabilize one's identity, this time to take into account declining potency or fertility, expanding abdomen, and approaching retirement and death (Levinson, 1978). Whether such stages are as clearly identifiable for every person in a particular culture is moot; a person who may be continually altering, in small dosages, his concept of himself through the thirties and early forties may never suddenly encounter the so-called mid-life crisis. I do not find the stage concept, in other words, to be a compelling scientific way of conceptualizing the growth process. Except for irreversible biophysical changes of the system which are universal within certain defined periods (e.g., pubertal endocrine changes), I am not persuaded that the more sociopsychological stages are necessarily invariant or universal. The fact that different theorists do not agree about naming their stages and identify different sequences to their stages (e.g., Erikson's "autonomy" stage is in early childhood, and Loevinger's "autonomy," defined somewhat differently, is in adulthood) and the fact that the sexes may differ in the sequence (e.g., Erikson's crisis of intimacy precedes rather than follows the crisis of identity for American girls but not for boys; Douvan and Adelson, 1966) suggest to me that a genuinely transcultural, invariant psychosocial stage view of personality development may be quite illusive. Others like Holt (1974) will disagree. They claim there is enough correspondence among the different views of stages to posit a universal sequence. The concept of "stage" has its heuristic value, however, for it identifies the types of normative adaptive problems that members of a particular social and sex group may have to resolve at very roughly comparable age periods in their lives. The more critical questions for those interested in adaptation, actualization, or other similar concepts are, I suggest, two. How does the person adapt and fashion a new equilibrium to whatever the changing biological and/or social demands are that confront him? Perry's stage model of cognitive maturation during late adolescence at least describes in some detail one plausible adaptive sequence (1970). The second question is, What are the factors that predict how maturely a person will adapt to a stage's crisis? Erikson, more than most theorists, has sought to relate his "stages" to the continued psychological health of the system. For example, he claims that an adult's mental health requires that he resolve the generativity stage and that fulfilling a parental or caretaking role with respect to the young contributes to that resolution and hence to his continued mental health.

The "stage" concept is more a descriptively normative than a powerfully analytic concept, particularly as we see in Levinson's (1974, 1978), Loevinger's (1976), and Gould's (1972) categorizations of adult development. However, both the Piagetian and psychoanalytically derived stage models do have some analytic power. Piaget and Kohlberg, as well as Freud and Erikson, agree that a person has difficulty adapting to a subsequent stage if he has not successfully adapted to an earlier stage. Loevinger seemingly does not make such an assumption for she has not related her stages to the quality of a person's adaptation (1976). Perhaps because of the paucity of longitudinal studies of adults throughout any significant section of their lives, the "stage" theorists have little to say about continued adult maturing as well as about the determinants of that growth. Erikson's idea that parenting contributes to psychological health is one of the few examples of a hypothesized determinant. Incidentally, recent evidence about the continued maturing of professional fathers suggests that fatherhood may not in and of itself be a particularly powerful contributor to their continued psychological health (Heath, 1978). Instead, the demands of a person's occupation and the kind of spouse that he marries are far more influential determinants (Heath, 1977d). Neither is included specifically in any "stage" model of healthy development.

Ironically, the analytic power of Piaget and Kohlberg's cognitive, Freud's psychosexual, and Erikson's psychosocial stage models of maturing depends, in part, on their underlying dimensional assumptions about growth. Piaget's cognitive stages are dependent upon the underlying dimensional development of formal operations like reversibility and combinativity (1947). Kohlberg's moral stages can be alternatively viewed as variations on an underlying theme of increasing complexity and allocentricism, i.e., growth from self-centered to more socialized modes of thought and identifications (1964). Implied in psychosexual stage development are assumptions about increasing integration, stabilization, and reality differentiation. Finally, of the four theorists, Erikson's stages are the most clearly dimensionally based, for each finds its roots in early infancy, becomes psychologically salient as a "crisis," and persists throughout life.

The dilemma that I as a researcher find in these stage theories is that I do not know what attributes of psychological health or maturity they actually predict. As influential and well known as are Erikson's and Kohlberg's stages, a systematic review of the research literature has identified remarkably few independent personality traits that are predicted by any measures of their stages. We have been unable to confirm that men who are more morally advanced, according to Kohlberg, are any more psychologically mature in a wide range of other aspects of their lives than men who are less morally mature (Miller and Moser, 1977). The failure to anchor such stage theories within a broader systemic understanding of the person means we do not know how to interpret the contribution such a stage theory may make to our knowledge about maturing.

Value-free

The last desirable characteristic of a scientific model of maturing is that it be *as free as possible* of parochial value assumptions and judgments. I emphasize "as free as possible" because, of course, any scientific study involves a host of value judgments, as Holt (1974) and others have perceptively identified. Behavioral scientists disagree about the possibility of ever achieving such value neutrality when studying complex human behaviors, like intelligence or mental health, that seem to involve evaluative judgments (Holt, 1974; Smith, 1961, 1974; Wechsler, 1975). In the past decade, others have been moving toward the belief that objective adaptational criteria that are transculturally universal may eventually be generated (Cattell, 1973; Opler, 1969; Sarbin, 1969). I would argue that it may be possible to identify from longitudinal developmental studies of random samples in different cultures, systemic dimensions that are transculturally general (e.g., increasing capacity for symbolization) which predict adaptive effectiveness in those cultures. Judgments about competence or effectiveness in fulfilling a role do, at this stage in our understanding of competence, involve value judgments. However, as we learn more about the specific qualities that define, for example, competent fathers or vocational adaptation, we may be able to progressively, though not perfectly, purify our adaptational criteria of more blatant value judgments. For example, if we learn how children develop cognitively and socially, we might be able to assess more objectively parental competence in terms of how well the parent has furthered such cognitive and social maturation in his child. We are making, however, the value judgment that furthering someone else's development is a fundamental criterion of parental competence.

SOME METHODOLOGICAL GUIDELINES FOR STUDYING MATURING SCIENTIFICALLY

Use of Exemplars

Since psychological research has yet to produce a widely accepted, valid, comprehensive measure of any of the terms with which this chapter began, we must rely on the judgments of judges to identify exemplars of different degrees of psychological maturity. When such judgments are made independently of the theory or hypothesis that we seek to test, the judgments can serve as the criterion variable we wish to predict. That is, do our model of maturing and its measures actually differentiate the judge-identified mature from the immature person?

Initially, such judgments will inevitably be colored by the judges' assessment of how effectively a person is adapting to the various demands of the situation in which he is being judged. Personal as well as cultural biases and values undoubtedly affect such choices. How might we reduce their more obvious effects? Certainly the use of very diverse judges who have intimate knowledge of how well the members of the population adapt to a wide range of different types of demands can bring a wide perspective to the selection process. For this reason, when studying mature and immature exemplars transculturally, I sought out small residential institutions in which all members could be known well in their different roles by many different judges. The use of a large number of judges dilutes the impact of a particular judge's more personal prejudices. It is of considerable methodological interest that when such selection precautions are taken, it is possible to secure agreement from the independent judges about who has and who has not adapted effectively to the varied demands of the situation within which the persons are functioning.

How might we escape being mired in the tautological quagmire of rediscovering in our assessment of the exemplars only those criteria which were the reasons for their initial selection? We can assess broadly for characteristics not contained in the initial criteria for selection. For example, the model of maturing that I will describe shortly predicts that mature in contrast to immature persons will more accurately predict what other persons think of them. Few judges would have such a criterion in mind when asked to compare several hundred young adults with respect to their effectiveness in living their lives.

How can we moderate the pervasive effects that different cultures have in shaping the judges' definitions of who is and who is not effective in living their lives? American judges are likely to identify a young male adult as more mature if he has demonstrated his independence from his family, is self-sufficient, adventurous, and enterprising. Italian judges do not rate such qualities as highly (Heath, 1977c). We can gradually free our understanding of maturity from such parochial cultural limitations by testing the generality of our findings in varying situations and cultures. We can progressively objectify the means of selection as we identify the more powerfully predictive psychological measures of maturity. Thus we can gradually abstract out of the particularistic biases that inevitably affect such research in its initial phases those more universal recurring themes that describe the mature person in increasingly diverse cultures. The hope is that out of this winnowing process will emerge a core set of qualities that distinguish more mature from less mature persons in most cultures.

Multifaceted Assessment

A second methodological guideline that follows from the assumption about systemic organization is that the assessment of its healthiness must be multifaceted and tap into different "levels" of organization. It is not sufficient to assess the degree of a system's integration by relying on one measure that taps only one "level" or sector of the personality. Just as one sub-test score of an intelligence test is a very limited index of the quality of the person's intelligence, so is one focused measure of a trait an inadequate guide to a person's maturity. I do not know how to interpret the findings of the typical research study of psychological health that relies exclusively on one test, most frequently a self-report questionnaire like the Minnesota

Multiphasic Personality Inventory (MMPI) or the Personal Orientation Inventory (POI). Such tests provide little information about the actual integration of a person. For example, two persons may value similarly the aesthetic way of life as measured by the Study of Values (Allport, Vernon, and Lindzey, 1960); but for one, the value may be a compensatory defensive reaction for inadequate intimacy relations, while for another, the value may be congruent with his temperament and talents. Unless we assess how integrative such a value is with other aspects of a person's personality (e.g., compare the value pattern with the person's actual temperamental similarity to persons in aesthetic fields), we do not know if the value pattern is healthily integrative or not. Studies of Sicilian and Istanbul males found both to score highly on autonomy. However, the pattern of the validity correlates of each group was radically different, indicating that autonomy meant something quite different to the men of each culture. The Sicilian men's autonomy was very integrative with their authoritarian machismo-dominated culture; the Istanbul men's autonomy manifested a defensive rebelliousness against their culture's authoritarianism. The autonomy measure of the Sicilians predicted every measure of maturity given them; the autonomy measure of the Istanbul men predicted poor ego strength, compulsive self-doubts, lack of social adaptability, and increased wariness in their interpersonal relationships (Heath, 1977c). Unless we assess comprehensively to reflect the contextual richness of the human personality, we risk misinterpreting the meaning of our individual test scores and do not know their ability to predict the psychological healthiness of the person.

Longitudinal

Another methodological implication of the criteria defining an adequate model of healthy growth is that persons should be studied at different periods in their lives. Although a healthy system adapts in response to new information, its changes are not random. Its existing structure responds selectively to that which it can assimilate and determines the kinds of responses made. Thus, there is continuity in change but relative stability to personality organization over extended time periods. To assess the healthiness of a person we need to know how he adapts to varying life experiences as well as whether such growth has been integrative. My study of men from 17 to 32 clearly shows that psychological health continues to improve, that maturing can continue, during young adulthood, and that persons who were quite mature relative to others when in college were similarly quite mature relative to the same group 10 or 12 years later. The data also suggest that there is relative stability in many other qualities that are components of, or contribute to, a person's psychological health. Since such data are rare in the behavioral sciences and have not been previously reported, I list in decreasing order in Table 6–1 the 15 most stable qualities of the 57 test scores for which adolescent and adult measures were available.

Although such stability described the sample as a whole, some men showed considerable change relative to other men on the various test scores. To predict the quality of a person's future growth, it becomes important to understand *which* traits most powerfully predict such relative improvement. While the analyses are not complete, we now know, for example, that the adolescent who had a more integrative and autonomous self-concept and was judged on 26 traits to be more mature is more likely to be a happier adult 10 to 12 years later than the adolescent who was not as maturely developed in these ways. The results also confirm Ernest Jones' claim that the more mature adult has the capacity for creating a happier life (1942). To know which specific attributes of an adolescent's psychological health predict subsequent healthy growth and happiness will greatly increase our

Table 6–1. Stability of Adult Personality Traits over a 12–15 Year Period.

Trait	Test Score	Correlation Coefficient	Number of Subjects
Masculinity	Strong Vocational	713	68
Inconsistency, lack of integration	MMPI F	688	39*
Reflective control	MMPI K	642	39
Social intraversion	MMPI Si	623	59
Anxiety, tension	MMPI At	597	49
Values aesthetic life	Study of Values	596	68
Tolerance for others	MMPI To	590	48
Clinical rating of psychological health	Rorschach	574	68
Maturity of interests	Strong Vocational	574	68
Imaginal productivity	Rorschach (# responses)	562	68
Social impression of good adjustment	MMPI Sr	532	49
Frequency of aggressive images in fantasy	Rorschach (% Aggression)	525	68
Domination by primary process mode-images	Rorschach (Holt % PriPro)	514	68
Masculinity-femininity	MMPI Mf	508	48
Domination of fantasy by benign socially acceptable libidinal-aggressive fantasies	Rorschach (Holt % L2)	504	68

*Original MMPI test blanks either not scored or not available for rescoring.

understanding of what potentials to search for when assessing adolescents. Only longitudinal studies can provide that information.

The implications of these methodological guidelines may trouble many researchers. They suggest much more intensive in-depth studies over longer time periods than is fashionable in mental health research. The longitudinal study of adult men that I just referred to has taken 15 years and involved numerous measures of their adolescent and adult mental health status and competence. The myriad methodological problems that plague such studies have been perceptively described by Block (1971); we probably can expect few similar studies in the future given their complexity and duration. The consequence is that there is little likelihood that the necessary replication studies will be done to assess both the reliability and the generality of the findings.

MODEL OF THE MATURING PERSON

To study the maturing of a person, we must ask, "What are the attributes of a person most critical to comprehend his systemic complexity?" and "What is the most economical number of dimensions to faithfully portray the process of maturing?" The model of maturing proposes to study the maturation of a person's cognitive skills, self-concept, values, and interpersonal relationships. It postulates that in each of these sectors, growth occurs on five interdependent dimensions: increasing symbolization, allocentricism, integration, stability, and autonomy. Figure 6–1 illustrates the model which provides 20 basic hypotheses about how more and less mature exemplars differ. It suggests, for example, that increasing interpersonal maturity is directly associated with increasing ability to become aware of one's relationships which become increasingly more allocentric, integrated, stable, and

DIMENSION OF MATURING

PERSONALITY SECTORS	Symboli-zation	Allocen-tricism	Integra-tion	Stability	Autonomy
Cognitive skills					
Self-concept					
Values					
Personal relations					

Figure 6-1. The model of maturing.

autonomous. The systemic equilibrating principle suggests that too extended development in autonomy, for example, may limit development in other sectors, like allocentricism, thus eventually braking the overall maturation of the system. Excessive autonomy may be seen in the self-sufficient individualist or narcissist who is incapable of understanding other person's view-points. Eventually such limited allocentric development adversely affects the ability to communicate empathically, to understand accurately how others think of one; it accentuates self-centered values which may block one's understanding and appreciation of the values of persons quite different from oneself; and it prevents the development of understanding, warm, tolerant interpersonal relationships.

Different societies encourage differential development on the dimensions. Women may be raised to be very accommodating to the demands of men and so score high on allocentricism, frequently at the expense of comparable development on autonomy. The consequence is that some women may be intellectually conforming. They may seldom challenge, argue, or take an independent position. They may be hypersensitive to the opinions that others have about them, so they shrink from asserting their own values. They may be unusually tactful and interpersonally sensitive but unable to create mature interdependent personal relationships because of conflicts about becoming independent and autonomous. The net potential effect of such socialization practices is to limit the integration into the personality of the positive potentials associated with increasing autonomy and independence.

I will briefly define each dimensional sector of the maturing person by drawing upon the research and thought of behavioral scientists, educators, and philosophers, and the principal religious traditions.* I will then briefly summarize some of the empirical data that most directly support the hypotheses that such qualities define maturing. The main empirical support for the validity of this conception of psychological health comes from several sources: (1) intensive studies of mature and immature exemplars, selected following the guidelines outlined earlier, in five diverse cultural areas, including Mid-Atlantic United States, Sicily, Northern Italy, Anatolia, and Istanbul; (2) longitudinal study of random samples of students developing in college and of several decades of alumni, and a second longitudinal study of other groups of students initiated when they were freshmen, retested as upperclassmen, and then again as adults in their early

---

*I have reported elsewhere content analyses of the views (1) of 35 behavioral science experts about the qualities that define a mentally healthy person (1965), and (2) of 20 educators and philosophers about the developmental goals of a liberal education (1968). For information about the developmental goals implied in many of the principal religious traditions, I rely on the analytic commentaries of Bellah et al., 1976; Bouwsma, 1976; Deikman, 1977; Goleman, 1975, 1976; Lapidus, 1976; Neki, 1975; Owens, 1975; Pederson, 1977; Rohlen, 1976; Tart, 1975; Tseng, 1973; Wei-Ming, 1976. I have found no similar analysis of Judaism.

thirties;* (3) focused personality studies designed to assess hypotheses other than those of the model of maturing but whose findings are congruent with the model's hypotheses. Although we will be examining each dimension separately, summary measures of the overall level of maturity or psychological health of a person have been devised against which to validate measures designed to assess more specific hypotheses of the model. For example, the Rorschach ink blot test, given to each person in the principal studies, was blindly analyzed and rated with respect to the degree of his psychological healthiness. A Perceived Self Questionnaire (PSQ) was designed to measure the dimensional maturity of a person. It consisted of 50 bipolar eight-point scales that measured each person's self-assessed maturity in each of the dimensional sectors of the model. The scales can be summed to yield a score of systemic maturity. A typical item, measuring the integration of the self-concept, is:

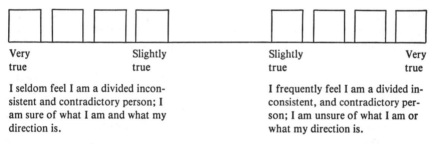

Very
true   Slightly
true   Slightly
true   Very
true

I seldom feel I am a divided inconsistent and contradictory person; I am sure of what I am and what my direction is.

I frequently feel I am a divided inconsistent, and contradictory person; I am unsure of what I am or what my direction is.

Persons who complete the PSQ are not aware of its theoretical rationale or that it measures maturity. The transcultural and longitudinal research suggests that the PSQ predicts a wider range of measures of maturity and competence more consistently than any other test used in the research, thereby indirectly confirming the validity of the model of maturing from which it was derived. Other summary measures of a person's overall psychological maturity include self- and judge-rated evaluations of 26 trait scales empirically found to differentiate between mature and immature persons, e.g., apathetic-energetic, strong convictions–weak convictions. A variety of other measures of the maturity of the person are described elsewhere (1977c).

DIMENSION OF SYMBOLIZATION

Man's ability to symbolize, to imaginally represent his experience with the external environment and his internal world, brings him great adaptive

---

*Throughout the rest of the chapter, when a finding is not referenced by name, it will refer either to my transcultural (1977c), college (1968), or adult longitudinal (1976a, b, c,; 1977a, b, d; 1978a, b, c; 1979; 1980) studies.

power, as Piaget has told us (1947). He is able to learn from his past experience as well as to anticipate the consequences of his acts. He can represent the possible, even the improbable. Symbolization, by freeing one's mind of the constraints of time and space, is a central human growth potential. The model of maturing hypothesizes that a psychologically healthy person has realized such potential in more sectors of his life than has the less healthy person.

Cognitive Skills.   That the more mature person is more capable of symbolizing is widely accepted by clinicians, educators, and religionists. Freud, for example, assumes that the person with a stronger ego has more developed secondary processes, and therefore greater conscious access to his memories, than the person whose thought is organized by fleeting, vague, primary process modes of organization (1900, 1923). Dewey claims that education furthers healthy growth and that central to that maturing is the development of the capacity to reflect about one's own experience, to stand outside of one's own ongoing thought and monitor it (1933a). For Zen Buddhists, progress toward enlightenment and zazen, the integration of all opposites, is by way of increasingly differentiated states of consciousness (Owens, 1975).

However, to test such a proposition empirically is forbiddingly difficult because psychology has no adequate measure by which to assess reflective ability, for example, let alone different states of consciousness. More, in contrast to less, mature exemplars from several diverse cultures do report on the PSQ that they have more information accessible to them. They are more imaginative in creating alternative stories to pictures, they see more differentiated details, and they are more introspective in the Rorschach (1977c). Haan has found that increasing symbolic ability to make discriminations is directly related to coping skills, presumably more developed in healthier persons (1963, 1965).

Values.   Most clinicians agree that psychological health is associated with potentially greater awareness of one's motives and values. A goal of insight therapy is to further such awareness. Educators like Bode (1927), Hook (1946), and Dewey (1903, 1928) also claim that the process of growth involves the increasing ability to articulate one's own values and to know how one's desires influence one's decisions. Also implied in the meditative religions, as well as in Islam (Lapidus, 1976), is the expectation that a person will become more aware of his emotions in his pursuit of their control.

The empirical evidence is only suggestive that awareness of one's own motives and values is associated with psychological health, again partially as a result of lack of adequate measures of the ability to symbolize accurately one's values. I was able to confirm only weakly that mature exemplars in five cultural areas were more able to articulate and represent their values than immature exemplars (1977c). College seniors have been found to be more aware of their values than freshmen (1968). Finally, increased awareness of their values was the second most important maturing change that occurred to men maturing in their twenties and early thirties, as measured by the number of statements they made in regularized interviews about how they had changed since graduation from college (1977d).

Self-concept.   From Socrates on, philosophers and clinicians claim that the more psychologically healthy person is more accurately aware of himself (c.f. Jahoda for a review of mental health specialists' views prior to 1958). For the great religious traditions, increasing self-knowledge leads to greater honesty about one's strengths and weaknesses, a growth highly prized by the Sikhs (Neki, 1975), Confucians (Tseng, 1973), Zen Buddhists (Owens, 1975), and other groups.

Empirically, we are on firmer ground, for considerable research supports the hypothesis about the accuracy of self-insight and its relation to maturity. When the men in the five cultural areas were asked to rate themselves on a variety of scales and when judges who knew them well independently rated them on the same scales, the self-ratings of the mature men in every cultural group agreed significantly more with the ratings of their judges than did those of the immature men with their judges (1977c). The second most salient maturing effect of one college upon its students was found to be the increase in their awareness of themselves (1968). Increased self-understanding was one of the four most salient effects of maturing since college for another sample of men in their early thirties (1977d). Numerous other studies, not shaped by the model of maturing, have confirmed that psychological health is directly associated with accuracy of self-insight (Barron, 1963; Chodorkoff, 1954; Kogan, Quinn, Ax, and Ripley, 1957; Westley and Epstein, 1969).

Personal Relations.   A content analysis of the writings of 35 experts on mental health and maturity revealed that interpersonal awareness and sensitivity ranked eighth in terms of the number who asserted that it was a trait of a mature person (1965). Among educational philosophers, Hook (1946) and Dewey (1937) urge that in promoting growth, schools should enhance interpersonal insight and understanding of social problems. In my reading of the psychological interpretations of the principal religious traditions, I found only one reference to increased interpersonal awareness as a goal of development, i.e., Japanese spiritualism's emphasis on *ki* as sensitivity to another's feelings and intentions (Rohlen, 1976).

I have found no adequate psychological measure of this attribute of maturing. By use of self-report indices from the PSQ and the number of different interpersonal interactions that men of five cultural areas interpretively attributed to pictures, it was possible to only weakly confirm that mature men were more interpersonally aware and sensitive than immature men (1977c). Interestingly, such growth during college, as evaluated from interviews and the PSQ, ranked fourth for graduating seniors (1968). Fragmentary evidence suggests that well-functioning persons may make more accurate identifications of emotional states of others than psychotics (Piat, 1975). The absence of any stronger confirmatory evidence suggests that we must remain cautious about claiming that interpersonal sensitivity is a central quality of psychological health.

DIMENSION OF ALLOCENTRICISM

Human beings as open systems are dependent upon a ceaseless flow of information and support from sources outside of themselves. From birth on, a growing person encounters such information and support through the medium of other persons who nurture his potentials for social communication and relationships with others. Although not a very elegant or precise term, allocentricism refers to the progressive movement of an infant away from his self-centered view of the world to an increasing empathic capacity to take, in Dewey's words, the multiplicity of perspectives that other persons have toward himself and toward others. Allocentric growth reflects the humanizing, socializing influence that others have in furthering one's own development.

Cognitive Skill. The development of more logical, realistic judgment is the foremost quality of a psychologically healthy person according to the ranked judgments of 35 mental health experts (1965). Growth from egocentric to socialized thought (Piaget, 1947), primary to secondary process (Freud, 1900), and prototaxic to syntactic thought (Sullivan, 1953) describes the maturation of cognitive skills. Such allocentric growth is also central to the process of becoming educated, as held by Newman (1852), Dewey (1933a), and Whitehead (1916), among others. For such philosophers, logical ordered thought is the consequence of the ability to project oneself into the thought of another, to be able to order consistently one's thought while communicating with the other. The great religious traditions do not identify such cognitive growth as central to their ideal of healthy growth.

Using Rorschach measures of realistic judgment and socialized thought, I was able to confirm only weakly that mature persons of diverse cultures were more realistic and logical in their thought than immature men, possibly because the available measures of allocentric cognitive skills were not as adequate as they should have been (1977c). Allocentric cognitive development, however, was one of the more salient effects of becoming liberally educated (1968). Studies by others of self-actualized and personally sound persons found that their thought was more realistic and objective and that they were more able to entertain alternative possibilities than was the case for the less sound person (Barron, 1963; Brown, 1960; Foxman, 1976).

Values and Interpersonal Relations. Mental health experts, educators, and religionists tend to fuse values and personal relationships when discussing their allocentric quality. The 35 mental health experts ranked social feeling and compassion, love and friendship for others, as the second most important quality of a mature person. There is a broad consensus from Abraham (1925) to Sullivan (1953) that valuing and experiencing affectionate and sympathetic feelings for others are distinguishing traits of healthy persons. A content analysis of the ideas of the 20 educational philosophers and educators that I surveyed revealed almost unanimous agreement that a liberal education promotes other-centered values and personal relationships. Qualities like tolerance, social interest, social conscience, and communal identification were recurring traits used to describe the educated person. The good life, the ideal person, was defined similarly by all of the principal religious traditions analyzed.

Despite the centrality of allocentric values and interpersonal relationships to ideas about mental health, liberal education, and religious growth, the behavioral sciences do not have very adequate measures of allocentric growth, especially of compassionate interpersonal relationships and of social feeling. Relying on the PSQ and a specially designed scale that measured the maturity of a person's values, we were able to confirm, though not strongly, that mature in contrast to immature Americans, Italians, and Turks had more allocentric values (1977c). One of the most well-established effects of becoming liberally educated is the increased liberalization of a student's values (Newcomb and Feldman, 1969). Mature persons have also been found to contribute more to charity than immature persons do (Heath, 1965; Vaillant and McArthur, 1972).

Interpersonally, the mature men of the three cultures we studied tended to be more socially responsible and affectionate than the immature men, but the differences were not as striking as we had expected, given the importance that allocentric relationships had for the theorists. However, we did find that allocentric interpersonal maturing was a major growth during college and that it was the most important kind of growth that occurred to professional men during their twenties and early thirties as they described their personality changes in interviews (1977d).

Self-concept. A long behavioral science tradition sparked by William James (1890) and Mead (1934), and empirically grounded by Rogers (1959) and his associates, has recognized that our ideas of ourselves find their origin in the reflected appraisals of others and that in development we gradually extend the boundaries of ourselves to identify with and incorporate others. The healthy person is able to understand empathically how others think and feel, even their thoughts about himself. Such understanding leads to self-insight, acceptance, and respect, qualities that are ranked as very important by mental health experts (1965). Educators like Hutchins (1936), MacLeish (1920), and Van Doren (1943) also agree that a growing person does not think of himself as unique but, by virtue of his allocentric growth, deepens his identification with the human community. The Confucian emphasis on the goodness of each person and Zen's view that enlightenment expands a person's identity to be "one with the All and the 'vast expanse of universal life' " (Owens, 1975, p. 167) also identify healthy growth to involve the progressive extension and acceptance of one's own humanness.

The transcultural empirical support of this hypothesis is very strong. Not only do mature exemplars from several cultures predict more accurately than immature exemplars what other persons think of them, but they also have more positive concepts of themselves (1977c). The longitudinal college and young adult studies, however, did not identify the development of more allocentric self-concepts to be a distinctive growth, relative to that of other types of maturing (1968, 1977d). Other researchers have consistently reported that more psychologically healthy persons have greater self-esteem and feelings of worth (Duncan, 1966; Seeman, 1966). Psychotherapy research consistently has demonstrated that therapeutic improvement is accompanied by increasing feelings of positive self-regard (Hart and Tomlinson, 1970).

DIMENSION OF INTEGRATION

An open evolving system becomes progressively more differentiated and complex in its interactions with others. Economy and effectiveness in adaptation require some internal coherence, consistency, integration. Theorists, like Lecky (1945), hypothesize that we have a basic need to create such internal consistency. Certainly, a pervasive theme that courses through the writings of most behavioral scientists, educators, and religionists is that the progressive integration of a person is the hallmark of psychological health. The mental health experts ranked it fifth in importance (1965); the educators, influenced by the Greek ideal of wholeness, insist that developmental integration is a major effect of becoming liberally educated

(1968); and every major religious tradition has created symbols of wholeness, harmony, and inner serenity as the ideal toward which to strive.

Cognitive Skill. As Piaget has demonstrated, cognitive development becomes progressively more differentiated, ordered, hierarchical, and organized (1947). Thought becomes less syncretic, juxtaposed, inflexible (1928). The developing ego secures increasing control of, and is able to synthesize, its component secondary processes (Freud, 1923; Nunberg, 1931). There is near unanimity among the educational philosophers surveyed that a liberal education should further integrative, relational thinking, the cultivation of the skills of generalizing (Hutchins, 1936; Newman, 1852), reflective synthesizing (Wriston in Thomas, 1962), and "understanding human endeavors . . . in their relations to one another" (Meiklejohn, 1920). The religious traditions, at least from my reading, remain silent about this aspect of integrative development.

I was able to confirm only weakly the hypothesis that maturing is directly related to increasing integrative cognitive development in the transcultural studies, and the principal supporting evidence came primarily from self-report statements such as, "I constantly try to relate and integrate intellectual ideas and facts into more comprehensive patterns." The mature American, Turkish, and Sicilian men's thought, as revealed on the Rorschach, was more logically and sensibly organized than that of the immature men (1977c). Studies of maturing in three different colleges (Fieselmann, 1973; Heath, 1968) and of the effects of graduate-professional school (1976c) identify increasing cognitive integration generally to be the foremost effect of higher education. Other researchers confirm that increasing cognitive flexibility is a principal effect of becoming liberally educated (Chickering, 1969; Newcomb and Feldman, 1969). Some evidence suggests that differences between mature and immature persons in integrative skill functioning may more likely be found when the content of the material has personal and emotional implications to the person (Wexler, 1974).

Values. Although few behavioral scientists speak as explicitly as Allport (1961) does about the development of a unifying philosophy of life as an attribute of maturity, many assume an underlying developmental trend toward integration when talking about self-actualization or the emerging organizing control of genital over pregenital instincts (Freud, 1915). Educational philosophers like Dewey talk about the integrative effect of an ideal and the importance of "consistency and harmony in belief" (1933b, p. 226); Hook urges students to learn how to interrelate their values (1946). The religious traditions also have as their ideal the integration of values. The ideal

Muslim, according to Lapidus, is one "who possesses a wholeness of being in which knowledge, virtue, and action have been wholely integrated" (1976, p. 97).

The strongest evidence for the relation of maturing to the progressive integration of one's values comes not from the transcultural studies, which only weakly confirmed the hypothesis, but from the longitudinal studies of college students and adults. Several different groups of alumni independently but retrospectively identified in their focused interviews that a principal enduring effect of their liberal education had been the integration of their values (1968, 1976c). The adult study strongly confirmed that men who had more coherent and integrated values were much more well-adjusted psychologically (MMPI); were more dimensionally mature (PSQ); had more stable, well-integrated, autonomous self-concepts as measured experimentally; rated themselves to be more mature on 26 traits that have been found to define mature persons; made a larger percentage of statements in interviews about having matured since college; and were rated by their wives, closest friends, and professional colleagues to be more psychologically healthy, as well as to be better adapted on 28 qualities that define vocational adaptation (1976a). The principal research on value maturation has been that of Kohlberg, who on the basis of transcultural developmental research, found that values become increasingly more differentiated, integrated as well as universal (1968). However, as I have said, we have not been able to confirm that increasing value integration as measured by Rest's test of Kohlberg's theory is related to psychological maturity generally (Miller and Mosher, 1977).

Self-concept. The hypothesis that the psychologically healthy person has a well-integrated concept of himself, while widely implied by mental health experts, receives its most forthright support from Rogers who has identified the increasing congruence of a person's view of himself with his experience to be the important growth that occurs in therapy (1959). Educational philosophers make a similar assumption about educational development, though it is Dewey who most sharply defines a goal of liberal education to be the development of a more "coherent and integrated self" (1928, p. 177). However, it is the religious traditions that are most explicit about the centrality of achieving self-integration through religious growth. The Eastern religious concept of *sahaja* emphasizes seeking harmony of the self (Neki, 1975), and zazen claims that the goal of living is to transcend opposites. The Christian finds his integration through the acceptance of his creatureness and dependence on God's will.

Transculturally, mature in contrast to immature exemplars were very consistently more integrated in their self-concepts as measured by the concordance of their private with their social selves. The person with a well-integrated sense of his own self was found in all cultures to be psychologically well adjusted, to be more dimensionally mature, and to have a greater sense of self-worth, and was judged by others to be more mature (1977c). Self-integration has also proved to be a consistently powerful index of a person's maturity in the longitudinal studies of students and adults as well. Other researchers have also confirmed the hypothesis, using the discrepancy between the private and the ideal self as the index of integration (Rogers and Dymond, 1954; G. M. Smith, 1958; Turner and Vanderlippe, 1958). More self-actualized persons, indexed by the POI, also have more congruent private and ideal selves (Mahoney and Hartnett, 1973). Some recent evidence suggests that the progressive integration of a man's self-concept continues throughout adulthood but that of a woman may not (Lowenthal, Thurnher, and Chiriboga, 1976).

Interpersonal Relations. Ideas like mutuality, intimacy, and loving, deep relationships are commonly identified by mental health experts to define psychological health (1965). Jourard has shown that interpersonal mutuality and trust that facilitate self-disclosure are keys to healthy development (1974). Educational philosophers, understandably, do not mention reciprocally mutual I-thou relationships to be a goal of education as frequently as the religious traditions do, particularly Christianity, which values loving identification with all persons and union with God.

Because I did not have adequate objective behavioral measures of interpersonal mutuality, I have not been able to confirm or disconfirm the hypothesis of a positive relation between maturity and mutuality transculturally. The longitudinal studies identified integrative interpersonal maturing to be the third most frequently reported growth of students in one college (1968). Indirect and very persuasive evidence about the relationship of mutuality and maturity comes from a measure of the marital sexual compatibility of the adult men that I have studied. The measure defined in part by the faithfulness of the men to their spouses, similarity in basic sexual values, and degree to which they were well mated sexually was, quite remarkably, significantly associated with ten diverse measures of the men's psychological adjustment and maturity (1978b). Other researchers like Vaillant have also found that psychologically healthy persons have warmer, more loving friendships and closer relationships with their children and spouses (1975, 1977). A transcultural study also confirmed that degree of personal adjustment was directly related to desires for intimate relationships with others (Scott and Peterson, 1975).

DIMENSIONS OF STABILITY AND AUTONOMY

The progressive integration of a system increases its resiliency, stability, and ability to be self-regulating or more autonomous. I discuss the two dimensions together. Although they can be distinguished theoretically, I have had difficulty separating them empirically for some sectors of the personality. A persistent theme in the writings of mental health experts is that a mature person has a sense of identity, is self-reliant, and has control over his emotions, as Jahoda induced also from her review of the mental health literature (1958). Educational philosophers have more to say about the development of autonomy, the growing "command over . . . [one's] powers" (Newman, 1852) and oneself (Hyde in Thomas, 1962), and increasing freedom from "external tutelages" (Dewey, 1933a, 1934). Yet again it is the religious traditions that focus most explicitly on these two dimensions. Bouwsma says of the Christian faith that it "is the necessary condition of true autonomy, of freedom not from the constraints of experience . . . but freedom to grow" (1976, p. 86). The good Muslim "subordinates passion and impulse to reasonable and ethical self-restraint. He faces life's trials with patient endurance and fortitude" (Lapidus, 1976, p. 96). Confucianism highly values self-control, internal regulation, freedom from covetousness, and self-sufficiency (Tseng, 1973).

Cognitive Skills.   A key insight of Freud was that the core of healthy ego functioning was the ability to maintain the stability of secondary processes, even when thinking about very personally disruptive issues (1900). Hartmann also says that the ego of a mature person can resist disorganization and maintain its autonomy (1960). Educators like Newman claim that an educated person can maintain "steadiness of intellect" (1852). Phrases like "capacity to weigh evidence dispassionately" (Gardner, 1956, p. 6), "freed intelligence," or "intellectual courage" regularly appear as developmental goals of educators. The religious traditions are quiet about this aspect of maturation.

When Americans, Italians, and Turks were given conceptual, analytic, and judgmental problems to solve that contained emotionally disturbing content, the mature men from every culture were cognitively more efficient and showed greater resiliency in their thinking, thus consistently confirming the hypothesis (1977c). The longitudinal studies have neither confirmed nor disconfirmed it. Researchers using other methods for assessing cognitive skill autonomy, such as measures of field-independence (Witkin et al., 1974), find that those who do not depend upon external distractions and irrelevant cues are more self-actualized (Doyle, 1975) and have higher self-esteem (Witkin et al., 1954).

Self-concept.   Much has been written by behavioral scientists, particularly Erikson, about a stable self-concept or sense of identity and its contribution to psychological health. Jahoda noted that the sense of identity was one of the few themes that organized the largest number of viewpoints. She suggested that "a healthy person knows who he is and does not feel basic doubts about his inner identity" (1958, p. 29). Such inner certainty provides the psychological basis, according to Maslow, for increasing independence of the influence of one's environment and culture (1954). The consequence of becoming liberally educated, according to many philosophers, is greater inner freedom and control. The Sikhs identify equipoise, self-confidence, and a state of serene blissfulness as resulting from the achievement of *sahaja* (Neki, 1975); the Christian and most other religious traditions I surveyed value the development of self-discipline and control and the elimination of carnal desires. Wei-Ming interprets Confucianism to say that "so long as one's self-image is mainly dependent upon the external responses of others, one's inner direction will be lost" (1976, p. 114), a thought also echoed by Zen Buddhists.

When the stability of the self-concept of mature and immature exemplars was assessed transculturally by the degree to which their self-ratings changed over time, we very consistently confirmed that maturity was directly associated with a stable sense of identity. The men of the five cultural areas studied who had more stable self-concepts were more well adjusted psychologically (MMPI), were more dimensionally mature (PSQ), and had higher self-esteem. They were also independently judged to be more mature (1977c). When persons are growing over time, both in college and during their twenties and early thirties, their sense of self has been found to become increasingly more stable (1968). Other studies have also confirmed that the more well-adjusted person has a more stable concept of himself (G. M. Smith, 1958) and thinks of himself more favorably (McGehee, 1957). Furthermore, mature persons are *selectively* accessible to influence, but immature ones indiscriminately resist any information that contradicts their conscious images of themselves (Tippett and Silber, 1966). The self-concepts of women have been found to be more dependent on the views of others than the self-concepts of men, so the relation between autonomous self-concepts and maturity may vary for the sexes (Lowenthal, Thurnher, and Chiriboga, 1976).

Values.   There is less agreement among mental health experts about the centrality to one's psychological health of having strong values and standing up for one's convictions, i.e., only 5 of the 35 experts identified such qualities to be necessary (1965). Melanie Klein, for example, identified strength of character and willingness to sacrifice oneself for one's convictions to be one of four cardinal traits of maturity (1960). Educators like McGrath talk of encouraging the development of a "provisionally firm set of convictions" (1959, p. 6). Van Doren claims an educated person is prepared to "meet resistance" to his values (1943) with courage (Russell, 1931), even rebelliousness (F. H. Sanford, 1966). Among the religious, the witness of the Christian martyrs testifies to the importance of commitment to, and courage in, defending what one believes.

Transculturally, the mature men of most of the five cultural areas tended to have more stable and autonomous values as measured by the Valuator Test and other indices (1977c). While value autonomy rather than value stability moderately increased in undergraduates during college, the stabilization of the values of alumni of several different groups emerged as a prominent type of growth during the early twenties and thirties, as indexed most clearly in the 32-year-old men's interviews about the types of changes experienced since graduation from college (1976c). Very little other research has been done on either the stability or autonomy of a person's values and their relation to mental health.

The relation of autonomous value choices to maturity may differ more for men than for women. Duncan reports that psychologically healthy men value making more independent value choices (1966), but Seeman found that psychologically healthy women did not differ from randomly selected women on tests of the autonomy of their judgments (1966).

Personal Relationships. Although many behavioral scientists describe the mature person's relationships as caring, affectionate, and loving, few, except for Clausen (1968), mention that such relationships persist and endure over long periods of time. However, implied in Erikson's (1963) and Sullivan's (1963) views of interpersonal intimacy is the idea of stable relationships. More mention independence, e.g., from one's parents (Saul, 1960), but generally the behavioral scientists' claims for interpersonal stability and autonomy are decidedly muted. The educators and religious that we surveyed also failed to ascribe such qualities to their ideal adult.

No very convincing relationship was found between either the stability or autonomy of one's personal relationships and psychological health in our transcultural, student, and adult longitudinal studies. I have already reported that men who are more sexually faithful to their spouses—one component of marital sexual compatibility—were more psychologically healthy than less faithful men (1978b). Because our measures of interpersonal maturing generally have not been very adequate, the most cautious conclusion is that the interpersonal hypotheses have been neither confirmed nor disconfirmed. Vaillant's longitudinal studies of Harvard men provide some support, however, for he has discovered that psychologically healthy adult males are more independent in their personal relations, have more stable marriages, and have more close friends (1974, 1975).

CRITIQUE OF MODEL OF MATURING

The model of maturing comprehended most of the traits attributed to mentally healthy, self-actualized, and mature persons by clinicians and theoreticians, as well as those qualities identified by educational philosophers to describe liberally educated persons. Although I have had no difficulty mapping most of the ideas of the great religions about healthy development, as interpreted by others, into the model (1977c, p. 218), my lack of expertise makes such an effort only a playful exercise to be checked by others.

More persuasively, the model has comprehended the principal types of changes that persons undergo when they are being liberally educated and when they are maturing during their twenties and early thirties. Three independent judges scoring interviews about personality change since college could not identify any frequently mentioned changes that could not be mapped into the model's categories. Similarly, no consistent major findings based on the extensive and varied psychological test findings in either the transcultural or the longitudinal studies emerged that could not also be mapped into the model's categories. To achieve such comprehensiveness may be a Pyrrhic victory, however. In searching for developmental dimensions that are genotypic and universal, we risk creating categories that are too abstract to be tested with any reasonable degree of precision and reliability. Triandis (1972a) admits that this is an unavoidable risk when transcultural universals are sought among phenotypically diverse cultures. However, the methodological challenge remains for any researcher who wishes to test such frequently cited qualities of a mature person as Erikson's concept of integrity (1963), Maslow's self-actualization (1962), and Jung's integration (1939). The problem is how to define a trait so clearly and sharply that it can be measured objectively but not so narrowly that its measure trivializes the quality and no longer predicts a wider range of other qualities. I have tried to resolve this dilemma, one not unique to those studying terms like psychological health, by using redundant but diverse measures of the same concept and embedding the research within a rich, multifaceted assessment battery. By so doing, it is possible within one, though intensive, study to generate the validity context for each measure. When that same context of correlates is replicated across several diverse groups, as regularly occurred in the transcultural and longitudinal studies, one has more confidence that a measure has some ecological validity as well as connotative generality.

Although the transcultural test of the model's validity confirmed 40 percent of the model's hypotheses and weakly confirmed another 50 percent, we are only approaching the threshold of valid knowledge about such terms. Not only are some of the dimensions (e.g., symbolization and autonomy) and personality sectors (e.g., interpersonal relations) too diffusely defined to provide clear guidelines about how to construct more precise measures, but the model may theoretically need to be extended or reshaped. Other dimensions or personality sectors may be required to make the model fully comprehensive. Some of the categories combine both process and product type variables; e.g., allocentric self-concept has been indexed by the skill of accurately predicting other's ratings of oneself as well as by defining oneself in self-acceptant, self-worthy terms. Rather than continue to recite the numerous methodological hurdles that assessment specialists have undoubtedly already recognized in such exploratory research, I will now examine how fruitful our budding knowledge about maturing may be for understanding the meaning of adult effectiveness, its relation to adaptation, and its related sociological concept of modernism.

MATURITY AND ADULT EFFECTIVENESS

Although the concept of competence had hovered on the periphery of the consciousness of behavioral scientists for years (Foote and Cottrell, 1955), not until Robert White (1963) used it as an organizing focal point for his insightful critique of the motivational assumptions of psychoanalytic theory did it stimulate more sustained theoretical interest and some research (M. B. Smith, 1966; B. L. White, 1971). Educators, influenced in part by the term's resurrection and in part by the effort to state educational goals in terms of more functional behavioral objectives, are now reshaping their curricular and assessment procedures to educate more explicitly for specific competencies. The Alverno College faculty, for example, has restructured its primary goals in an impressively thoughtful and insightful way to teach for, and explicitly assess, the development of eight competencies that it identifies to be the core of the liberal educational process and which are necessary for adapting as effective adults to the demands of the twenty-first century. These competencies are effective communication ability, analytic capability, problem solving ability, facility in forming value judgments, effective social interaction, understanding of individual-environmental relationships, understanding the contemporary world, and educated responsiveness to the arts and humanities (1976).

Such value choices need to be informed by knowledge about what defines an effective adult and what are the determinants of that effectiveness, particularly those determinants that societal institutions may be able to affect. Despite the obvious importance of the issue, few behavioral scientists have studied effectively functioning adults either with the depth necessary or over sufficient periods of time. Consequently, few behavioral scientists are able to contribute much informed knowledge to faculties like that of Alverno College, to admissions officers of professional schools, or to numerous other persons who must make decisions about who is and who is not likely to be an effectively functioning adult in their setting or in society.

The longitudinal study of adult males in their early thirties is one of those few that may open up new insights about the meaning of adult effectiveness and its relation to the maturing process (Block, 1971; Cox, 1970; Grinker, 1962, 1974; Vaillant, 1974, 1977; White, 1952). Its technical details have been reported elsewhere (1976a, b, c; 1977a, b, d; 1978a, b, c; 1979). Briefly, the men who were studied when they were freshmen and upperclassmen in college and again when they were typically 32 are primarily professionals and managers. In one sense, they are exemplars of liberally educated persons. Of the 68 men who participated in the three assessment phases, 81 percent had received post-college degrees by the time they were 32. Sixteen percent were lawyers, 16 percent medical specialists, 22 percent had received their Ph.D.'s and were teachers and researchers; 26 percent had received degrees in other fields and were in theology, social work, business. Several were presidents or managers of their firms; one was a poet, one a singer, one associated with opera. More than 100 measures of their adolescent mental health and competence are available. More than 400 measures were also secured about their adult mental health status, including the measures given when they were adolescents, and about every possible adult competence that could be objectively assessed, if not by psychological tests, then by the judgments of their wives, closest friends, and professional colleagues who knew them most intimately.

In addition to the findings I have mentioned earlier in this chapter, there are others that may enrich our understanding of the relation of maturity to adult effectiveness. The men not only significantly improved in their psychological health since their graduation from college but they became more homogeneous in mental health, primarily because of the improvement of some men who as adolescents had been very disturbed and immature. Generally, mental health status when an adolescent predicted mental health status when an adult.

A core set of *generalized competencies* seems to have contributed to the effectiveness of the men in their various adult roles. Men who had created happy, mutually satisfying marriages were also better adapted to their vocations (also reported by Vaillant, 1977), were more effective fathers, enjoyed sexual relations more, and generally, were happier persons.

Happiness seems to be mediated by two qualities: one's psychological maturity and, more specifically, one's interpersonal maturity. The happy man was more well adjusted psychologically and more dimensionally mature; was judged by his wife, closest friend, and a professional colleague to be more mature on a variety of traits; and had matured more in the decade than had the less happy person. Happiness is associated with continued growth, in other words. Happiness was also directly associated with closer interpersonal relationships, more satisfying marriages in which communication was excellent, enjoyment of sexual relations, and excellent personal relationships at work. No measure of academic excellence in high school or college or of income was associated with adult happiness.

Within the range of incomes of a professional-managerial group, *income* did not predict any measure of effectiveness, except possibly the quality of relations at work. However, the men with high incomes had dismal relationships with their families. They were dissatisfied with their marriages, had tense and conflictual relations with their oldest child, and while they rated their wives to be good hostesses, mothers, and managers of the household, they did not rate them to be good companions or friends. Sexual relations seemed to be incidental in importance. Generally, the families of the high-income men seemed to be instrumental to furthering the success of the men at work. Income level was not related to any measure of mental health.

We need to distinguish between technical vocational competence and *vocational adaptation*. A person may be quite technically competent in his work but not find it fulfilling, may have dismal colleaguial relationships, and may find that his work demands so much energy and time that it impedes his own sense of fulfillment. Recall that successful adjustment to the demands of a role is not equivalent to adaptation, particularly if such adjustment is at the expense of self-fulfillment. The vocational adaptation of the men was measured by a 28-item scale which was completed by the men themselves and independently by their wives, friends, and professional colleagues (1976a). The most pervasive predictor of the men's vocational adaptation was their psychological maturity when they were adolescents and adults. The variety of specific competencies the men identified to be essential for "success" in their vocations could be readily mapped into the model of maturing. I mention the competencies in terms of the frequency with which they were cited by the men: symbolized cognitive skills (e.g., anticipatory planning, imaginativeness, reflective monitoring), stability of values (e.g., commitment, persistence), allocentric interpersonal skills (e.g., empathy, tolerance, caring, allocentric cognitive skills (e.g., entertain alternatives, logical analysis, communication skills), and integrative cognitive skills (e.g., organizing, scheduling, contextual knowledge).

The men who rated themselves and were rated by their wives to be *competent fathers* were psychologically well adjusted as adolescents and psychologically healthy and mature as adults; they had happier marriages, communicated more adequately with their spouses, were more sexually compatible, and had wives who were highly competent as mothers (1976b).

Finally, *marital sexual compatibility* was directly and very consistently related to every measure of psychological maturity used in the study, to interpersonal maturity and the mutuality of the marital relationship, to marital happiness, and to effectiveness in fulfilling other adult roles (1978a).

What have we learned about the predictors of the effectiveness or competence with which an adult fulfills his diverse roles as a worker, spouse, sexual partner, and parent? Within the range of talent represented in our sample, the evidence is quite clear that traditional academic measures do not predict much of anything 10 to 15 years later. Men of high quantitative aptitude, for example, were neither more nor less well adapted vocationally, or competent as fathers, or good marital or sexual partners. Actually, the men with high quantitative SAT scores were more interpersonally immature. Their relations with their occupational colleagues were tense and distant, as rated by the judges; their relations with their spouses were not warm and close; they felt that their spouses did not understand them. They were not able to be self-disclosing with their spouses with whom they did not feel it important to be a close friend or companion anyway. They had not anticipated that sexual relations would be enjoyable. Whether we use as measures of academic excellence scholastic aptitude or achievement test scores, faculty ratings of the men's intellectual caliber, academic grades, or the receipt of college honors, the general pattern was similar: within a sample of highly talented and academically competent men, increasing academic competence was related to subsequent interpersonal immaturity (1977a). These findings are consistent with those of other studies of academically talented and achieving students as reported elsewhere (1979). The early emergence of high talent may lead to social isolation from one's peers which may only be reinforced by schools that emphasize individualistic and competitive rather than social and cooperative modes of learning.

The central theme that organizes the findings about what predicts who will be an effective adult is a person's psychological maturity. The more mature person is happier, more well adapted vocationally, has a more satisfying marriage, is sexually compatible with his spouse, enjoys sexual relations, and is a more effective parent (1978b).

Why? What is the relation of maturity or psychological health to adult effectiveness? To be an effective adult means one must be able to adapt to many demanding roles and be open to continued growth and development. Psychological maturity is, I suggest, its own condition for further maturing. Psychotherapy research has shown that those who grow most in therapy are those who initially were more psychologically healthy. I have mentioned that the transcultural findings, confirmed by the longitudinal studies, demonstrated that the Perceived Self Questionnaire, which was theoretically derived from and assessed the model of maturing, consistently predicted a wider range of other measures of the men's effectiveness and mental health status than even psychology's two most widely used measures, the MMPI and the Rorschach.

MATURITY AND THE PROCESS OF ADAPTATION

I propose that the model of maturing identifies the skills, values, and interpersonal traits that are the core qualities that facilitate adaptation. By educating in ways to further a youth's maturing, as the educational philosophers intuited, we are enhancing his potential for adapting to varying situations in the future. Let us first analyze the adaptive sequence in terms of the model of maturing and then examine some of the evidence from which my interpretation of the adaptive process was induced.

What initiates the process of adaptation? A disturbance to the equilibrium of a system. The source may be an internal change, like menopausal symptoms, or the desire to shake oneself up by changing one's job, or an external change, such as a challenge to a prized value, the demands of a new role, or the arrival of the first child. Previously stabilized and autonomous modes of action become less effective or efficient. We are now under stress. We may seek to avoid, defend, or reinstitute our formerly secure ways, or we may seek to create a new adaptation, either by altering the demands made of us and/or fashioning a different response to them. Disequilibrium initiates what I call the adaptive sequence. The process of adapting may persist for months and years, may be short circuited or aborted, may be simultaneously occurring at different stages while resolving different problems. A person may be in the midst of a long-term struggle to alter his relations with a spouse while concurrently adapting to the changing demands of his work, for example.

The adaptive sequence is ordered by the model of maturing. The initial response in reaction to a disequilibrium is to *symbolize* the problem, to identify the difficulty, to reflect about oneself, one's values, and one's interpersonal relationships to determine what may be contributing to or affected by the problem. This stage rapidly moves into the *allocentric* phase when a person begins to seek alternative viewpoints about the difficulty. He analyzes it from his boss's or spouse's perspective; he may try to understand how his colleagues or patients feel about him; he tries to understand their values and motives and in the process may become more open and tolerant.

At some point, he begins to search for and create possible alternative lines of resolution that take into account the complex factors involved. This *integrative* phase is similar to the hypothesis formation phase of the scientific process, which is, at its core, a model of the adaptive process. The next phase of the adaptive sequence is initiated when the hypothesis is tested, acted upon, tried out in order to determine its feasibility. Repetition of the test or act leads eventually to its consolidation or *stabilization*. In time, the stablized pattern of new habits, like the one so arduously developed when we first learned how to drive, becomes increasingly *autonomous,* as when we drive to work quite oblivious to the complicated patterns that we are performing. The autonomous pattern becomes increasingly more "mobile," in Piaget's words (1947), that is, freed of the initial learning conditions. We can almost instantaneously switch from driving on the right-to driving on the left-hand side of the road when in England. In the language of educators, the autonomous pattern becomes more transferable. This adaptive sequence results in a new equilibrium which is now more economical and efficient in its use of the system's energy. Freed energy becomes available for other adaptive purposes. The release of energy, the resultant sense of mastery, even of joy, combined with the knowledge of a new level of competence provide a sense of power and efficacy to a person. I find that the degree of expressive, affirmative enthusiasm which a person has available to commit for sustained periods of time toward some goal provides a direct glimpse into his psychological healthiness. A frequently reported consequence of a mystical and/or religious conversion experience is the feeling of transcendence, of unity, of serenity and greater energetic power (Pahnke and Richards, 1966). Such character transformations in which long-standing unresolved doubts and crippling inhibitions are resolved and new integrations occur, sometimes quite suddenly, may be so profoundly liberating of such great stores of energy that the experience is subjectively felt to be caused by some external, even divine, force.

Although folklore suggests that those who make creative or original adaptations are maladjusted and neurotic, the analysis of the adaptive process suggests the opposite. The creative process involves what Kris (1952) calls "regression in the service of the ego," the ability to abandon one's self-control or ties to reality to explore less symbolized modes and contents of thought. Such exploration risks discovering emotionally charged ideas, taboo wishes, provocative intuitions, and hunches that may defy conventional ways of adapting. The mature person has the stability, resiliency, and autonomy to control that regression to recover his former level of organization and reinstate his ties to reality. He also has the allocentric and integrative maturity to translate what he has discovered into a language or form that communicates to others.

Although data are scarce to support these hypotheses about the relation of maturity to creativity, Barron's (1963) and MacKinnon's (1960, 1965) studies found that highly creative persons are in fact sound and well organized, and have good control of their impulses. They are less repressed and defensive, more intuitive and open to admitting to turbulent inner conflicts. Creative persons are more curious, have wide-ranging interests, and have integrated the stereotypic qualities of the opposite sex into their lives. They are also more maturely autonomous and so less dependent upon the views that others have of them. The determinants of creative adaptations or products are more complex than my analysis of the adaptive process suggests. The contribution that psychological maturity makes probably varies greatly depending upon the type of creative product being produced.

That the model of maturing could provide the basis for a theory of adaptation was an unanticipated and surprising consequence of noting the process of becoming liberally educated, a process that I have described in detail elsewhere (1968, pp. 174–176). Since that initial induction, accumulating informal and formal evidence confirms that in general the process of adaptation is ordered as the model suggests. The Alverno College faculty constructed instructional sequences or levels for developing and assessing the educational competencies that they identified to be critical to adult effectiveness. What is intriguing is that without any knowledge of the scientific studies of the adaptive sequence, as far as I know, the faculty intuitively ordered the levels in terms of qualities remarkably similar to those of the model of maturing. For example, six objective instructional goals and criterion levels for nurturing students' communication skills were identified:

Level 1: Becoming aware of and learning how to assess one's own communication skills (symbolization).

Level 2: Analyzing the communication performances of others and comparing them to one's own (allocentricism).

Level 3: Learning to communicate in a variety of roles, whether as writer, speaker, listener (allocentricism), and developing self-assurance about one's abilities (stabilization of self-concept).

Level 4: Sharpening one's communication abilities, applying them to more complex material, and integrating the different communication skills by applying them to new situations (integration, autonomy).

Level 5: Deepening and extending the skills learned earlier to a specific discipline (stabilization).

Level 6: Applying one's communication skills to different situations and audiences that require different purposes and means (autonomy); explaining the relationship of one's presentation to the theory of one's discipline (symbolization, allocentricism, and integration).

Although the educational parallels to the adaptive sequence are not quite isomorphic, what is of interest is the faculty's independent judgment that there is an order to the process of learning competencies and that that process can be systematically nurtured. Parenthetically, it would be very exciting to discover if the students matured in the ways the model predicts by educating in this way.

Other more formal evidence supporting the general adaptive sequence, for which the model of maturing identifies the principal skills, values, self-attitudes and interpersonal qualities, comes from analyses of vocational decision making (Ginzberg et al., 1951; Tiedeman, 1961) and from Cantril's study of the stages through which developing countries pass. Cantril (1965, p. 308) has hypothesized an invariant, irreversible sequence that begins with increasing national frustration; creating a national dream (symbolization), usually by a charismatic leader; expanding a sense of loyalty from one's family or region to include the nation (allocentricism); developing coordinated realistic ways to realize the dream (integration); increasing national confidence as the dreams are realized (stabilization); and "heightening of the feeling that self-direction is possible through responsible action" (autonomy).

The sociological studies of modernity—the process by which persons from traditional cultures, typically rural peasants and workers, become more modern—are essentially studies of how persons adapt to the educational, industrial, and societal changes of contemporary times (Doob, 1967; Inkeles and Smith, 1970, 1974). Inkeles assumes that the adaptive process is similar for different cultures, that there is a "potential psychic unity of mankind" in its "inner 'rules' of organization" (which I would redefine to mean "inner dimensions of systemic maturing"), such that when a person is becoming more modern, the emerging qualities will be similar irrespective of the specific culture within which he is adapting (1969, p. 212). The traits that define "modern" man are readily mapped into the model of maturing, e.g., increasing ability to anticipate and plan (symbolization); expanding identifications beyond immediate familial and tribal ones (allocentricism); increasing cognitive flexibility and curiosity (integration); more self-confidence in ability to adapt (stabilization of self-concept); more independence of traditional authorities (autonomy of values). If the model of maturing comprehends the core qualities that facilitate adaptation, it may suggest other qualities that define modernity which Inkeles failed to assess.

SOME IMPLICATIONS AND CONTRIBUTIONS OF SCIENTIFIC RESEARCH ON MATURING

For Behavioral Scientists

Within the past decade, the behavioral sciences have seen the burgeoning of what is now called life-span psychology—an effort to order the developmental process from birth to death for the purpose of more deeply understanding the continuities as well as the stages that mark human growth. The construct of "stage" has been the favored organizing schema for developmental psychologists. It is a concept even found in certain religious traditions like Confucianism and Zen Buddhism that mark out landmarks to pass in religious development. As I have stated, the "stage" concept does not have sufficient analytic power to help me understand the details of healthy growth, perhaps because I have not studied large enough chunks of maturing to learn firsthand the organizing power of a specific stage. However defined, a stage sets the adaptive task, one might say; it is a time of disturbance, of disequilibrium, of "crisis" in Erikson's language. The model of maturing may provide a theoretical framework for understanding and predicting the course of the adaptive process that the "crisis" precipitates, as well as the maturing and immaturing effects that the response to the "crisis" produces.

If we wish to understand healthy growth, the critical issue may not be the content of the "crisis," which is not unimportant since it does "set the stage," so to speak. The more searching issues to explore are to identify those factors that influence how a person adapts to the crisis and the enduring effects that his response has on how he responds to future crises. Evidence from the transcultural study showed that psychologically healthy persons did not differ from unhealthy persons in their anxiety thresholds for personally conflictual crises; they differed in the way that they adapted to the crises, a conclusion that Vaillant has also come to from the longitudinal study of Harvard men (1977).

Another important developmental question to ask, which has not received the systematic attention that it deserves, is: What are the maturing and immaturing effects that different crises produce? Or put differently, What are the principal determinants of increasing mental health and how can we comprehensively map their effects? Let us examine some of the significant crises that most persons encounter during their adulthood that may profoundly affect them. Work, marriage, and parenthood are three potentially disrupting events. Yet, the research literature about the maturing and immaturing effects of each is like a barren desert, and the oases are more often mirages, because of their too limited conception of healthy growth. Take, for example, the largest national sample study of which I am aware, namely, the effect of occupation on personality (Kohn and Schooler, 1973). Despite its impressive resources and sophisticated analyses, it was flawed by a singularly atheoretical and inadequate conception of personality. The researchers assessed the effects of different occupational attributes on only ten personality traits (e.g., cognitive flexibility) and concluded that "the central fact of occupational life today is . . . the opportunity . . . to direct one's own occupational activities" (1973, p. 116). Such a comparative statement cannot be made in the absence of a comprehensive assessment of all of the major effects that occupations may have upon subsequent healthy growth. Using the model of maturing to organize a much less ambitious, more exploratory study, I found that professional occupations, for example, furthered, in declining order of magnitude of effect: the stabilization of the self-concept, allocentric cognitive skill development, allocentric nonfamilial relationships, and then the autonomy of the self-concept that Kohn and Schooler reported to be the principal effect (1977d). Some of these principal effects were not even assessed by them.

I have reported elsewhere how the relative importance of different types of determinants of healthy growth and the most likely types of maturing effects such determinants are likely to have might be very crudely assessed. For example, the data from the longitudinal adult study show very clearly that the type of spouse one marries and one's type of occupation affect maturing in most sectors of a person's life. Adult sexual relations, on the other hand, affected healthy growth in only two of the personality sectors, i.e., integration and stabilization of the self-concept (1978a). To take another example: being a father for professional men apparently may not be as powerful a determinant of continued maturing as some studies suggest; it had only limited effects on a minority of the fathers that I studied (1978c).

Do the model and its associated research have anything to contribute to counselors? The definition of the goals and the determination of the actual outcomes of psychotherapy have been persistent sources of dispute among clinicians and researchers (Malan, Heath, Howard, and Balfour, 1975; Malan and London, 1973). Since the model organizes what mental health specialists have claimed are qualities of psychological health, some of which are represented in current psychiatric diagnostic procedures like the Health-Sickness Rating Scale (Luborsky, 1962; Luborsky and Bachrach, 1974) and the Global Assessment Scale (Endicott, Spitzer, Fleiss, and Cohen, 1976), the model may provide a more systematic framework for assessing the effects of therapy (1980).

The application of the model of maturing for understanding sexuality illustrates how another mental health topic could become more accessible to scientific research. Masters and Johnson's most comprehensive summary of their work on sexual pleasure (1974) identified numerous qualities of maturity that contributed to sexual enjoyment, e.g., sense of identity, ability to create other-centered and integrative relationships, autonomy, self-regard. However, their failure to be systematic in identifying the personality variables to assess, to use any psychological assessment procedures at all, and to report their detailed evidence makes it impossible to evaluate the comparative validity of their rich and insightful hypotheses. The model of maturing and its measures have provided the means to verify and extend their hypotheses. We now have the supporting data to claim that the psychological maturity of a person is directly and very consistently related to his capacity to enjoy his sexuality (1978a,b,c).

For Educators

Increasing knowledge about healthy growth may have direct implications for educators in a number of ways. I mention only four to be illustrative.

One contribution is that as educators struggle again to clarify their purposes, a model that explicitly organizes the developmental goals historically associated with a liberal education may help clarify future value choices. For example, several college faculties have been very provoked to discover from mapping their catalogue statements of goals into the model of maturing that their colleges' distinctive strengths were not represented in their goals. The goals of one college exclusively emphasized cognitive skill development and autonomy, but failed to assert its concern for the value and interpersonal maturation of its students, goals deeply embedded within its religious tradition. Another faculty was shocked to discover, when confronted with the map of its goals, that it had not mentioned any cognitive skill growth in its catalogue. Now college catalogues have not been known to play much of a role in affecting how faculty teach, but such statements of goals may in the future have greater impact as faculties begin to hold themselves to more explicit standards of accountability.

A second implication of the model is that educators need to understand the equilibrating nature of healthy growth which, recall, states that excessive development in one personality sector may induce resistance to further development until compensatory growth occurs in other parts of the system. A poignant illustration of this principle is the following anxiety dream of a brilliant mathematics senior who had been urged the previous day by his professor to apply for graduate school.

> Walking up and down in a skyscraper looking for where math class is held on the first day of the new semester, I was leading Bill (who impresses me as grinding in physics to show he can do it). Up at the very top is the math class. I begin walking into the clean, well-ordered room where someone is writing math on the blackboard. Then I am following Henry (he has done a lot of hitchhiking, traveling to South America and around) through a series of attics, filled with old furniture, interesting knickknacks, exotic but dusty rugs. We are tunneling through the stuff, over junk and under tables.

He interpreted his dream to tell him not to continue in mathematics but to develop the less differentiated social and emotional parts of himself, which he sought to do by way of psychotherapy several years later after hitchhiking "around." Unfortunately, he never returned to mathematics where his gifts so obviously lay. The implication is that education that cultivates too narrow a range of human potentials risks creating in the long run less mature, less educable, and eventually less adaptable adults. That is one of my interpretations of the findings that I reported earlier about high-aptitude and academically achieving students. Despite their exceptional gifts, the men who had received college honors, for example, were no more effective, competent, or happy persons than those who had stumbled through college with average grades. Unfortunately, such honor students rated themselves to be less mature and were so judged by others in their interpersonal relationships.

A third contribution that research on healthy growth may make to educators is to deepen their understanding of the process of becoming liberally educated. Research that has been guided by an understanding of healthy growth has shown that the first weeks of college is the period during which students are most educable, that is, their former equilibrium has been disrupted and they are open to new types of growth. The pattern of maturing effects initiated during that time is similar to the pattern of effects that the college will be strengthening during the remaining three and a half years. If faculties wish to create powerful maturing environments, they then need to pay particular attention to the freshman's first semester, particularly to his values which are the entry point into his educability, so to speak. We are learning that a powerful, liberally educating college intensely affects a wide sector of a student's personality and that its effects may persist long past graduation. We are also learning that the short-term effects, those that occur while a student remains within the college environment, are not necessarily the same effects that become internalized, become more autonomous, and persist once the student leaves the supporting college environment. In other words, to assess the power of a college to have maturing effects, we must examine which effects have become stabilized and autonomous by follow-up studies of its alumni (1976c). What little comparative data we have also suggest that colleges differ not only in their explicit goals but also in the pattern of their effects. It is not infrequent for the actual effects of a college to be quite different from those that the faculty has stated are its goals, as well as different from the effects that the faculty believes that it is having. Finally, the model has enabled us to secure information about the differential maturing and immaturing effects of different aspects of a college, e.g., residential living patterns, specific faculty members. We are now beginning to learn what may be the de facto institutional attributes that have specific types of maturing effects.

Another related contribution that an understanding of healthy growth may make to educators is that it may deepen their awareness of, and sensitivity to, the complexity of the types of effects that an educational intervention has. I make the same critique of the research on educational outcomes as I do of the vocational study that I cited. Too narrow a conception of growth may distort and blind us to the actual pattern of effects that may occur. For example, I do not know how to assess the "Sesame Street" studies. Although the TV show may accelerate letter recognition by several months in certain types of children, failure to assess its effects more comprehensively over a longer time span does not tell us whether it may be enhancing immature stabilization of letter recognition, inhibiting student interest, limiting attention span, and furthering interpersonal autocentricism. More generally, might not such programs predispose a youngster to be more bored when he gets to school and finds that education is not as entertaining as the Cookie Monster? As another example, I do not know how to assess the cumulative research which suggests that most colleges have very limited impacts on their students. Colleges seem to increase cognitive integration, allocentric values, aésthetic sensitivity (Newcomb and Feldman, 1969), possibly the stabilization of moods (King, 1973), and a few other effects. Since the full range of possible effects of which educational philosophers talk has not been studied (behavioral measures do not even exist for many of them), we can make no justifiable generalization about the overall power of a liberal education to further a youth's maturing.

For the Religious

Implied in my discussion has been a potentially arrogant claim that needs to be made explicit, namely, it is possible to provide an empirical basis not only for the goals of a liberal education but also for the meaning of the "good life." More baldly, if one makes the key value choice to live the "good life," to grow healthily, to become fulfilled, then such a choice predetermines the values which define that mature life. In Maslow's terms, fact and value can become the same. Since I skirt close to committing the naturalistic fallacy—particularly when implying that once the basic value choice is made, there are universally shared values that are not relative—I must defend my stance.

If it is possible to create eventually a transculturally general set of developmental dimensions that empirically distinguish more mature from less mature persons and if such dimensions predict their adaptability in diverse cultures, then maturing results in the nurturing of qualities that philosophers and religionists have valued as central to the good life.

As a person matures on the dimension of symbolization, he increases his knowledge of the world and of himself, and as the Confucian text *Great Learning* suggests, in the words of Tseng, "when one acquires knowledge he can be honest with himself about his own motivations; when one can be honest with himself, he can purify and stabilize his own mind; when the mind is purified, then one can cultivate his moral character . . ." (1973, p. 193). Increasing symbolization increases the possibility that a person will become progressively more *honest*.

When a person develops the allocentric ability to enter deeply the interior lives of others, to share with them their joys and pains, to empathize with those who differ in sex, sexual orientation, color, and cultural values, and to expand the circumference of the boundaries of the self, he is potentially becoming a more understanding and *compassionate* person. From the Christian view of development, the individual grows into a "close and organic community with others," marked by a spontaneous "loving unity" (Bouwsma, 1976, p. 88).

To become more integrated; to live, as the Sikhs suggest, a natural life "unaffected by the artificiality of keeping up appearances" (Neki, 1975, p. 2); to become a *halim,* a wise Muslim—this is to possess "a wholeness of being" that brings *integrity* or "harmony of inner faculties and outer actions" (Lapidus, 1976, p. 97). With integrity comes spontaneity.

Increasing stability of mind, of character; developing a grounded sense of self, or as Confucius says of the great man, holding "fast to his cherished principles" (Tseng, 1973, p. 198); striving for *samadhi,* that is, the capacity to be fully absorbed, to experience "one-pointedness" (Goleman, 1975) for as long as one chooses to—these facets of stability increase the likelihood that a person can commit, devote himself *steadfastly*.

Finally, as Bouwsma defines the ideal Christian adult, he becomes "freed of bondage to the self, to the anxieties and the false absolutisms embedded in human culture, by which . . . [he] is otherwise imprisoned . . . [this] is the necessary condition of true autonomy" (1976, p. 86). *Sahaja* is "freedom from desire" (Neki, 1975, p. 5). Such autonomy from imperious desires and the claims of culture leads to the *courage* that Confucianism identifies with the wise man, "to want to keep and follow his ideal . . . even when he has to face many thousands of enemies by himself alone" (Tseng, 1973, p. 197).

I suggest that honesty, compassion, integrity, commitment, steadfastness, and courage are universally valued among the great religious traditions, that they are the behaviors–virtues we educate for when we are furthering the maturing of youth, and that they are values central to the "good life."

Why might the religious traditions of East and West share common values? My hypothesis is that as societies have evolved, their survival as well as the psychological well-being of their members has depended upon the quality of adaptations that the group and its leaders made. We have seen that the attributes of maturity are consistently related to the effectiveness with which adults adapt to diverse and varying situations and roles. Might not the different religions have identified and valued as virtues those core universal qualities found to be desirable for the psychological survival and well-being of their society's members? The values that we identify with the good life—enlightenment, the great man, the wise person, *samadhi, sahaja,* salvation—find their roots in the collective experience of mankind, the facts of living fully and happily. These adaptive facts are human virtues.

THE FRONTIER EDGES FOR RESEARCH ON MATURITY

Our Western scientific understanding of healthy growth, becoming, maturing has made only a small step, particularly when one places what we may now know against the backdrop of the other views of human potential reported in this book. Our current knowledge is grounded on a very, very narrow empirical base; it has little breadth in terms of independently confirming evidence. Few researchers have been interested in pursuing the issues of this chapter or book; the contemporary Western psychological zeitgeist suggests to me that it will be the clinicians, educators, and religious—not the personality researchers or other behavioral scientists—who will continue to illumine the edges of our current understanding. Yet to those who wish to explore and set such intuitions on firmer public, objective, and empirically disciplined grounds, what are some of the pathways more open to explore these days?

Certainly, the tedious but indispensable task of replicating the reported findings about healthy growth and its relation to subsequent adult effectiveness is a promising pathway that has implications for more fully understanding and predicting who may become a competent person in contemporary Western society. Certainly, the replication should extend over more social classes and, hopefully, cultures to test the generality of our knowledge. Certainly, too, we need to determine if the empirical relationships found for 17 to 33 year olds hold for other age groups. We may be able to ask and now test more sophisticated questions like, Will the more developmentally mature person of 30 adapt more effectively at the time of the alleged mid-life crisis, or will he not encounter such a "crisis" just because he has been a continually growing, adaptive person? What specific qualities that define healthy growth during the early adult years predict healthy growth during the sixties and seventies?

Another research problem is how to relate dimensional with "stage" views of development empirically. Can we begin to talk more objectively about different stages of symbolization, as the Sufis (Deikman, 1977) and Zen Buddhists (Shultz, 1975) do about the development of consciousness? Can we begin to identify developmental regularities, in other words, for each dimension of systemic growth? One effort to do just this (i.e., formulate and assess a developmental dimension labeled the objectification of the awareness of self and of others) was, however, not successful (Brehm, 1974). Erikson raised and responded to this neglected but important question when he was analyzing identity and its different phases throughout the life span. Also, what are the relationships between different phases of autonomy or stability and one's psychological well-being? I have found that the typical self-sufficient, individualistic form of autonomy that many males parade during late adolescence may actually block their subsequent maturing. The men, to continue to grow more wholely, need to be more open to allocentric growth, even its emotional dependencies, during early adulthood if they are to develop the foundations for the integrative mutuality that defines more mature modes of relationships. We know little about the qualities that predict which persons will continue to grow and fulfill themselves healthily, though the evidence is accumulating that one's psychological health is a principal determinant of continued growth (Dworken and Widom, 1977).

A related question is, What are the environmental (e.g., societal role or educational) determinants that provoke what types of growth? Just as we are beginning to learn what aspects of a liberal education have powerful maturing effects, so do we need to know what attributes of an occupation promote continued symbolization or integration. For example, Kohn and Schooler identified complexity of a job to encourage the integration of cognitive skills (1973). I have found it increasingly fruitful to ask, "What are the different educational principles, in contrast to techniques, that further development on each dimension, and what do such principles imply for our teaching and curricular organization?" (1971, 1980).

My judgment is informed more by intuition and hunch than by knowledge or expertise, but may it not be time to return to the issue that Maslow earlier raised about the possibility of developing a scientifically based value system (1959)? Just as Kohlberg's stage model of moral development is stimulating thought about the relation of science to values, perhaps a dimensional understanding of concepts like healthiness and maturity may provoke other types of questions. As Campbell (1975) urged in his presidential address to the American Psychological Association, perhaps the time is now ready for behavioral scientists to become more open to the wisdom embedded in the historically great religions about the qualities that facilitate the survival of our species.

CONCLUSION

Human development, the study of man as a whole, appears to be best able to facilitate the unification of the sciences and the humanities and to open up the perspectives we need to view the best as well as the future evolution of ourselves and our society.

Robert Aldrich (1977)

By drawing liberally from the behavioral sciences and from educational, philosophical, and religious traditions—just those most intimately concerned with the development of persons—I have suggested that there may be a genotypic understanding of healthy growth implied in each tradition that may provide a common basis on which such unification may occur. Each tradition differs in its emphases and methods, its language and its insights. However, the striking correspondences that we have seen between the more scientific and the more humanistic views of what it means to develop healthily and to fulfill one's *potentia* provide a fragment of hope that someday a deeper understanding of how a human being develops healthily may illumine the direction of "the future evolution of ourselves and our society" (Aldrich, 1977, p. 1).

REFERENCES

Abraham, K. Character-formation on the genital level of the libido (1925). In *Selected Papers of Karl Abraham*, London: Hogarth Press, 1949, Ch. 25.

Aldrich, R. A. The early antecedents of aging. Quotation from *Major Transitions in the Human Life Cycle* (H. Spierer, Ed.). N.Y.: Academy for Educational Development, 1977.

Allport, G. W. *Pattern and Growth in Personality*. New York: Holt, Rinehart, and Winston, 1961.

Allport, G. W., Vernon, P. E. and Lindzey, G. *Study of Values* (Manual, 3rd ed.). Boston: Houghton Mifflin, 1960.

Alverno College faculty. *Liberal Learning at Alverno College*. Milwaukee, Wis: Alverno College, 1976.

Ashton, P. T. Cross-cultural Piagetian research: an experimental perspective. *Harvard Educational Review*, 1975, *45*, 457–506.

Barron, F. *Creativity and Psychological Health*. Princeton, N.J.: Van Nostrand, 1963.

Bellah, R. N. et al. Adulthood. *Daedalus*, 1976, *105*, No. 2.

Binswanger, L. *Being-in-the-world. Selected Papers*. New York: Basic Books, 1963.

Block, J. *Lives through Times*. Berkeley, Calif.: Bancroft, 1971.

Bode, B. H. *Modern Educational Theories*. New York: Macmillan, 1927.

Bouwsma, W. J. Christian adulthood. In Adulthood, *Daedalus*, 1976, 77–92.

Brehm, S. S. Developmental aspects of objective self awareness. *Dissertation Abstracts International*, 1974, 34(9-B), 4654–4655.

Brown, D. R. Non-intellective qualities and the perception of the ideal student by college faculty. *Journal of Educational Sociology*, 1960, *33*, 269–278.

Campbell, D. T. On the conflicts between biological and social evolution and between psychology and moral tradition. *American Psychologist*, 1975, *30*, 1103–1126.

Cantril, H. *The Pattern of Human Concerns*. New Brunswick, N.J.: Rutgers University Press, 1965.

Cattell, R. B. The measurement of the healthy personality and the healthy society. *The Counseling Psychologist,* 1973, *4,* 13–18.

Chickering, A. W. *Education and Identity.* San Francisco: Jossey-Bass, 1969.

Chodorkoff, B. Adjustment and the discrepancy between the perceived and ideal self. *Journal of Clinical Psychology,* 1954, *10,* 266–268.

Clausen, J. A. Values, norms, and the health called "mental": purposes and feasibility of assessment. In *The Definition and Measurement of Mental Health* (S. B. Sells, Ed.). National Center for Health Statistics, U.S. Public Health Service, 1968.

Cox, R. D. *Youth into Maturity.* New York: Mental Health Materials Center, 1970.

Deikman, A. J. Sufism and psychiatry. *Journal of Nervous and Mental Disease,* 1977, *165,* 318–329.

Dewey, J. Logical conditions of a scientific treatment of morality (1903). In *John Dewey on Education* (R. D. Archambault, Ed.). New York: Modern Library, Random House, 1964.

Dewey, J. Progressive education and the science of education (1928). In *John Dewey on Education* (R. D. Archambault, Ed.). New York: Modern Library, Random House, 1964.

Dewey, J. The process and product of reflective activity (1933a). In *John Dewey on Education* (R. D. Archambault, Ed.). New York: Modern Library, Random House, 1964.

Dewey, J. Why reflective thinking must be an educational aim (1933b). In *John Dewey on Education* (R. D. Archambault, Ed.). New York: Modern Library, Random House, 1964.

Dewey, J. The need for a philosophy of education (1934). In *John Dewey on Education* (R. D. Archambault, Ed.). New York: Modern Library, Random House, 1964.

Dewey, J. Democracy and educational administration (1937). In *John Dewey on Education* (R. D. Archambault, Ed.). New York: Modern Library, Random House, 1964.

Dohrenwend, B. P. and Dohrenwend, B. S. Social and cultural influences on psychopathology. *Annual Review of Psychology,* 1974, *25,* 417–452.

Doob, L. W. Scales for assaying psychological modernization in Africa. *Public Opinion Quarterly,* 1967, *31,* 414–421.

Douvan, E. and Adelson, J. *The Adolescent Experience.* New York: Wiley, 1966.

Doyle, J. A. Field-independence and self-actualization. *Psychological Reports,* 1975, *36,* 363–366.

Duncan, C. B. A reputation test of personality integration. *Journal of Personality and Social Psychology,* 1966, *3,* 516–524.

Dworken, R. H. and Widom, C. S. Undergraduate profiles and the longitudinal prediction of adult social outcome. *Journal of Consulting Clinical Psychology,* 1977, *45,* 620–624.

Endicott, J., Spitzer, R. L., Fleiss, J. L. and Cohen, J. The Global Assessment Scale. A procedure for measuring overall severity of psychiatric disturbance. *Archives of General Psychiatry,* 1976, *33,* 766–771.

Erikson, E. H. *Childhood and Society* (2nd ed.). New York: Norton, 1963.

Fieselmann, A. The college environment as an affector of maturity. Unpublished thesis, Hanover College, 1973.

Foote, N. N. and Cottrell, L. S., Jr. *Identity and Interpersonal Competence: A New Direction in Family Research.* Chicago: University of Chicago Press, 1955.

Foxman, P. Tolerance for ambiguity and self-actualization. *Journal of Personality Assessment,* 1976, *40,* 67–72.

Freud, S. *The interpretation of dreams* (1900). New York: Basic Books, 1956.

Freud, S. Instincts and their vicissitudes (1915). In *Collected Papers,* Vol. IV. London: Hogarth, 1949.

Freud, S. *The Ego and the Id* (1923). New York: Norton, 1960.

Gardner, J. W. *Fifty-first Annual Report 1955–56.* New York: Carnegie Corporation of New York, 1956.

Ginzberg, E. et al. *Occupational Choice: An Approach to a General Theory.* New York: Columbia University Press, 1951.

Goleman, D. The Buddha on meditation and states of consciousness. In *Transpersonal Psychologies* (C. T. Tart, Ed.). New York: Harper and Row, 1975, Ch. 5.

Goleman, D. Meditation and consciousness: An Asian approach to mental health. *American Journal of Psychotherapy,* 1976, *30,* 41–54.

Grinker, R. R., Sr. with collaboration of Grinker, R. R., Jr. and Timberlake, J. "Mentally healthy" young males (homoclites). *Archives of General Psychiatry,* 1962, *6,* 405–453.

Grinker, R. R. and Werble, B. Mentally healthy young men (homoclites) 14 years later. *Archives of General Psychiatry,* 1974, *30,* 701–704.

Gutmann, D. Parenthood: a key to the comparative study of the life cycle. In *Life-span Developmental Psychology* (N. Datun and L. H. Ginsberg, Eds.). New York: Academic Press, 1975.

Haan, N. Proposed model of ego functioning: coping and defense mechanisms in relationship to IQ change. *Psychological Monographs: General and Applied,* 1963, *77*(8), 1–23.

Haan, N. Coping and defense mechanisms related to personality inventories. *Journal of Consulting Psychology,* 1965, *29,* 373–378.

Harmon, D. K., Masuda, M. and Holmes, T. H. The Social Readjustment Rating Scale: a cross-cultural study of Western Europeans and Americans, *Journal of Psychosomatic Research,* 1970, *14,* 391–400.

Hart, J. T. and Tomlinson, T. M. (Eds.). *New Directions in Client-Centered Therapy,* New York: Houghton Mifflin, 1970.

Hartmann, H. Towards a concept of mental health. *British Journal of Medical Psychology,* 1960, *33,* 243–248.

Heath, C. W. *What People Are; A Study of Normal Young Men.* Cambridge, Mass.: Harvard University Press, 1945.

Heath, D. H. *Explorations of Maturity.* New York: Appleton-Century-Crofts, 1965.

Heath, D. H. *Growing Up in College.* San Francisco: Jossey-Bass, 1968.

Heath, D. H. *Humanizing Schools: New Directions, New Decisions.* Rochelle Park, N. J.: Hayden, 1971.

Heath, D. H. Adolescent and adult predictors of vocational adaptation. *Journal of Vocational Behavior,* 1976a, *9,* 1–19.

Heath, D. H. Competent fathers: their personalities and marriages. *Human Development,* 1976b, *19,* 26–39.

Heath, D. H. What the enduring effects of higher education tell us about a liberal education. *Journal of Higher Education,* 1976c, *47,* 173–190.

Heath, D. H. Academic predictors of adult maturity and competence. *Journal of Higher Education,* 1977a, *48,* 613–632.

Heath, D. H. Maternal competence, expectation, and involvement. *Journal of Genetic Psychology,* 1977b, *131,* 169–182.

Heath, D. H. *Maturity and Competence: A Transcultural View.* New York: Gardner (Wiley), 1977c.

Heath, D. H. Some possible effects of occupation on the maturing of professional men. *Journal of Vocational Behavior,* 1977d, *11,* 263–281.

Heath, D. H. Marital sexual enjoyment and frustration of professional men. *Archives of Sexual Behavior,* 1978a, *7,* 463–477.

Heath, D. H. Personality correlates of the marital sexual compatibility of professional men. *Journal of Sex and Marital Therapy,* 1978b, *4,* 67–82.

Heath, D. H. What meaning and effects does fatherhood have for the maturing of professional men? *Merrill-Palmer Quarterly of Behavior and Development,* 1978c, *24,* 265–278.

Heath, D. H. Marital sexuality and the psychological health of professional men. *Journal of Sex and Marital Therapy,* 1979, *5*(2) 103–116.

Heath, D. H. Wanted: A comprehensive model of healthy development. *Personnel and Guidance Journal,* 1980, *58,* 391–399.

Holt, R. R. The problem of values in the science of personality development. Invited address, Michigan Psychological Association, October 25, 1974.

Hook, S. *Education for Modern Man.* Toronto: Longmans, 1946.

Hutchins, R. W. *The Higher Learning in America.* New Haven: Yale University Press, 1936.

Inkeles, A. Making men modern: on the causes and consequences of individual change in six developing countries. *American Journal of Sociology,* 1969, *75,* 208–225.

Inkeles, A. and Smith, D. H. The fate of personal adjustment in the process of modernization. *International Journal of Comparative Sociology,* 1970, *11,* 81–114.

Inkeles, A. and Smith, D. H. *Becoming Modern. Individual Change in Six Developing Countries.* Cambridge, Mass.: Harvard University Press, 1974.

Jahoda, M. Current Concepts of Positive Mental Health (A report to the staff director, Jack R. Ewalt). New York: Basic Books, 1958.

James, W. *The Principles of Psychology,* Vol. 10, New York: Henry Holt, 1890, Ch. 10.

Jones, E. The concept of a normal mind. *International Journal of Psychoanalysis,* 1942, *23,* 1–8.

Jones, M. D., Bayley, N., Macfarlane, J. W. and Honzik, M. P. (Eds.). *The Course of Human Development.* Waltham, Mass.: Xerox College Publ., 1971, pp. 451–461.

Jourard, S. *Healthy Personality: An Approach from the Viewpoint of Humanistic Psychology.* New York: Macmillan, 1974.

Jung, C. G. *The Integration of the Personality.* New York: Farrar and Rinehart, 1939.

Kagan, J. and Moss, H. A. *Birth to Maturity. A Study in Psychological Development.* New York: Wiley, 1962.

King, S. H. *Five Lives at Harvard: Personality Change during College.* Cambridge, Mass.: Harvard University Press, 1973.

Klein, M. On mental health. *British Journal of Medical Psychology,* 1960, *33,* 237–241.

Knapp, R. R. and Comrey, A. L. Further construct validation of a measure of self-actualization. *Educational and Psychological Measurement,* 1973, *33,* 419–425.

Kogan, W. S., Quinn, R., Ax, A. F. and Ripley, H. S. Some methodological problems in the quantification of clinical assessment by Q array. *Journal of Consulting Psychology,* 1957, *21,* 57–62.

Kohlberg, L. The development of moral character and ideology. In *Review of Child Development Research* (M. L. Hoffman and L. W. Hoffman, Eds.), Vol. 1. New York: Russell Sage Foundation, 1964.

Kohlberg, L. The child as a moral philosopher. *Psychology Today,* 1968, *2*(4), 25–30.

Kohlberg, L. Moral development and the education of adolescents. In *Adolescents and the American High School* (R. F. Purnell, Ed.). New York: Holt, Rinehart, and Winston, 1970.

Kohlberg, L. The development of moral stages. Uses and abuses. *Proceedings of the Individual Conference on Testing Problems,* 1973, 1–8.

Kohn, M. L. and Schooler C. Occupational experience and psychological functioning: an assessment of reciprocal effects. *American Sociological Review,* 1973, *38,* 97–118.

Kris, E. *Psychoanalytic Explorations in Art.* New York: International University Press, 1952.

Lapidus, I. M. Adulthood in Islam: religious maturity in the Islamic tradition. In Adulthood, *Daedalus,* 1976, 93–108.

Lecky, P. *Self-consistency; A Theory of Personality.* New York: Island Press, 1945.

Levinson, D. J. *Seasons of a Man's Life.* New York: Knopf, 1978.

Levinson, D. J., Darrow, C. M., Klein, E. B., Levinson, M. H. and McKee, B. The psychosocial development of men in early adulthood and the mid-life transition. In *Life History Research in Psychopathology* (D. F. Ricks, A. Thomas, and M. Roff, Eds.), Vol. 3. Minneapolis, Minn: University of Minnesota Press, 1974, pp. 243–258.

Loevinger, J. *Ego Development: Conceptions and Theories.* San Francisco: Jossey-Bass, 1976.

Lowenthal, M. F., Thurnher, M. and Chiriboga, D. *Four Stages of Life.* San Francisco: Jossey-Bass, 1975.

Luborsky, L. Clinicians' judgments of mental health. *Archives of General Psychiatry,* 1962, *7,* 407–417.

Luborsky, L. and Bachrach, M. Factors influencing clinicians' judgments of mental health: eighteen experiences with the Health Sickness Rating Scale. *Archives of General Psychiatry,* 1974, *31,* 292–299.

MacKinnon, D. W. The highly effective individual. *Teachers College Record,* 1960, *61,* 367–378.

MacKinnon, D. W. Personality and the realization of creative potential. *American Psychologist,* 1965, *20,* 273–281.

MacLeish, A. Professional schools of liberal education. *The Yale Review,* 1920, *10,* 362–372.

Mahoney, J. and Hartnett, J. Self-actualization and self-ideal discrepancy. *Journal of Psychology,* 1973, *85,* 37–42.

Malan, D. H., Heath, S. E., Bacal, H. A. and Balfour, F. H. G. Psychodynamic changes in untreated neurotic patients. *Archives of General Psychiatry,* 1975, *32,* 110–126.

Malan, D. H. and London, D. M. The outcome problem in psychotherapy research. *Archives of General Psychiatry,* 1973, *29,* 719–729.

Maslow, A. H. Self-actualizing people: a study of psychological health. *Personality,* 1950, Symposium No. 1, 11–34.

Maslow, A. H. *Motivation and personality.* New York: Harper & Row, 1954.

Maslow, A. H. (Ed.). *New Knowledge in Human Values.* New York: Harper, 1959.

Maslow, A. H. *Toward a Psychology of Being.* Princeton, N. J.: Van Nostrand, 1962.

Maslow, A. H. Fusions of facts and values. *American Journal of Psychoanalysis,* 1963, *23,* 117–131.

Masters, W. H. and Johnson, V. E. *The Pleasure Bond. A New Look at Sexuality and Commitment.* Boston: Little, Brown, 1974.

McGehee, T. P. The stability of the self-concept and self-esteem. *Dissertation Abstracts,* 1957, *17,* 1403–1404.

McGrath, E. J. *The Graduate School and the Decline of Liberal Education.* New York: Bureau of Publications, Teachers College, Columbia University, 1959.

Mead, G. H. *Mind, Self and Society from the Standpoint of a Social Behaviorist.* Chicago: University of Chicago Press, 1934.

Meiklejohn, A. *The Liberal College.* Boston: Marshall Jones, 1920.

Miller, K. and Mosher, G. Maturity and moral development. Unpublished senior research theses, Haverford College, 1977.

Murphy, L. B. *The Widening World of Childhood.* New York: Basic Books, 1962.

Neki, J. S. *Sahaja:* an Indian ideal of mental health. *Psychiatry,* 1975, *38,* 1–10.

Newcomb, T. M. and Feldman, K. A. *The Impacts of Colleges on Students.* San Francisco: Jossey-Bass, 1969.

Newman, J. C. *The Idea of a University, Defined and Illustrated* (1852). New York: Longmans, Green, 1891.

Nunberg, H. The synthetic function of the ego. *International Journal of Psychoanalysis,* 1931, *12.*

Opler, M. K. Anthropological contributions to psychiatry and social psychiatry. In *Changing Perspectives in Mental Illness* (S. C. Plog and R. B. Edgerton, Eds.). New York: Holt, Rinehart and Winston, 1969, pp. 88–105.

Osgood, C. E., May, W. H. and Miron, M. S. *Cross-cultural Universals of Affective Meaning.* Urbana, Ill.: University of Illinois Press, 1975.

Owens, C. M. Zen Buddhism. In *Transpersonal Psychologies* (C. T. Tart, Ed.). New York: Harper & Row, 1975, Ch. 4.

Pahnke, W. N. and Richards, W. A. Implication of LSD and experimental mysticism. *Journal of Religion and Health,* 1966, *5,* 175–208.

Pedersen, P. Asian personality theories. In *Current Personality Theories* (R. Corsini, Ed.). Ithaca, Ill.: F. E. Peacock, 1977.

Perry, W. G., Jr. *Forms of Intellectual and Ethical Development during the College Years.* New York: Holt, Rinehart, and Winston, 1970.

Piaget, J. *Judgment and Reasoning in the Child.* New York: Harcourt, Brace, 1928.

Piaget, J. *The Psychology of Intelligence* (1947). New York: Harcourt, Brace, 1950.

Piat, J. L. Factor analytic investigation of the ability to symbolize emotions: a comparison of children, college students, and hospitalized psychiatric patients. *Dissertation Abstracts International,* 1974, *34*(8–B), 4055.

Rogers, C. R. A theory of therapy, personality, and interpersonal relationships as developed in the client-centered framework. In *Psychology: A Study of a Science* (S. Koch, Ed.), Vol. III: Formulations of the person and the social context. New York: McGraw-Hill, 1959, 184–256.

Rogers, C. R. *On Becoming a Person.* Boston: Houghton Mifflin, 1961.

Rogers, C. R. and Dymond, R. F. (Eds.) *Psychotherapy and Personality Change.* Chicago: University of Chicago Press, 1954.

Rohlen, T. P. The promise of adulthood in Japanese spiritualism. In Adulthood, *Daedalus,* 1976, 125–143.

Rosenhan, D. L. On being sane in insane places. *Science,* 1973, *179,* 250–258.

Russell, B. *Education and the Good Life.* New York: Liveright, 1931.

Sanford, F. H. A faculty's goals for its students. In *The Challenge of Curricular Change.* New York: College Entrance Examination Board, 1966, pp. 118–126.

Sanford, N. What is a normal personality? In *Writers on Ethics: Classical and Contemporary* (J. Katz et al., Eds.). Princeton, N. J.: Van Nostrand, 1962.

Sarbin, T. R. The scientific status of the mental illness metaphor. In *Changing Perspectives in Mental Illness.* (S. C. Plog and R. B. Edgerton, Eds.). New York: Holt, Rinehart, and Winston, 1969.

Saul, J. *Emotional Maturity* (1947, 2nd ed.). Philadelphia: Lippincott, 1960.

Scott, W. A. and Peterson, C. Adjustment, Pollyannaism, and attraction to close relationships. *Journal of Counseling and Clinical Psychology,* 1975, *43,* 872–880.

Seeman, J. Personality integration in college women. *Journal of Personality and Social Psychology,* 1966, *4,* 91–93.

Shostrom, E. L. A test for the measurement of self actualization. *Educational and Psychological Measurement,* 1964, *24,* 207–218.

Shostrom, E. L. and Knapp, R. R. The relationship of a measurement of self actualization (POI) to a measure of pathology (MMPI) and to therapeutic growth. *American Journal of Psychotherapy,* 1966, *20,* 193–202.

Shultz, J. Stages on the spiritual path: a Buddhist perspective. *Journal of Transpersonal Psychology,* 1975, *7,* 14–28.

Sinnott, E. W. The creativeness of life. In *Creativity and Its Cultivation* (H. H. Anderson, Ed.). New York: Harper & Row, 1959, Ch. 2.

Smith, G. M. Six measures of self-concept discrepancy and instability: their interrelations, reliability, and relations to other personality measures. *Journal of Consulting Psychology,* 1958, *22,* 101–112.

Smith, M. B. "Mental health" reconsidered: a special case of the problem of values in psychology. *American Psychologist,* 1961, *16,* 299–306.

Smith, M. B. Explorations in competence: a study of Peace Corps teachers in Ghana. *American Psychologist,* 1966, *21,* 555–566.

Smith, M. B. On self-actualization: a transambivalent examination of a focal theme in Maslow's psychology. *Journal of Humanistic Psychology,* 1973, *13,* 17–33.

Smith, M. B. *Humanizing Social Psychology.* San Francisco: Jossey-Bass, 1974.

Sullivan, H. S. *The Interpersonal Theory of Psychiatry.* New York: Norton, 1953.

Szasz, T. S. *The Myth of Mental Illness. Foundations of a Theory of Personal Conduct.* New York: Dell, 1961.

Szasz, T. S. *Ideology and Insanity.* Garden City, N. Y.: Doubleday, Anchor, 1970.

Tart, C. T. (Ed.). *Transpersonal Psychologies.* New York: Harper & Row, 1975.

Thomas, R. *The Search for a Common Learning: General Education 1800–1960.* New York: McGraw-Hill, 1962.

Tiedeman, D. V. Decision and vocational development: a paradigm and its implications. *Personnel and Guidance Journal,* 1961, *40,* 15–21.

Tippett, J. S. and Silber, E. Autonomy of self-esteem. *Archives of General Psychiatry,* 1966, *14,* 372–385.

Triandis, H. C. An approach to the analysis of subjective culture. In *Transcultural Research in Mental Health* (W. P. Lebra, Ed.). Honolulu: University Press of Hawaii, 1972, Ch. 16.

Tseng, W-S. The concept of personality in Confucian thought. *Psychiatry,* 1973, *36,* 191–202.

Turner, R. H. and Vanderlippe, R. H. Self-ideal congruence as an index of adjustment. *Journal of Abnormal Social Psychology,* 1958, *57,* 202–206.

Vaillant, G. E. Theoretical hierarchy of adaptive ego mechanisms. *Archives of General Psychiatry,* 1971, *24,* 107–118.

Vaillant, G. E. Antecedents of healthy adult male adjustment. In *Life History Research in Psychopathology* (D. F. Ricks, A. Thomas, and M. Roff, Eds.), Vol. 3. Minneapolis, Minn.: University of Minnesota Press, 1974, pp. 230–242.

Vaillant, G. E. Natural history of male psychological health. III. Empirical dimensions of mental health. *Archives of General Psychiatry,* 1975, *32,* 420–426.

Vaillant, G. E. Natural history of male psychological health. V. The relation of choice of ego mechanisms of defense to adult adjustment. *Archives of General Psychiatry,* 1976, *33,* 535–545.

Vaillant, G. E. *Adaptation to Life.* Boston: Little, Brown, 1977.

Vaillant, G. E. and McArthur, C. C. Natural history of male psychological health. I. The adult life cycle from 18–50. *Seminars in Psychiatry,* 1972, *4*(4).

Van Doren, M. *Liberal Education.* New York: Henry Holt, 1943.

Warren, J. R. and Heist, P. A. Personality attributes of gifted college students. *Science,* 1960, *132,* 330–337.

Wechsler, D. Intelligence defined and undefined. A relativistic appraisal. *American Psychologist,* 1975, *30,* 135–139.

Wei-Ming, T. The Confucian perception of adulthood. In Adulthood, *Daedalus,* 1976, 109–123.

Werner, H. *Comparative Psychology of Mental Development* (1948). Chicago: Follett, 1957 (rev. ed.).

Westley, W. A. and Epstein, N. B. *The silent majority.* San Francisco: Jossey-Bass, 1969.

Wexler, D. A. Self-actualization and cognitive processes. *Journal of Consulting and Clinical Psychology,* 1974, *42,* 47–53.

White, B. L. Fundamental early environmental influences on the development of competence. *Third Western Symposium on Learning: Cognitive Learning.* Bellingham, Wash.: Washington State College, 1971.

White, R. W. Ego and reality in psychoanalytic theory. *Psychological Issues,* 1963, *3,* #3, Mono. 11.

White, R. W. *Lives in Progress: A Study of the Natural Growth of Personality* (2nd ed.). New York: Holt, Rinehart, and Winston, 1966.

Whitehead, A. N. The aims of education (1916). In *The Aims of Education and Other Essays.* New York: Macmillan, 1929.

Witkin, H. A., Lewis, H. B., Hertzman, M., Machover, K., Meissner, P. B. and Wapner, S. *Personality through Perception: An Experimental and Clinical Study.* New York: Harper, 1954.

Wohlwill, J. F. *The Study of Behavioral Development.* New York: Academic Press, 1973.

In the deeper reality beyond space and time, we may all be members of one body.

Sir James Jeanes

This book provides several views about the nature of individual well-being, but what would an extremely healthy intimate relationship be like? Johanna and Deane Shapiro point out that most traditions are surprisingly silent on this point. Indeed, a few seem somewhat disparaging, suggesting that the heights of psychological development may best be reached alone, through the forsaking of special intimate relationships in order to devote all one's energies to self-mastery. Only then, these traditions suggest, is it most profitable to return to full engagement in the world, and even then the ideal may not be one of a few exclusive relationships, but rather a selfless and nonexclusive service of all. This model is by no means true of all traditions, and some embrace intimate and sexual relationships as beautiful and joyous vehicles of learning and liberation. It is this latter perspective which the Shapiros describe, suggesting a balance between personal and interpersonal, inner and outer work, and in so doing they provide a useful balance to the other contributions in this book.

Dr. Johanna Shapiro received her Ph.D. in 1975 from Stanford University. She is currently Director of the Behavioral Science Program and Assistant Professor, Department of Family Medicine, University of California at Irvine. Dr. Shapiro has maintained a long-standing personal and professional interest in dual-career marriage and in issues of combining family, adult intimacy, and career. She has coordinated and facilitated several groups addressing these issues for professional women, including women engineers and physicians. Dr. Shapiro has published in the areas of both the psychology of women and behavioral medicine, and her research and writing reflect a continued interest in various clinical and descriptive aspects of the family.

In the context of their committed, intimate (sometimes more and sometimes less) relationship, the Shapiros travelled and lived in Asia for 15 months studying Eastern disciplines; simultaneously pursued professional careers in the field of psychology; and for a period of two and a half years exemplified a commuter marriage, with Johanna working in Southern California and Deane in Northern California. The Shapiros currently have three children and live together as a family in Laguna Beach.

206

7

Well-Being and Relationship

Johanna Shapiro, Ph.D.

and

Deane H. Shapiro, Jr., Ph.D.

A quick review of the contents of this book reveals an implicit assumption about the nature of exceptional psychological well-being. This assumption is that exceptional psychological well-being, whether it be called enlightenment, satori, personal power, path of heart, developing the third eye, or uncovering the sacred unconscious, is primarily a personal task. For example, Globus and Globus describe the man of knowledge as a *solitary* bird. Further, when intense interpersonal relationships are mentioned, they are generally those between teacher and pupil (e.g., Rajneesh, Deikman, Globus and Globus).

The pursuit of transcendent or transforming experiences is often posited as antithetical to relationship. Indeed, great lovers of humanity in the abstract, such as Mahatma Gandhi or Albert Schweitzer, have not always been overly successful in their most intimate family relationships. In the meditative tradition, it is generally described as the task of the *individual* to cultivate right living, right thoughts, and right habits. In the Sufi tradition, it is again an *individual* task to develop the intuitive seeing eye of higher consciousness. The meditative and spiritual traditions emphasize the importance of each individual following the path of moral purity; they talk about nonattachment, a letting go of fear and greed and ego, but little mention is made of how this is manifest in intimate relationship.[1]

The environment of a monastery also focuses on the personal worth of the *individual*. For example, in Vipassana meditation retreats, eye contact and talking with others are prohibited. The mere presence of a significant other is often seen as a distraction to spiritual pursuits.

In many of these self-actualizing and spiritual traditions, there is an explicit proscription against intimate relationships.[2] For example, Gandhi, a Hindu, became an ascetic in order to give more selflessly of himself. In Catholicism, becoming a priest still requires strict celibacy. Renunciation of one's sexuality and living an ascetic life are often seen as ways to further develop one's "higher consciousness" and thus have complete energy to contribute to one's inner work and to society. Sexuality in the chakras of kundalini yoga is seen as a lower form of consciousness. In another example, Herman Hesse's Siddhartha must renounce the pleasures of the flesh to attain enlightenment. The arahat, a person of extreme psychological well-being in the Buddhist tradition, renounces the world in order to first attain enlightenment. The bodhisattva, who may have reached a similar level of well-being, chooses not to renounce the world, but to help humanity. However, even this is a helping of humanity in general rather than involvement with, and service to, one specific other.

The task of trying to be a bodhisattva, i.e., offering selfless service to all humanity, involves compassionate giving to many individuals. By comparison, cultivation of an intimate relationship may be seen as of lesser value. A single intimate may be perceived as more frustrating, more demanding, less rewarding then giving impartially to all humanity. It is almost as if the spiritual traditions seduce one into thinking, "How much easier to be a wise saint, compassionate and full of knowledge while living alone, than to be a mediocre human, living and struggling within the daily foibles of a relationship."

For some, less developed than a bodhisattva or an arahat, an experience of heightened psychological well-being may somehow be marred or reduced by trying to explain it to another, especially when that other is an intimate supposedly in tune with one's innermost feelings. Experiences of this nature are difficult to put into words and are often termed ineffable.[3] There may be an ensuing sense of frustration that the partner is not able to participate in or understand one's own altered state experience. There may also be the controlling urge to force one's partner along one's own path. Two members of a couple may even begin to compete to see who is most enlightened!

Thus, it is by no means automatic that extreme personal psychological well-being will be transformed into relational intimacy. Indeed, as we have seen, the two may appear to be directly threatening to each other. The question must be raised: What is the connection between the path of the warrior attempting to live an impeccable personal life and the path of closeness, trust, and love between two individuals? Must the images of extreme psychological well-being be only those of individuals struggling alone or in relationship to a teacher? Are passion and sexuality antithetical to spirituality integrity? Is intimacy itself unrelated to extreme psychological well-being, or is it something which can allow the expression and even foster the development of well-being?

What is the Value of Relationship?

Most individuals, regardless of their social class, occupation, sexual preference, and religious or political beliefs, agree on the value of an intimate relationship, a close and loving relationship with one special person.[4-5] Despite changing sexual mores, a soaring divorce rate, and a cultural emphasis on the importance of one's own professional and personal growth, most people still value the cultivation of interpersonal relationships.

A recent survey[6] did a cluster analysis of some of the rewards of intimacy between two people. On a personal level, subjects reported the feeling of being loved and needed, an inner sense of harmony and well-being, a sense of fulfillment, completion, and wholeness, a sense of personal freedom and liberation, and an opportunity for growth, change, and maturation. Interpersonally, subjects noted the importance of unconditional acceptance and understanding from another, the experience of sharing and trust, authentic and deep friendship, and being able to give and nurture as well as recieve. Finally, subjects reported that such intimacy at times led to feelings of transcendence, of being at one with the world. This last is similar to Bhakti, in which one reaches the transcendent through relationship, and to the Kabbalah or to Tantric Buddhism, in which sexual practice provides a door to the transcendent.

The benefits of such intimate relationships have been extolled by poets and philosophers for ages and need not be elaborated here. Fromm[7] points out that true love and intimacy can unlock the human potential of both participants and stimulate them to increasingly creative and meaningful living. It has also been pointed out that such relationships, nourished and expanded over time, may provide both safety and mutual understanding as a context for exploration and growth.[8]

Sullivan notes that valuing and experiencing affectionate and sympathetic feelings for others are distinguishing traits of the healthy person.[9] Characteristics such as mutuality, intimacy, loving, and ability to form deep and lasting relationships, are commonly identified as defining psychological health. Researchers such as Vaillant [10-11] have found that psychologically healthy persons have warmer, more loving friendships and closer relationships with their children and spouses than do psychologically unhealthy persons.

Further, there is now a well-substantiated research literature suggesting that there are negative medical consequences for social isolation, such as protracted rehabilitation or convalescence, and increased risk of illness and death. James Prescott maintains that parents who are physically affectionate with their children may decrease chances of later violence in their offspring. Ethology research suggests that intimate bonding is biologically derived, implying that intimacy may be part of our genetic makeup. [12]

Thus, we would suggest that intimacy is an important value on a variety of dimensions and that the skills of learning intimacy, what Heath refers to as allocentrism, are important for the development of the individual. In addition, as has been confirmed by some of the sources cited above, we believe that in fact the pursuit of extreme psychological well-being need not be anthithetical to developing deeper intimacy. Emotion and compassion are, of course, a part of the spiritual traditions. Certainly they can be applied to the committed intimate relationship as well as to humanity as a whole. As Kahlil Gibran noted in his now-classic poem *The Prophet,* love consists of two individuals who are strong enough to be able to come together and to respond to this experience as a personal and spiritual opportunity. Indeed, it can be through the daily struggle of an ongoing relationship that self-actualization occurs. It can also be the final challenge to a self-actualizing being, the final risk of applying one's spiritual lessons to that part of life closest to one's personal, psychological core.

We would suggest that personal psychological growth, often through individual retreat, introspection, or physical withdrawal, may be a necessary first step toward the development of exceptional relational health. However, as an end in itself, we believe that withdrawal or purely personal self-cultivation, without an element of engagement, a returning to the world, resembles narcissim in a vacuum—empty and meaningless. We prefer a more activist philosophy based on the assumption that a prime way to actualize a truly exceptional state of psychological health is through living in the world, in relation rather than in isolation. Of course, there are many ways of relating to, and being engaged in, the world. Here we are discussing only the way of intimate and enduring relationship with a significant other.

Limitations

In attempting to write about exceptional levels of health and relationship, we encounter several problems. The first and foremost problem derives from a shared belief system that one can only teach what one knows and experiences. However, as we look to our own relationship—for insights and problems—we are aware of the significant discrepancies between current reality and the vision to which we aspire. Therefore, we acknowledge a certain self-consciousness and humility at our limitations in attempting to discuss exceptional relational well-being.

A second difficulty is that when we look to the literature (or to life!) we find few examples of individuals who provide models of relationship mirroring extreme psychological health. The thoughts we are offering here must necessarily then be a suggesting of the importance of this dimension and a sharing of our beliefs and hopes about the forms it might take, rather than a detailed description or analysis.

Our Vision

We would suggest that exceptional levels of relational well-being will be found to be the product of two individuals who have been able to reach an extremely high state of individual psychological health. Further, we would suggest that without individual work, people who on a personal level are controlled by attachments, greed, insecurity, and ego, have little hope of moving beyond these problems when working within the context of a relationship. Paradoxically, by developing one's true self, one may be able to become like the mirror in Zen—more selfless, empty, and giving. This selfless self might be able to move beyond both traditional and liberated, male and female identities and roles, resulting in forms of androgyny in which both individuals could act with equal scope and flexibility.

Relationships in this stage would be seen not as a means for aggrandizing the ego, but as an opportunity for giving and service. The relationship might be pursued less for what one could get, and more for what one could give. Further, this loving closeness with another would also serve to stimulate the personal process of awakening oneself to new heights of psychological health and well-being. Each interaction would be perceived as containing a lesson to be appreciated and absorbed. Thus, difficulties and conflicts within the relationship, which undoubtedly would still exist in some sense, nevertheless would be transformed. Instead of representing struggles for ego enhancement—power, control, status—they would be perceived as opportunities for growth and a source of feedback about one's own behavior and intentions. Indeed, in this sense, the relationship would be valued by both partners as a kind of miracle, like the life of a growing child, which one realizes one cannot take credit for, but to which one must contribute to the utmost of one's ability, which one marvels at and is privileged to be a part of.

This stage is one which can be seen as a type of karma yoga, in which the individual engages in relationship to mutually facilitate awakening and service. This context and purpose transform the meaning of all interpersonal difficulties; anger and sadness are seen as feedback to both the individual and the relationship; power struggles are seen as gifts. While it may be easier to love humanity in the abstract than in the specific, to serve the poor rather than to serve our spouse, to guide and teach rather than to be led and learn, the healthy individual might well want to attempt both. Indeed it might even be that such a relationship could provide a foundation from which both partners could more effectively love, serve, and teach at a universal level. For the majority of us, this remains only a vision, but one which we may all be able to consciously move toward.

A Concluding Parable

In conclusion we would like to offer a short parable about the seeker after knowledge Naciketas:

Naciketas, bereft of heart after separating from his love of many years, sought solace and wisdom from a master. He set out on long pilgrimage to the mountains of Nepal, where it was rumored that a person wise in the ways of love and relationship could be found.

Many tears were shed along the path; many blisters formed as the pilgrim sought this wise one to ask the truth about the self, how to be strong and powerful and also able to develop a truly mature relationship—accepting, compassionate, nurturing, and caring.

The wise one had lived within his small cave nestled deep in the Himalayas for many years, cultivating a deep sense of compassion and love for other human beings, learning to still the mind and cultivate a warmth of heart.

One day the young pilgrim passed the cave, and only by chance looked in and saw the wise one sitting peacefully and staring in a fixed yet kindly fashion at a small candle.

Now, after so long a pilgrimage, and so close to the goal, the young pilgrim felt fear. Summoning all the courage possible, leaning his arm against the entrance of the cave, the pilgram peered in and said, "Excuse me for interrupting you."

"No interruption, I am pleased you came, come in," said the wise one, almost as if he were expecting this individual.

"I had difficulty finding you," said Naciketas. "The air is thin, the weather cold and there is no other person for miles around. Why, master, you who are so famous, do you endure such hardships in this cave? And why, if I may be so bold, why do you live up here alone"

The master thought for a moment and said, "To cultivate deep wisdom and compassion for others."

"But why don't you share that compassion?"

"I am, now, with you."

"But why not where more people can be near you? Or with another in a deep and enduring relationship?"

The wise one smiled, looked over at Naciketas, and said, "Let me share with you the secret of true compassion and relationship."

The young pilgrim sat near the master, watching the candle flame, feeling cold and yet with a sense of excitement as the master began to talk.

"First, for there to be love and true intimacy, you must learn to control your own mind, to silence its fears and doubts. This task is yours and no one else's, and you can ask or demand, but no one can do it for you."

"But what happens when this mind is still?"

"When your mind is sufficiently stilled, you will hear the sound of your own heart. Listen to it. For, until you hear your own heart, how can you hear the heart of another?"

The student spent many years studying with the master, and finally felt prepared to return to the world. Naciketas felt the lessons were learned and on the day of departure recited to the master a summary:

Love requires the clarity of a polished mirror, self-aware, but not self-preoccupied—able to attend to what is around.

Love requires the fearlessness of a samurai warrior going into battle but not afraid of death.

Love requires the wisdom of the Taoist sage who is willing to trust the process, let the stream flow without trying to alter its progress.

Love requires the precision of a scientist; and the endurance of an ascetic who can patiently travel miles through a burning desert, bare soles on hot sand.

And finally, love requires the softness and gentleness and freshness of a smile in a child's eye.

The master smiled graciously and said, "You have learned much, you have practiced hard, and there is only one more ability which you need have. As you go forth, realize the delicate humanness in us all, remember our frailty, hold your knowledge lightly, hold your own self lightly, and keep a sense of delicate joy and humor, a cosmic chuckle, along your path, for love requires this also.

"Now go, and bless you. . . ."

REFERENCES

1. Goldstein, J. *The Experience of Insight.* Unity Press: Santa Cruz, CA: 1977.
2. Franks, J. D. Nature and functions of belief systems: Humanism and transcendental religion. *American Psychologist,* 1977, 32, (7) 555-9.

3. Shapiro, D. Precision Nirvana. New Jersey: Prentice-Hall, 1978.
4. Peplau, L. A. What homosexuals want. *Psychology Today,* March, 1981, pp. 28–38.
5. Branden, N. *The Psychology of Romantic Love.* Los Angeles: J. P. Tarcher, 1981.
6. Shapiro, J. and Shapiro, D. Perceived rewards of intimacy: An investigation of males and females. Manuscript in preparation. University of California Irvine Medical Center.
7. Fromm, E. *The Art of Loving.* New York: Harper and Row, 1962.
8. Bardwick, J. *In Transition.* New York: Holt, Rinehart and Winston, 1979.
9. Sullivan, H. S. *The Interpersonal Theory of Psychiatry.* New York: W. W. Norton, 1953.
10. Vailliant, G. E. Natural history of male psychological health: correlates of successful marriage and fatherhood. *American Journal of Psychiatry,* 135:653–659 (1978).
11. Vailliant, G. E. and Milofsky, E. Natural history of male psychological health: Empirical evidence for Erickson's model of the life cycle. *American Journal of Psychiatry,* 137:11, 1980, 1348–1359.
12. Lynch, J. *The Broken Heart: The Medical Consequences of Loneliness.* New York: Basic Books, 1979.

III
NON-WESTERN
PERSPECTIVES

And yet there were the exalted figures of the sages and holy men themselves, each one of them a living example of the possibility of human growth and maturity and of the attainment of an imperturbable inner peace, a joyous freedom from guilt, and a purified, selfless goodness and calmness. . . . No matter how carefully I observed the waking lives of the holy men, no matter how ready they were to tell me about their dreams, I could not detect in the best of them a trace of selfish action or any kind of repressed or consciously concealed shadow life.

Medard Boss

Buddhist psychology is a gold mine of carefully categorized information on psychological well-being, and provides a particularly detailed and systematic description of both relevant theory and practices. The Buddha was clearly a man of extraordinary psychological and philosophical insight who 2500 years ago gave detailed descriptions of concepts which Western psychology has recognized only within recent decades, such as altered states of consciousness, state dependent learning, meditation, and cognitive behavior modification. Across the centuries Buddhism has profoundly influenced the cultures it has permeated, and no less a historian than Arnold Toynbee is said to have remarked that he considered its introduction to Western cultures to be one of the most significant events of our time.

In "The Ten Perfections," Roger Walsh describes in Western psychological terms the qualities said to characterize the highest levels of psychological development. Taken together they point to an individual of prodigious self-mastery who, through a life-style of impeccable commitment, ethicality, and mental training, has effectively eradicated all traces of egocentric motivation, leaving a profound understanding of the mind, the ways in which suffering is created, and a central desire to use this understanding for the well-being of all.

8

The Ten Perfections: Qualities
of the Fully Enlightened Individual
as Described in Buddhist Psychology

Roger Walsh

Such was the Buddha's impact that people sometimes felt he must be something more than human.
"Are you a God?" they wondered.
"No," replied the Buddha.
"Are you an angel?"
"No."
"Then what are you?" they asked.
"I am awake."

Huston Smith[1]

Like all branches of the perennial psychology, Buddhism is very much an applied psychology, aimed at training the mind and bringing it to optimal levels of functioning. The means for this are laid out in the eightfold path, a prescription for ethical living and meditation training, the meditative component of which will be described in Chapter 9 by Goleman and Epstein. The aim is the cultivation of certain mental qualities and attributes said to characterize the highest levels of enlightenment, qualities which can be recognized as the goals of all the great religious and consciousness disciplines.[2] In

218

Buddhist psychology, certain of these have been labeled as the ten "param-itas or perfections."[3]

While an individual may cultivate any one or more of these qualities, it is held that the simultaneous perfection of all ten was first attained by the Bud-dha, whose self-imposed training and discipline were extraordinarily ar-duous and broad ranging. He began his formal practice with concentrative meditation, and over a period of two years mastered all the higher levels of concentration, known as the jhanas, an extraordinarily rare achievement (for a discussion of these states, see Chapter 9). Not satisfied with the tem-porary nature of the relief of suffering which these states permitted, he next turned to the path of asceticism with a severity which almost killed him. Recognizing that extreme starvation and deprivation only impeded his men-tal faculties, he then relinquished asceticism and mastered the path of insight meditation among others, thus supposedly bringing to complete fruition all ten perfections.

The ten paramitas might be thought of as involving five overlapping cate-gories: effort (determination and energy), ethics (ethicality and truthful-ness), nonattachment (renunciation, patience, and equanimity), service to others (generosity and loving kindness), and wisdom. Although the refine-ment of these qualities to the degree described in Buddhist psychology may be exceedingly rare, all of us are said to possess them to varying extents and to be capable of cultivating them if we so choose.

1. Determination. Buddhist psychology is very explicit and repetitive about the need for intense determination and effort in attaining exceptional levels of well-being. "Oh Monks, rouse up yet more effort" is a familiar ex-hortation in the teachings of the Buddha, who was very explicit that

> It is you who must make the effort.
> The masters only point the way.
>
> The Buddha[4]

Buddhism makes no claims that the path to exceptional well-being is an easy one and regards the cultivation of unyielding determination as essential for overcoming the many difficulties that are encountered along the way.

2. Energy. One of the "five hindrances" which the practitioner must face and overcome is what the Buddhists have so picturesquely labeled "sloth and torpor".[5] Early in meditative practice there may be frequent experiences of low arousal, apathy, and sleepiness as the mind is deprived of its customary high levels of interaction, conversation, and stimulation. This claim has received recent support from empirical studies which show that beginning meditators may sometimes display electrical brain wave activity consistent with early stages of sleep.[6] The student must learn how to cultivate and control arousal and energy so as to reduce dependence on outside stimuli and bring the mind to an optimal level of activation freed from the extremes of both lethargy and agitation.

3. Ethicality.

> See yourself in others
> Then whom can you hurt?
> What harm can you do
>
> The Buddha[4]

Ethicality as it is implied in Buddhism and other consciousness disciplines has been much misunderstood in popular thinking and institutionalized religion. In the consciousness disciplines, ethicality is recognized as a functional and skillful device which is essential for mental training, not be confused with externally imposed moralism or sanctions. No one deeply involved in an intensive mental training program can long remain ignorant of the deleterious effects of unethical behavior on mental activity and control. The practitioner soon comes to recognize that unethical behavior is motivated by powerful emotions and states, such as greed, anger, or dislike, which grip the mind and render it hard to control.[5,7] Unethical behavior stems from such motives and at the same time conditions and reinforces them, thus leaving the mind more deeply entrapped in counterproductive conditioning, which in turn produces still more disruptive states such as agitation and guilt.

The practice of ethicality, on the other hand, is designed to reverse this process and to extinguish those attachments and emotions which produce it. The final result is the mind of the arahat (the fully enlightened individual), which is said to be totally freed of such states and hence to be quite incapable of unethical behavior.[3,8,9]

Ethicality is a particularly clear example of the synergistic nature of the paramitas. That is, they necessarily serve both the practitioner and others so that selfish or sacrificial, you or me, zero sum, win-lose dichotomies become meaningless.

4. Truthfulness.

The Buddha admonished his son to "never lie, even in jest." This stringent advice seems to reflect the Buddha's deep insight into the powerful influence of speech on our mental functioning and behavior.

Few of us are unaware of the effects of lying on our well-being. Like unethicality of which it is a part, lying reinforces the attachments, greed, and other unskillful behaviors which motivate us and result in further disrupting emotions such as guilt, agitation, and fear. Further lying and unethicality to protect the original lie frequently follow.

The impeccable practice of truthfulness, on the other hand, appears to serve many functions for the practitioner. It encourages ethicality, requires precise awareness of speech and motivation, enhances clear perception and memory of events which might otherwise be distorted by lying, frees the mind of guilt and fear of discovery, and consequently reduces agitation and worry.

The fully enlightened individual, freed from greed, attachment, anger, and other unskillful mind states, has neither desire nor need to distort the truth or act unethically. Those who are fully ethical have nothing to hide, and truthfulness, like all the other perfections, ultimately becomes a spontaneous and continuous expression of the arahat's essential nature.

Like a lovely flower,
Bright and fragrant
Are the fine and truthful words
Of the man who says what he means.

The Buddha[4]

5. Renunciation. Renunciation is an attribute somewhat foreign to our Western thinking and calls up images of asceticism, sacrifice, and the relinquishment of pleasure. However, a deeper understanding of the term as it is used in Buddhist psychology suggests that it implies the voluntary relinquishment of one source of pleasure in order to gain access to pleasures of a deeper and more permanent nature.

Contrary to our traditional Western models, Buddhist psychology recognizes four types of pleasure: sensory pleasures, pleasures arising from states of extreme concentration such as the jhanas, the pleasures of insight (i.e., the pleasure which arises as a result of training in insight meditation), and the pleasure of nirvana.[10,11] These pleasures are supposedly of increasing refinement, sensitivity, and degree.[5] The pleasures recognized by our Western models are confined to the first type, the sensory realm, which in Buddhist psychology includes mental pleasures such as memory and fantasy since in Buddhist psychology these are regarded as sensory inputs.

Renunciation can be viewed as a relinquishment of attachments to sense pleasures in order to cultivate the remaining three. This choice can also be seen in terms of Maslow's hierarchy of needs. Lower-order needs are primarily concerned with material objects and sensory stimulation, whereas higher-order needs are more concerned with internal self-produced stimulation and are held to be inherently more satisfying to the individual who has experienced them.[12-14] Thus renunciation can be viewed as a voluntary relinquishment of lower-order needs in order to cultivate the higher ones.

Renunciation also facilitates a life-style of voluntary simplicity.[15] With deepening perceptual sensitivity, practitioners of the consciousness disciplines are said to recognize more clearly the disrupting effects of greed and attachment.[9] At the same time, they find themselves better able to generate a sense of well-being and positive emotions which formerly depended upon external possessions and stimuli. Greater pleasure is now found in a deepening sensitivity to the moment-to-moment flow of experience, and each moment, no matter what one is doing, becomes a source of rich and multifaceted stimulation. Thus from this perspective, renunciation is seen not as an ascetic practice demanding sacrifice and suffering, but rather as a skillful means for removing distractions to the attainment of higher pleasure.

In the individual who has perfected this quality the mind is said to be free of attachment and aversion, and therefore to no longer covet, grasp after, or avoid any experience. Rather, all situations and stimuli are viewed with equanimity, itself also one of the perfections, and the individual's sense of well-being is no longer so dependent on the environment.

> If you are filled with desire
> Your sorrows swell
> Like the grass after the rain.
> But if you subdue desires
> Your sorrows fall from you
> Like drops of water from a lotus flower.
>
> The Buddha[4]

6. Patience.

> At the end of the way is freedom.
> Till then, patience
>
> The Buddha[4]

Impatience reflects dissatisfaction with present experience and attachment to anticipated experience. The result is, as almost all of us are aware, an agitated mental state characterized by discomfort and fantasy. Yet the work of mental training is to open to, accept, and be fully aware of all experience, moment by moment, neither resisting what is present, fantasizing about what could be, nor comparing the two.[5] Brought to fruition, patience removed preoccupation with anticipated experience, thus allowing the mind to fully experience the present moment while remaining calm, full of equanimity, and fantasy free. In the words of the Tibetan yogi Milarepa,[16] "The shortest road to freedom is the path of patience." In Buddhism patience also applies particularly to patience with others, a kind of nonjudgemental acceptance and forebearance. The person who can accept the present moment as it is can also accept others as they are.

7. Equanimity. The mind which responds with conditioned, automatic likes and dislikes is dominated by reactive pleasure and pain. Such a mind is at the mercy of its environment and is said to be turbulent, hard to control and concentrate, inconstant in purpose and direction, and insensistive in perception and insight.[3] With training, this conditioned reactivity and elaboration of strong affective responses is reduced, and the mind gradually becomes less reactive and more calm. As such, it becomes more easy to control and remains unperturbed in the face of an increasingly broad range of experience. Finally, it is said to be able to encompass all experiences and to allow "the one thousand beatific and one thousand horrible visions" to pass before it without disturbance. Of such a mind it is said,

Pleasure-pain
praise and blame
fame and shame
loss and gain
are all the same.

8. Generosity. The Buddha said that if we understood the power of generosity as deeply as he did, we would never sit down to a meal without sharing it.[5] Generosity has long been recognized as both means and end in all the major consciousness disciplines and great religions. It appears to be a powerful inhibitor of such unskillful mental habits as greed, attachment, and hatred. Buddhism describes three levels of generosity: beggarly, brotherly, and kingly. In beggarly giving, we give—with great hesitation and consideration—the worst and least valued of what we have. In brotherly giving, we share equally. In kingly giving, we unhesitatingly offer that which we most value for the pleasure and enjoyment of others.[5]

The fully enlightened individual, it is said, is no longer driven by egocentric motives of any kind. Rather, behavior is said to emerge spontaneously and appropriately in any situation in such a way as to most effectively serve and contribute to others. For such an individual, freed of unhealthy mental factors,[17] generosity is now the only possible response. As such, giving is no longer experienced as a sacrifice of any kind but rather as a natural and joyful expression of the perfections of loving kindness, renunciation, and ethicality which usually accompany it.

9. Loving Kindness.   Buddhist psychology describes several practices for the cultivation of loving kindness. Some appear to be almost perfect analogues of certain behavior modification techniques such as systematic desensitization. However, instead of replacing anxiety with calm as desensitization usually does, the Buddhist practices of loving kindness replace unskillful states such as anger and hatred with loving kindness.[3,18] This suggests that some of the principles of behavior modification were identified 2500 years earlier than has usually been recognizd.[19]

One family of practices for the cultivation of this quality is described for use by advanced practitioners with extreme powers of concentration. Such people are said to be able to completely fill all awareness with the experience of loving kindness or other desired qualities. Four such qualities are particularly recommended, namely, universal loving kindness, universal compassion, sympathetic joy (joy which derives from the well-being of others), and another of the ten perfections, equanimity.[3,5] When these qualities are held alone and without fluctuation in the fully concentrated mind, they are said to result in extremely positive and beneficial states which are labeled the four "divine abodes." When the extreme concentration is released, the qualities tend to dissipate in part though they do result in certain trait changes including readier access to them in the future and restraint of inhibiting factors such as anger. When perfected, the quality of loving kindness is no longer dependent on entering specific states of consciousness, but rather arises spontaneously.

10. Wisdom.   Like the other perfections, wisdom has many levels. A certain amount of it is considered necessary even to begin some type of mental training. Through this training, the mind is gradually brought under greater control, and perceptual distortions, unskillful habits, disruptive affects, and unskillful behavior of any type are gradually pared away. This leads to clearer perception and greater concentration, which in turn allow the recognition of still more subtle levels of unskillful habits that are pared away in their turn. The result is said to be a positive feedback cycle in which wisdom leads to the recognition of the need for removing unskillful habits and cultivating skillful ones, which in turn leads to greater wisdom.

One of the results is a deep insight and understanding, born of direct experience of what are called "the three marks of existence"—dukkha, anicca, and anatta. *Dukkha* is the recognition of the extent to which dissatisfaction and suffering pervade the untrained mind and of the fact that no possession or stimulation can completely or permanently remove it, a recognition analogous to the angst of the existentialists. *Anicca* is the recognition of impermanence—that everything is in constant flux, that nothing remains the same, and hence that there is no ultimate source of security in the world on which one can rely. *Anatta* refers to an insight that there is no permanent unchanging self or ego. Rather, what the advanced practitioner is said to recognize is that in the psyche there exists only an impersonal continuously changing flux of thoughts, emotions, and images.[9,11] The untrained mind identifies with these mental components and illusorily perceives them as evidence of the existence of a solid ego, much as a moviegoer perceives an illusory sense of continuity and motion even though there actually exists only a succession of still frames.

The deep recognition of these three marks of existence is said to result in a radical wrenching of one's cognitive system. Seeing the transitory and ultimately less than fully satisfying nature of sensory pleasures, as well as the illusory nature of our usual egoic identification, undermines egocentric motivation, thus enhancing renunciation and equanimity. Out of this wisdom springs a compassionate understanding of the counterproductive nature of the means by which people usually seek happiness but all too often only sow the seeds of further discontent. This in turn is said to lead to the desire to serve others and alleviate suffering wherever possible and the recognition that the perfection of the paramitas may be a strategic way of best fitting oneself for the task. With this realization, the individual has become a bodhisattva, one committed to both full enlightenment and selfless service to others.

Discussion

For ease of discussion the paramitas have been talked about as though they were separate and independent. Yet each largely rests upon and facilitates the others. Not one can be practiced and cultivated without thereby enhancing the others. Taken together, the *paramitas* point to an individual of prodigious self-refinement and mastery. To most of us in the West, the perfection of these qualities probably seems somewhat idealistic at best, if not totally unrealistic. The lack of any reference in our Western psychologies to the possibility of such attainments, together with a certain degree of cultural cynicism about human nature, makes such descriptions seem suspect. On the other hand, the perennial psychology has claimed for millennia that through mental training, such perfections not only are possible but are the highest goals to which any person can aspire and are also the most beneficial in terms of contributing to others.

The ten perfections as described here are taken from Buddhist psychology, yet similar qualities could be found at the esoteric core of most consciousness disciplines and great religions. As such they point to "the transcendent unity of religions," the fact that the highest goals of these traditions coverge on a common range of qualities and experiences, and a common picture of the fully actualized individual: the prototype saint of all traditions, the arahat of Buddhism, the sage of Taoism, the jivanmukti of Hinduism, or the master of Zen.

In any case, whether or not we think such qualities are fully perfectable, they can act as signposts and guiding values for our own lives. In addition, a certain inspiration, humility, and appreciation come from knowing that over thousands of years, up to and including the present time, there have been literally millions of our fellow human beings who have chosen to commit their lives at the deepest possible level to the cultivation and perfection of these qualities and who have done so as a means of contributing to us all.

For the unified mind in accord with the Way all self centered striving ceases.

Sengtsan[20]

REFERENCES

1. Smith, H. *The Religions of Man*. New York: Harper & Row, 1958.
2. Kornfield, J. Meditation: Aspects of theory and practice. In *Beyond Ego: Transpersonal Dimensions in Psychology*. (R. Walsh and F. Vaughan, Eds.). Los Angeles: J. Tarcher Press, 1980, pp. 150–153.
3. Buddhagosa. *The Path of Purity* (P. M. Tin, translator). Sri Lanka: Pali Text Society, 1923.
4. Byrom, T. (Translator) *The Dhammapada: The Sayings of the Buddha*. New York: Vintage, 1976.
5. Goldstein, J. *The Experience of Insight*. Santa Cruz, Calif.: Unity Press, 1976.
6. Shapiro, D. *Meditation: Self Regulation Strategy and Altered States of Consciousness*. New York: Aldine, 1980.
7. Walsh, R. Initial meditative experiences: I. *Journal of Transpersonal Psychology*, 1977, *9*, 151–192.
8. Goleman, D. *The Varieties of the Meditative Experience*. New York: E. P. Dutton, 1977.
9. Goleman, D. and Epstein, M. Meditation and well-being: An eastern model of psychological health. This book.
10. Mahasi Sayadaw. *Practical Insight Meditation*. Kandy, Sri Lanka: Buddhist Publication Society, 1976.
11. Mahasi Sayadaw. *The Progress of Insight*. Kandy, Sri Lanka: Buddhist Publication Society, 1978.
12. Maslow, A. H. *The Farther Reaches of Human Nature*. New York: Viking, 1971.
13. Roberts, T. Beyond self actualization. *ReVision*, 1978, *1*, 42–46.
14. Walsh, R. and Vaughan, F. Toward an integrative psychology of well-being. This book.
15. Elgin, D. *Voluntary Simplicity*. New York: Morrow, 1981.
16. Evans-Wentz, W. (Ed.). *Tibet's Great Yogi Milarepa* (2nd ed.). New York: Oxford University Press, 1951.
17. Goleman, D. Mental health in classical Buddhist psychology. In *Beyond Ego: Transpersonal Dimensions in Psychology* (R. Walsh and F. Vaughan, Eds.). Los Angeles, J. Tarcher Press, 1980, pp. 131–134.

18. Vimalo, B. Awakening to the truth. *Visaka Puja: Annual Publication of the Buddhist Association,* 1974, 53–79.
19. Shapiro, D. *Precision Nirvana: An Owner's Manual for the Care and Maintenance of the Mind.* New Jersey: Prentice Hall, 1978.
20. Sengtsan. *Verses on the Faith Mind* (R. B. Clarke, translator.). Sharon Springs, N. Y.: Zen Center, 1975.

To study Buddhism is to study the self.
To study the self is to forget the self.
To forget the self is to be one with others.

Zen master Dogen

One of the most detailed and descriptive accounts of the Eastern vision of psychological health is embodied in the classical text of the Abhidhamma. *This is a long and complicated text, and is very difficult for Western readers to understand, although the message it contains is one which may have a great deal of significance for our discussion of extreme psychological well-being. Daniel Goleman and Mark Epstein perform an invaluable service in this chapter by describing the Eastern concept of exceptional psychological health based on that text.*

Goleman and Epstein introduce the concept of mental factors and suggest that well being is defined by the balance between healthy and unhealthy ones. Healthy factors, by definition, are those which reduce our suffering, and unhealthy factors are those which increase it, and the Buddhist aim is to increase the healthy an decrease the unhealthy.

Meditation is described as a technique which can facilitate the increase of healthy mental factors. The authors describe the different types of meditation, including concentrative and insight practices as well as the factors which hinder and facilitate them. The chapter concludes by defining the Buddhist ideal of personality, and discussing Eastern and Western models of mental well-being.

Daniel Goleman, Ph.D., is a Senior Editor of Psychology Today. *He studied meditation and Asian psychologies while spending two years in India and Ceylon, first as a Harvard Travelling Fellow, and then as a Postdoctoral Fellow of the Social Science Research Council. He has published two dozen articles on meditation and Eastern psychologies, and is the author of* The Varieties of the Meditative Experience *(New York: E.P. Dutton, 1977) and coeditor of* Consciousness: The Brain, States of Awareness, and Mysticism *(New York: Harper & Row, 1979). While on the faculty of Harvard University, he supervised an honors thesis by Mark Epstein, M.D., on which this article is based in part.*

Mark Epstein, M.D., is a magna cum laude graduate of Harvard University in social relations and is a graduate of Harvard Medical School. He has been a student of Vipassana meditation, both in India and America, since 1974, has published papers on Buddhist psychology and is a psychiatrist.

228

9

Meditation and Well-Being: An Eastern Model of Psychological Health

Daniel Goleman and Mark Epstein

Attempts to forge a systematic understanding of human personality and mental health did not originate with contemporary Western psychology. Our formal psychology, about a hundred years old, is merely a recent version of an endeavor probably as old as human history. Western models of health and normality are the product of European and American culture, and are only one set of the innumerable ideals and norms that people in many times and places have articulated.

Some of the richest alternative sources of well-formulated psychologies and visions of human possibilities are Eastern religions. Quite separate from the vagaries of cosmology and the dogma of beliefs, most major Asian religions have at their core a psychology little known to the masses of adherents to the faith, but quite familiar to the appropriate "professionals," be they yogis, monks, or priests. This is the practical psychology that people apply to discipline their own minds and hearts in order to attain an ideal state of being.

Just as there are multitudes of personality theories in Western civilization, there are numerous Eastern psychologies. However, while there are major differences of belief and world view among the religions that contain the Eastern psychologies, there is far less difference among the psychologies themselves. One common feature of these psychologies is that they find fault with man as he is, positing an ideal mode of being that anyone can attain who seeks with diligence to do so. The path to this transformation is always via a far-reaching change, so that these ideal qualities may become stable traits. The Eastern psychologies also agree that the main means to this transformation of self is meditation.

Abhidhamma: An Eastern Psychology

One of the most systematic and intricately laid out of these psychologies is that of classical Buddhism. Called in the Pali language of Buddha's day *Abhidhamma* (or *Abhidharma* in Sanskrit), which means "the ultimate doctrine," this psychology elaborates Gautama Buddha's original insights into human nature. Since it stems from Buddha's basic teachings, Abhidhamma, or a psychology very much like it, is at the core of all the various branches of Buddhism. From its fullest development during the first millennium after Buddha's death, it has been preserved largely unchanged by the Theravadan Buddhists as part of their scriptures, the Pali Canon.

Many Abhidhamma principles represent the psychological teachings common to all Eastern faiths rather than those limited to Buddhism. As a prototype of Asian psychology, Abhidhamma presents us with a set of concepts for understanding mental activity and an ideal for mental health that differ markedly from the concepts of Western psychology. Like other Eastern psychologies, Abhidhamma contains an ideal type of the perfected personality around which its analysis of the workings of the mind is oriented. As Bhikkhu Nyanaponika, a modern Buddhist scholar-monk put it, "In the Buddhist doctrine, mind is the starting point, the focal point, and also, as the liberated and purified mind of the Saint, the culminating point" (1962, p. 12). Abhidhamma students follow the avenue of meditation to reach the end point in this model of the healthy personality.

What we denote by the word "personality" equates most closely in Abhidhamma to a concept of *atta,* or self. However, a central premise of Abhidhamma is that there is no abiding self whatsoever, only an impersonal aggregate of processes that come and go. The semblance of personality springs from the intermingling of these impersonal processes. What appears to be "self" is the sum total of body parts, thoughts, sensations, desires, memories, and so on. While we may identify the self with psychological activities such as our thoughts, memories, or perceptions, all these phenomena are part of a continued flow. Each successive moment of our awareness is shaped by the previous moment and will in turn determine the following moment; it is *bhavanga*—the "life-continuum" consciousness that, for example, predominates in deep sleep. The human personality, says Abhidhamma, is like a river that keeps a constant form, seemingly a single identity, though not a single drop is the same as a moment ago. In this view, "there is no actor apart from action, no percipient apart from perception, no conscious subject behind consciousness" (Aung, 1972, p. 7). In the words of Buddha (*Samyutta-Nikaya*, 1975, I, p. 35):

> Just as when the parts are set together
> There arises the word "chariot,"
> So does the notion of a being
> When the aggregates are present.

The study of personality in Buddhism does not deal with a complex of postulated entities, such as "ego" or "unconscious," but with a series of events. The basic event is the ongoing relationship of mental states to sense objects—for example, a feeling of desire (the mental state) toward a beautiful woman (the sense object). A person's mental states are in constant flux from moment to moment; their rate of change is reckoned in microseconds. The basic method Abhidhamma offers for studying the mind's multitudinous changes is introspection, a close and systematic observation of one's own experience.

In Abhidhamma, the mind itself is counted as the sixth sense, supplying information to awareness, and so thoughts are lumped with the objects of the five senses. Thus, just as a sound or a sight can be the object of a mental state, so can a thought—for example, the thought "I should take out the garbage," might be the object of a mental state of aversion. Each mental state is composed of a set of properties, called mental factors, which combine to flavor and define that state. The Abhidhamma system discussed here enumerates 53 categories of such mental factors; in other branches of Buddhism the count varies up to 175. In any one mental state only a subset of the factors are present. The unique qualities of each mental state are determined by which factors it combines.

Mental states come and go in a lawful and orderly manner. As in modern psychology, Abhidhamma theorists saw that each mental state derives in part from biological and situational influences, in addition to a carry-over from the preceding psychological moment. Each state in turn determines the particular combination of factors in the next mental state.

Healthy and Unhealthy Mental Factors

The Abhidhamma distinguishes between mental factors that are pure, wholesome, or healthy and those that are impure, unwholesome, or unhealthy. Most perceptual, cognitive, and affective mental factors fit into either the healthy or the unhealthy category. The judgment of healthy or unhealthy was arrived at empirically, on the basis of the collective experience of large numbers of early Buddhist meditators. Their criterion was whether a particular mental factor was the cause of suffering. Those factors that led to suffering were designated as "unhealthy," those that relieved it as "healthy."

In addition to healthy or unhealthy factors, there are seven common properties present in every mental state. Apperception is the mere awareness of an object; perception is its first recognition as belonging to one or the other of the senses; volition, the conditioned reaction that accompanies the first perception of an object; feeling, the quality of pleasantness, unpleasantness, or neutrality in experience; one-pointedness, the focusing of awareness; spontaneous attention, the involuntary directing of attention because of attraction by the object; and psychic energy, that which lends vitality to and unites the other six factors. These factors provide a basic framework of consciousness in which the healthy and unhealthy factors are embedded. The particular combination of unhealthy and healthy properties that embeds in this framework varies from moment to moment.

Unhealthy Factors. The central unhealthy factor, delusion, is perceptual: delusion is defined as a cloudiness of mind that leads to misperception of the object of awareness. Delusion is seen in Abhidhamma as basic ignorance, the primary root of human suffering. This misperception of the true nature of things—the simple failure to see clearly, without bias or prejudice of any kind—is the core of all unhealthy mental states. Delusion, for example, leads to "false view" or misdiscernment. False view entails miscategorization, and so is the natural outcome of misperception. The working of these factors is clear in the case of the paranoid, who misperceives as threatening someone who wishes him no harm, and so categorizes the other person as part of a fancied conspiracy against himself. The Buddha is quoted as saying that while a man's mind is dominated by false view, whatever he might do or aspire to could only "lead him to an undesirable, unpleasant, and disagreeable state, to woe and suffering" (*Anguttara-Nikaya,* 1975, I, p. 23).

Perplexity denotes the inability to decide or make a correct judgment. When this property dominates a person's mind he is filled with doubt and, at the extreme, can become paralyzed. Other unhealthy cognitive factors are shamelessness and remorselessness; these attitudes allow a person to disregard the opinions of others and one's own internalized standards, respectively. When these hold sway, a person views evil acts without compunction, and so is apt to misbehave. Indeed, these factors are prerequisites for the mental states that underly any act of ill will. Another unwholesome property that might lead to wrong doing is egoism, comparing oneself to others. This attitude of self-interest causes a person to view objects solely in terms of fulfilling his own desires or needs. The concatenation of these three mental factors in a single moment—shamelessness, remorselessness, and selfishness—is undoubtedly often the basis for much human evil.

The rest of the unhealthy mental factors are affective. Agitation and worry are states of distractedness, remorse, and rumination. These create a state of anxiety, the central feature of most mental disorder. Another set relate to clinging: greed, avarice, and envy denote different kinds of grasping attachment to an object, while aversion is the negative side of attachment. Greed and aversion are found in all negative mental states, and always combine with delusion. Two final unhealthy factors are contraction and torpor; these lend a rigid inflexibility to mental states. When these negative factors predominate, a person's mind as well as his body is prone to sluggishness.

Healthy Factors.   Each of the unhealthy factors is opposed by a healthy one. The central healthy factor is insight, the opposite of delusion. Insight, in the sense of "clear perception of the object as it really is," suppresses delusion. These two factors cannot coexist in a single mental state: where there is clarity, there cannot be delusion; nor where there is delusion in any degree can there be clarity. Mindfulness is the continued clear comprehension of an object; this essential partner of insight steadies and holds clarity in a person's mind. Insight and mindfulness are the primary healthy factors; when they are present in a mental state, the other healthy properties tend to be present also. The presence of these two healthy factors is sufficient to suppress all of the unhealthy ones.

Some healthy factors require certain circumstances to arise. The twin cognitive factors of modesty, which inhibits shamelessness, and discretion, the opposite of remorselessness, come to mind only when there is a thought of an evil act. Modesty and discretion are always connected with rectitude, the attitude of correct judgment. Faith or confidence is a sureness based on correct perception. This group—modesty, discretion, rectitude, and confidence—act together to produce virtuous behavior as judged by both personal and social standards.

The cluster of unhealthy factors formed by greed, avarice, envy, and aversion is opposed by the healthy properties of nonattachment, nonaversion, impartiality, and composure, which reflect the physical and mental tranquillity that arises from diminishing positive and negative feelings of attachment. These four factors replace a grasping or rejecting attitude with an evenmindedness toward whatever object might arise in a person's awareness. They allow one to accept things as they are, but also to respond in whatever way seems appropriate.

Body and mind are seen as interconnected in Abhidhamma. While every factor affects both body and mind, the final set of healthy factors are the only ones explicitly described as having both physical and psychological effects. These are buoyancy, pliancy, adaptability, and proficiency. When these arise a person thinks and acts with a natural looseness and ease, performing at the peak of his skills. They suppress the unhealthy factors of contraction and torpor, which dominate the mind in states such as depression. These healthy properties enable one to adapt physically and mentally to changing conditions, meeting whatever challenges may arise.

The factors usually arise as a group, either positive or negative. In any given mental state the factors that compose it arise in differing strengths; whichever property is the strongest determines how a person experiences and acts at any given moment. Although all the negative factors may be present, the state experienced will be quite different depending on whether, for example, it is greed or torpor that dominates the mind. When a particular factor or set of factors occurs frequently in a person's mental states, then it becomes a characteristic trait. Table 9–1 lists the healthy and unhealthy factors.

Table 9-1. Healthy and Unhealthy Factors.*

UNHEALTHY FACTORS

Perceptual

Delusion (*moha*): cloudiness of mind that leads to misperception of the object of awareness. "Delusion has the characteristic of blindness . . . of unknowing. Its function is to conceal the individual essence of an object. . . . It should be regarded as the root of all that is unprofitable." (p. 530)

Cognitive

False view (*ditthi*): misdiscernment, miscategorization; opinions based on misperception of a situation. "Its characteristic is unjustified interpreting. Its function is to preassume. It is manifested as wrong interpreting. . . . It should be regarded as the most reprehensible of all." (p. 530)

Egoism (*mana*): conceit, arrogance, pride; comparing one's own qualities with those of another to one's own advantage. "That has the characteristic of haughtiness. . . . It should be regarded as like madness." (p. 531)

Perplexity (*vicikiccha*): doubt, indecisiveness; Inability to decide. "Its function is to waver." (p. 533)

Shamelessness (*ahirika*): absence of inner anxiety, or conscience, during the performance of unwholesome acts; inability to see the worthiness inherent in certain thoughts or actions.

Remorselessness (*anottappa*): inability to perceive the consequences of one's actions on others, or lack of anguish over those consequences; lack of scruples.

* All page numbers refer to *Visuddhimagga* (1975).

Affective

Greed (*lobha*): attachment, clinging, craving, desire, acquisitiveness directed at desirable objects. "Greed has the characteristic of grasping an object. . . . Its function is sticking, like meat put in a hot pan. It is manifested as not giving up. . . . Its proximate cause is seeing enjoyment in things that lead to bondage. Swelling with the current of craving, it should be regarded as taking beings with it to states of loss, as a swift flowing river does to the great ocean." (p. 529)

Aversion (*dosa*): ill will, hatred, anger; displeasure with regard to the object; pollutes all co-present mental factors. "It has the characteristic of savageness, like a provoked snake. Its function is to spread, like a drop of poison, or its function is to burn up its own support, like a forest fire. It is manifested as persecuting, like an enemy who has got his chance. . . . It should be regarded as like stale urine mixed with poison." (p. 532)

Envy (*issa*): the inability to endure the success and prosperity of others, leading to dissatisfaction with one's own condition. "It should be regarded as a fetter." (p. 532)

Avarice (*macchariya*): selfishness; concealing one's own success so as to avoid sharing it with others. "Its characteristic is the hiding of one's own success that has been or can be obtained. Its function is not to bear sharing these with others. It is manifested as shrinking, or . . . meanness. Its proximate cause is one's own success. It should be regarded as a mental disfigurement." (p. 532)

Agitation (*uddhacca*): restlessness. "It has the characteristic of disquiet, like water whipped by the wind. Its function is unsteadiness, like a flag or banner whipped by the wind. It is manifested as turmoil, like ashes flung up by pelting with stones. Its proximate cause is unwise attention to mental disquiet." (p. 530)

Worry (*kukkucca*): brooding or grieving over unwholesome acts already performed or over wholesome acts never done. "It has subsequent regret as its characteristic. Its function is to sorrow about what has and what has not been done. It is manifested as remorse. . . . It should be regarded as slavery." (p. 532)

Contraction (*thina*): stiffness, sloth, lack of vitality or motivating force. "Stiffness has the characteristic of lack of driving power. Its function is to remove energy. It is manifested as subsiding." (p. 530)

Torpor (*middha*): laziness, boredom—producing an inability to deal with the object of awareness. "Torpor has the characteristic of unwieldiness. Its function is to smother. It is manifested as laziness, or it is manifested as nodding and sleep." (p. 530) Activity of co-present mental factors is inhibited due to the smothering capacity of torpor.

HEALTHY FACTORS
Perceptual

Insight (*panna*): wisdom, nondelusion; clear perception of the object as it really is. "Nondelusion has the characteristic of penetrating things according to their individual essences, or it has the characteristic of sure penetration, like the penetration of an arrow shot by a skillful archer. Its function is to illuminate the objective field, like a lamp. It is manifested as non-bewilderment, like a guide in the forest." (p. 525) Insight is not necessarily present when the other healthy factors arise.

Mindfulness (*sati*): continued clear comprehension of an object. "It has the characteristic of not wobbling. Its function is not to forget. It is manifested as guarding, or it is manifested as the state of confronting an objective field. . . . It should be regarded as like a pillar because it is firmly founded, or as like a door-keeper because it guards the sense-doors." (p. 524)

Cognitive

Confidence (*saddha*): assurance based on correct perception; well-founded faith. "Its characteristic is trusting. Its function is to clarify, like a water-clearing gem, or its function is to enter into, like the setting out across a flood. It is manifested as non-fogginess, or it is manifested as resolution. . . . It should be regarded as a hand, because it takes hold of profitable things. . . . " (p. 524)

Modesty (*hiri*): inner conscience which creates an abhorrence for evil; functions in the present moment to prevent any evil action. "It has conscientious scruples about bodily misconduct. . . . It has the characteristic of disgust at evil. . . . It has the function of not doing evil. . . . Its proximate cause is self-respect. . . . " (p. 524)

Discretion (*ottappa*): anxiety over wrongdoing out of respect for others. It is ashamed of bodily misconduct. . . . It has the characteristic of dread of evil. . . . It has the function of not doing evil. . . . Its proximate cause is the respect of others. . . . (p. 524)

Rectitude (*ujakata*): correct judgment, decisiveness, uprightness, honesty, lack of insincerity. It has "the characteristic of uprightness. . . . Its function is to crush tortuousness. . . . It is manifested as noncrookedness. . . . It should be regarded as opposed to deceit, fraud, etc., which cause tortuousness in the mental body and in consciousness."

Affective

Nonattachment (*alobha*): nongreed or active generosity. "Non-greed has the characteristic of the mind's lack of desire for an object, or it has the characteristic of non-adherence, like a water drop on a lotus leaf. Its function is not to lay hold, like a liberated bhikku (yogi or monk)." (p. 525)

Nonaversion (*adosa*): may be absence of ill will or aversion, or active friendliness, sympathy, goodwill, or love. "Non-hate has the characteristic of lack of savagery, or the characteristic of non-opposing, like a gentle friend. Its function is to remove annoyance, or its function is to remove fever, as sandalwood does. It is manifested as agreeableness, like the full moon." (p. 525)

Impartiality (*tatramajjhattata*): balance of mind, equanimity; impartial view of the object. "Its function is to prevent deficiency and excess, or its function is to inhibit partiality. It is manifested as neutrality. It should be regarded as like a conductor (driver) who looks with equanimity on thoroughbreds progressing evenly." (p. 527)

Composure (*passaddhi*): tranquillity, calmness, serenity. "Its function is to crush disturbance of the mental body and of consciousness. It is manifested as inactivity and coolness. . . . It should be regarded as opposed to the defilements of agitation, etc., which cause unpeacefulness." (p. 525)

Buoyancy (*lahuta*): lightness, nonsluggishness; agility of mind and body.

Pliancy (*muduta*): elasticity, malleability. "They have the characteristic of quieting rigidity in the mental body and in consciousness. Their function is to crush stiffening. . . . They are manifested as nonresistance. . . . They should be regarded as opposed to the defilements of views, conceit, etc., which cause stiffening. . . . " (p. 526)

Adaptability (*kammannata*): wieldiness; allows object to be dealt with efficiently, as mind and body are prevented from being either too soft or tranquil or too rigid.

Proficiency (*pagunnata*): fitness, competence, skillfulness of function, healthiness. "They are manifested as absence of disability. . . . They should be regarded as opposed to faithlessness, etc., which cause unhealthiness. . . . " (p. 526)

THE HEALTHY PERSONALITY AND MENTAL DISORDER

The factors that form one's mental states from moment to moment determine one's mental health. The operational definition of mental disorder in Abhidhamma is simple: the continuing absence of healthy factors and the sustained presence of unhealthy factors. Each variety of mental disorder stems from the hold of certain unhealthy factors on the mind. The special character of each unhealthy factor leads to a particular disorder—egoism, for example, underlies the purely self-interested actions which we in modern psychology call "sociopathic" behavior; agitation and worry are the anxiety at the core of neuroses; aversion tied to a specific object or situation is a phobia.

The criterion for mental health is equally simple: the presence of the healthy factors, and the relative absence of unhealthy factors, in a person's psychological economy. The healthy factors, besides supplanting unhealthy ones, also provide a necessary mental environment for a group of positive affective states that cannot arise in the presence of the unhealthy factors. These include loving kindness and "altruistic joy" (i.e., taking pleasure in the happiness of others).

The normal person has a mixture of healthy and unhealthy factors in the flow of his mental states. Each of us probably experiences periods of wholly healthy or unhealthy mental states as our stream of consciousness flows on. Very few people, however, experience only healthy mental states, and thus all of us are "unhealthy" in this sense. Indeed, one scripture quotes the Buddha as saying of normal people, "All worldlings are deranged." The goal of psychological development in Abhidhamma is to increase the amount of healthy states and, correspondingly, decrease unhealthy ones. At the peak of mental health, no unhealthy factors arise at all in a person's mind. While this is the ideal that each person is urged to seek for himself, it is, of course, rarely realized.

Meditation: Means to a Healthy Personality.   As a catalogue of the mental properties we experience from moment to moment, the Abhidhamma list of mental factors is by no means exhaustive. The possibilities for categorizing mental states are countless; the Abhidhamma theorists do not pretend to offer a total compendium, but theirs is a purposeful analysis: their categories are designed to help a person through simple awareness to recognize key states of mind so that he may ultimately rid himself of unhealthy states. The practicing Buddhist embarks on a coordinated program of environmental, behavioral, and attentional control to attain his final goal, a plateau of purely healthy mental states. In the classical Buddhist path, a person who sought this plateau of health would enter the controlled surroundings of a monastery, regulate his actions by taking the 227 vows of a monk or nun, and most important, meditate.

Once a person has become familiar with the categories of healthy and unhealthy mental factors so that he can see them at play in his own mind, he will find that simply knowing a state is unhealthy does little or nothing to end it. For example, if a person resents the predominance of unhealthy factors in his mind, or if he wishes they would go away, he is merely adding aversion and desire to the psychological mix. The strategy the Abhidhamma offers for attaining healthy states is neither directly to seek them nor to be averse to unhealthy states. The optimal approach is noninterfering, clear awareness of them, a process best achieved through meditation.

Meditation is, technically speaking, the consistent attempt to maintain a specific attentional set. For example, in the effort to keep his attention on the sensations of breathing, the meditator tries to keep his mind concentrated. His mind will not actually stay concentrated, but will wander to other thoughts and feelings. In practice he spends most of his time trying to *remember* to return his wandering mind to his breath, the object of concentration. The important thing is his attempt to concentrate on the breath. In an alternate type of meditation, called "mindfulness," the meditator adopts a neutral stance toward whatever comes and goes in his stream of awareness, placing an equal value on whatever arises in his mind. No matter what might cross his mind, the meditator tries to maintain his mindfulness. His effort is not toward the generation of healthy factors per se. Because the healthy factors are the mental properites that keep his attention stable, they will come to .dominate his mind as a by-product of his success in meditation. By learning to meditate with greater proficiency, the meditator at the same time increases the amount of healthy factors in his mental states.

Opposites

The means in Abhidhamma for attaining a healthy mental state is by replacing the unhealthy factors with their polar opposites. The principle that allows this is akin to "reciprocal inhibition" as used in systematic desensitization, where relaxation inhibits its physiologic opposite, tension. For each negative mental facet there is a corresponding positive factor which overrides it. When a given healthy factor is present in a mental state, the unhealthy factor it suppresses cannot arise.

In the Abhidhamma psychodynamics, positive and negative mental factors are mutually inhibiting; the presence of one suppresses its opposite. However, there is not always a one-to-one correspondence between a pair of healthy and unhealthy factors; in some cases a single healthy factor will inhibit a set of unhealthy factors—nonattachment alone, for example, inhibits greed, avarice, envy, and aversion. Certain key factors will inhibit the entire opposite set; for example, when delusion is present, not a single positive factor can arise with it.

For each unwholesome factor there exists at least one wholesome factor that effectively blocks the entry of its negative counterpart into consciousness. In cases in which specific unwholesome factors are particularly intense, their oppositions must be repeatedly invoked in order to eradicate them. As the influence of the unhealthy factors dwindles, the strength of the corresponding healthy influences increases. Progress in meditation may be described solely in terms of which wholesome qualities are cultivated at the expense of which unwholesome ones, a process aiming at the *eradication* of all unwholesome factors from one's mental economy.

The dynamics of the wholesome-unwholesome duality clears the way for a mind cleansed of unwholesome factors. When a specific wholesome factor is present, its unwholesome counterparts cannot be—as that wholesome quality increases in strength, the likelihood that its negative counterpart will arise decreases accordingly. If the wholesome factor becomes a constant staple of the mind, the other will never find room to assert itself.

Wholesome factors cannot exist in the same mind moment as unwholesome factors because of specific antagonistic relationships between mental factors. The mind cannot be felt to be both heavy and light, both clear and hazy, at the same time. The existence of one at a given moment nullifies the other. Normal waking consciousness involves an oscillation between the two influences, but a complete absence of all of the unhealthy factors is rarely found in normal awareness for any great length of time. The Abhidhamma ideal of mental well-being, though, posits the total abeyance of unhealthy factors.

Methods of Eradicating Unwholesome Factors: Concentration versus Mindfulness

The *Visuddhimagga* spells out two distinct methods of reorganization of consciousness designed to lessen and finally eradicate the impact of the unwholesome factors. The first employs a meditative strategy of concentration; the second, one of mindfulness. Progress in one or the other form of meditation may be understood and explained solely in terms of the restructuring of roles played by various mental factors.

The Abhidhamma assumes as a starting point a person whose mind is bound by unwholesome factors. When the wholesome factors are weak, a person's psychological health is poor; as seen through the Abhidhamma lens, the mental state of a normal person is rather dour:

> A general heaviness and unwieldiness of the mental processes results: force of habit predominates; changes and adaptations are undertaken slowly and unwillingly, and to the smallest possible degree; thought is rigid, inclined to dogma. It takes long to learn from experience or advice; affections and aversions are fixed and biased; in general the character proves more or less inaccessible. (Nyanaponika, 1949, p. 67)

As a person's mindfulness and concentration are both assumed to be weak, very little control over perceptual abilities is expected of him at the outset. The initial steps aim to make the meditator's mind pliable and receptive to the influence of wholesome qualities while loosening the ingrained control of the unwholesome factors. Initial practice is often difficult and even painful since the meditator's mind is unaccustomed to the kind of mental discipline demanded.

Concentration

On the path of concentration the meditator strives to restrict his awareness solely to a single object. Such a limitation is virtually impossible in normal consciousness, for the neutral mental factor of concentration is undeveloped. Normally the mind constantly shifts objects of attention, a fact observed by William James (1910), who noted that it seemed impossible to hold a single object in his awareness for more than a few moments. Even when the meditator expends an enormous amount of effort in the attempt to keep his mind on the object, whatever it may be, his focus is apt to slip away. Thoughts, desires, feelings, and external sense perceptions all intrude upon consciousness; unwholesome factors do not easily lose their grip on the mind. Much practice is needed if the meditator's mind is to become capable of remaining on a single object beyond the normal limits of attention.

Five Hindrances versus Factors of Absorption

The meditator's progress in concentration is inhibited by a set of unwholesome factors collectively termed the five hinderances: lust (or greed), ill will, sloth and torpor, agitation and worry, and doubt. These factors are especially bothersome when a person attempts to develop concentration; as the *Visuddhimagga* (1975, p. 152) put it:

> The mind affected through lust by greed for varied objects does not become concentrated on an object consisting in unity, or being overwhelmed by lust, it does not enter on the way to abandoning the sense-desire element. When pestered by ill-will towards an object, it does not occur uninterruptedly. When overcome by stiffness and torpor, it is unwieldly. When seized by agitation and worry, it is unquiet and buzzes about. When stricken by uncertainty, it fails to mount the way to accomplish the attainment of jhana [a state of prolonged concentration].

As concentration develops, certain other factors develop; as they grow, concentration strengthens. In order for concentration to be strong enough to fix the mind on a single object, these factors—resolution, energy, willingness, attention, rapture, and one-pointedness—must all arise together, an event which does not occur except when concentration builds. Resolution allows the energy necessary for extended concentration, and willingness directs the mind to the one object. The other particular factors—initial and sustained attention (i.e., turning a focus toward the object and keeping it there) and rapture along with the joyful aspect of feeling and one-pointedness—counter the five hindrances mentioned above. Initial and sustained attention, rapture, joy, and concentration form a team which, when specifically cultivated, prevents any deviation from the single point of focus.

In moments of concentration, the strength of these normally innocuous factors is powerful enough to counter the otherwise potent influence of the hindrances. Specifically, initial application of the mind to the object overwhelms the activity of sloth and torpor, which avoid the object because it appears unwelcome. Sustained application, which keeps the mind on the object, suppresses the influence of doubt, which jumps from object to object in indecision. Joy, which is delight in the object, counters the agitation which exemplifies worry and restlessness. Rapture, which is fascination with the object, diminishes the influence of ill will, which rejects the object with a displeased state of mind. One-pointedness, which is the actual fixity of the mind in the object, counters the influence of greed and lust, which are continually seeking after novel objects to be enjoyed. When they arise together, these five factors—applied and sustained attention, joy, rapture, and one-pointedness—are called the "factors of absorption."

Access Concentration

When the factors of absorption dominate the meditator's consciousness, he experiences the first moment of what is termed "access" concentration. Access concentration is simply a moment of fixity on the object, the first direct experience of what is possible through concentration. This achievement is not lasting; the mind soon flits back into its habitual territory of random thoughts, feelings, and sensations. The factors of absorption at this point are nowhere near developed to their full capacity; the meditator remains vulnerable to external and internal distractions which constantly impinge upon his concentration. Access concentration comes and goes, since the meditator cannot yet remain immersed in an object of his own free will. Still this concentrative ability—precarious though it may be—marks the attainment of a level from which the mind may become absorbed in the object.

Jhana

With continued practice, the factors which were strong in access concentration become even stronger, to the point where the mind becomes totally absorbed in the meditation object for the first moment ever. This marks the attainment of the first level of *jhana,* a trance or absorption that is a total break with normal consciousness. At this moment the five factors of absorption are predominant. Each successive moment of consciousness focuses upon the same object, and absolutely no other objects—whether they be thoughts, feelings, or sense perceptions—intrude for the duration of the jhana. Most of the wholesome factors are strengthened, and most of the unwholesome factors are weakened, by the process that brings the meditator to the first jhana. The meditator's first attainment of jhana lasts for only an instant, but upon continued practice, the jhana may be mastered so that the meditator can enter it at will for as long as he desires. In the first jhana, the object of consciousness remains constant.

The meditator's strength of attention in jhana suppresses sloth, torpor, and doubt for the duration of the jhana path, a series of progressively more subtle states of concentration. In the place of sloth and torpor arise buoyancy, pliancy, adaptability, and proficiency of mind. In place of doubt arise faith, equanimity, tranquillity, and rectitude. The meditator in the first jhana experiences fixity in the object accompanied by joy, rapture, calm, mental agility, and equanimity.

One of the fruits of jhana mastery is the capacity to develop what are termed the four "illimitables," or measureless states. These include compassion, sympathetic joy, all-embracing kindness, and equanimity. Through a set of concentration exercises tailored to that purpose, the meditator can cultivate these attitudes toward all beings:

> Just as at the sight of a dear and agreeable person one may feel kindness, just so does he penetrate with his kindness to all living beings....

Just as, when seeing one man living in misery and distress, one may feel compassion: just so the monk penetrates all beings with compassion. . . .

Just as, when seeing a kind and dear person, one feels joy, just so the monk penetrates all beings with joy. . . .

Just as, when seeing somebody who to oneself is neither agreeable, nor disagreeable, one remains indifferent, just so the monk penetrates all living beings with equanimity. (Nyanatiloka, 1952, pp. 102–110)

Limits of Concentration

Despite the allure of such states, Buddhist tradition regards the jhanas as limited in usefulness. There is an afterglow from the jhanas, so that after the meditator emerges from these states, the unwholesome factors are weak. However, the effects of jhana are state dependent and sooner or later wear off; the state is an impermanent one which must be reentered in order for the meditator to reexperience its effects. The unwholesome factors are temporarily suppressed, but remain latent until they are able to reassert themselves. Proficiency of concentration does nothing to eradicate the influence of delusion; its suppression of the other unhealthy factors is only temporary.

The limitations of proficient concentration may be understood in another way. There are said to be three levels at which the unwholesome factors function: transgression in deeds or in speech, transgression in internal thought processes (where, for instance, hatred will be felt toward a person but not acted upon), and a latent potential for such factors to arise if the appropriate situation occurs. Eradication at the first two levels is not sufficient in the Buddhist view of psychological growth; the meditator achieves complete freedom from the unwholesome factors only with the elimination of their latent potential. The fixity of mind which concentration offers temporarily suppresses the unwholesome factors but does not itself get to the root of the problem. This deeper penetration can be accomplished only through the factor of insight, or wisdom. This demands a different meditative strategy from that employed for concentration, although it builds on concentrative skills.

Mindfulness and Insight

The meditator can achieve freedom from the unwholesome factors only through the cultivation of mindfulness, which blossoms into the establishment of insight. Insight finally can culminate in an altered state called "nibbana" (more commonly known by its Sanskirt name, *nirvana*), in which the unwholesome factors are permanently eradicated. Mindfulness and insight are different, though related. In mindfulness, the meditator notes successive moments of consciousness; with insight, the meditator examines the characteristics of those mind-moments. The meditator's mindfulness ripens into insight at the moment when it becomes strong enough that he remains attentive to the ever-changing flux of his consciousness without succumbing to a single distraction.

During mindfulness training the meditator notices whatever is most distinct in his consciousness. He may attend to a central object, such as the breath, but also notes thoughts, feelings, or sounds as they arise in his awareness. The aim is not to reduce awareness to a single object (as in concentration) but rather to remain attentive to the ebb and flow of consciousness. Gradually, the meditator calms his mind so that he observes stray thoughts or feelings from their outset, but is not carried away by them.

> To note mindfully, and immediately, the arising of one of the hindrances ... is a simple but very effective method of countering these and any other defilements of mind. By doing so, a brake is applied against the uninhibited continuance of unwholesome thoughts, and the watchfulness of mind against their recurrence is strengthened. This method is based on a simple psychological fact which is expressed by the commentators as follows: "A good and evil thought cannot occur in combination. Therefore at the time of *knowing* the sense desire (that arose in the proceeding moment) that sense desire does no longer exist (but only the act of knowing)." (Nyanaponika, 1963, p. 4)

Faculties

Five faculties emerge as dominant factors as the meditator cultivates mindfulness: faith, energy, wisdom, mindfulness, and concentration. These factors provide the meditator with the energy, skill, and confidence necessary to continue along the path of insight. There is a danger of loss of directive energy if the five faculties are out of harmony with each other. If the meditator develops one or several at the expense of the others, no further progress is possible. Mindfulness keeps the other faculties in balance.

Stages in the Development of Insight

Observation of whatever is most distinct in the mind marks the first stage in the development of insight. At the second stage, known as "purification of mind," there arise the development of moment-to-moment concentration, mindfulness sharpened to the point of instantaneous noticing of stray thoughts, and temporary relief from the unwholesome factors. Mindfulness matures into insight when contemplation continues without lag; the meditator notices each and every moment in the stream of awareness in unbroken succession.

The third stage, known as "purification of view," marks the beginning of insight into the moment-to-moment processes of mind. The meditator's experience of consciousness in this stage continually arises anew with each successive object. The meditator perceives consciousness and its object as clearly distinct phenomena arising and passing away together in each moment. This insight into the impermanence of consciousness deals a severe blow to the meditator's illusion that there is a "self"; he understands the "voidness of self." Insight can now penetrate into the true nature of the process of consciousness.

Overcoming of Doubt

This intensification of insight allows the fourth stage, "overcoming of doubt." At this stage the meditator develops insight into the cause-effect relationship in each moment of experience, i.e., how each mind-moment arises due to causes and vanishes when they dissipate. When still noticing one object, the next will appear; when noticing that one, another arises. As insight continues to intensify, the meditator notices both the arising and the passing away of objects, and sees that a new object cannot arise until the previous one has passed away. With this awareness he comprehends the three characteristics inherent in all phenomena: impermanency, insubstantiality, and suffering. This knowledge helps to overcome the meditator's latent store of doubt about how the mind works.

Through the overcoming of doubt and false view, chain reactions are set in motion which inhibit all three primary unhealthy factors—greed, hatred, and delusion. Weakening the unwholesome factors strengthens insight in every way. If a person reaches this stage of development in meditation, he is said to have the potential for enlightenment in this lifetime.

Pseudo-Nibbana

With the clarity of perception that allows the meditator to see clearly the beginning and end of each successive moment of awareness there may occur:

- the vision of a brilliant light or luminous form;
- rapturous feelings that cause gooseflesh, tremor in the limbs, the sensation of levitation, and the other attributes of rapture;
- tranquility in mind and body, making them light, plastic and wieldy;
- devotional feelings toward, and faith in, the meditation teacher, the

Buddha, his teachings—including the method of insight itself—and the spiritual community, accompanied by joyous confidence in the virtues of meditation and the desire to advise friends and relatives to practice it;

• vigor in meditating, with a steady energy neither too lax nor too tense;

• sublime happiness suffusing the meditator's body, an unprecedented bliss that seems never-ending and motivates him to tell others of this extraordinary experience;

• quick and clear perception of each moment of awareness: noticing is keen, strong, and lucid, and the characteristics of impermanence, nonself, and unsatisfactoriness are clearly understood at once;

• strong mindfulness so the meditator effortlessly notices every successive moment of awareness—mindfulness gains a momentum of its own;

• equanimity toward whatever comes into awareness: no matter what comes into his mind, the meditator maintains a detached neutrality; and

• a subtle attachment to the lights and other factors listed here, and pleasure in their contemplation.

As the wholesome factors become strengthened, the meditator experiences them so powerfully he may convince himself he has finally been enlightened. This stage, however, is called a "corruption" of insight because of the dangerous attractiveness for the meditator of this experience. These experiences are corruptions only because of the meditator's attachment to them.

Dissolution

This attachment is rectified by "knowledge and vision of what is and is not the path," whereby the meditator returns to his meditative practice, noting each of the "corruptions" mindfully as they enter his awareness. By turning the focus of insight on them, he severs attachment to them. He then progressively refines his insight so that finer and finer distinctions of mindmoments are made. As the precision of his insight intensifies, the ending of each moment of awareness is more clearly perceived than its arising. Finally the meditator perceives each moment only as it vanishes; consciousness and its object are seen as constantly dissolving. Says the *Visuddhimagga* (1975, p. 752) of this stage:

He disregards the arising, presence, occurrence and sign of all formations, which keep on breaking up, like fragile pottery being smashed, like fine dust being dispersed, like sesamum seeds being roasted, and he sees only their breakup.

Anyplace that the meditator looks for support he finds in a state of dissolution, and so he understands the inevitable impermanency of all that comes into being. This perception of all-pervasive impermanence leads the meditator to experience the misery, fearfulness, terror, and unsatisfactoriness of all phenomena.

The meditator's world of reality is in a constant state of dissolution. A dreadful realization flows from this; the mind becomes gripped with fear. All his thoughts seem fearsome. He sees becoming, that is, thoughts coming into being, as a source of terror. As the *Visuddhimagga* (1975, p. 753) puts it:

> As he repeats, develops and cultivates in this way the contemplation of dissolution, the object of which is cessation consisting in the destruction, fall and break-up of all formations, then formations . . . appear to him in the form of a great terror, as lions, tigers, leopards, bears, hyaenas, spirits, ogres, fierce bulls, savage dogs, rut-maddened wild elephants, hideous venomous serpents, thunderbolts, charnel grounds, battle fields, flaming coal pits, etc., appear to a timid man who wants to live in peace.

At this point, the meditator realizes the unsatsfactory quality of all phenomena. All of his awareness, every thought, every feeling, appears insipid. This includes any state of mind the meditator can conceive. In all the meditator perceives, he sees only suffering and misery. Feeling this misery in all phenomena, the meditator becomes entirely disgusted with them. The comfortless nature of mind stuff becomes more evident than ever; the desire for deliverance from it emerges at the root of his being.

The only solution to the terror which the meditator sees everywhere within is the complete cessation of all mental activity. So long as moments of awareness arise, so they must decay; if they can somehow be prevented from arising, the meditator could find peace. The idea of nibbana becomes immensely appealing to the meditator, as he sees its attainment as the only possible happiness in the face of the terror that he experiences. He is impelled by an urge for deliverance and so pursues his meditation with the goal of nibbana in mind.

Now the meditator's contemplation proceeds automatically, without special effort, as if borne onward of itself. The meditator's mind has abandoned both dread and delight. An exceedingly sublime clarity of mind and a pervasive equanimity emerge. The meditator need make no further deliberate effort; noticing continues in a steady flow for hours without his tiring. His meditation has its own momentum, and insight becomes especially quick.

Insight is now on the verge of its culmination: the meditator's noticing of each moment of awareness is keen, strong, and lucid. His detachment from them is at a peak. His noticing no longer enters into or settles down on any phenomena at all. A consciousness arises that takes as its object the "signless, no-occurrence, non-formation": nibbana. Awareness of all physical and mental phenomena ceases entirely.

This moment of penetration of nibbana does not, in its first attainment, last even for a second. This first moment, called "path consciousness," is said to uproot mental defilements (i.e., eradicate altogether certain unhealthy mental factors from the meditator's mind). The next moment is "fruition," where the meditator enters the peace of nibbana. Following fruition, the meditator's mind reflects on the experience of nibbana just past. That experience is a cognitive shock of deepest psychological consequence. Because it is of a realm beyond that of the commonsense reality from which our language is generated, nibbana is a "supramundane reality," describable only in terms of what it is not. Nibbana has no phenomenology, no experiential characteristics. It is the unconditioned state.

This moment marks the meditator's entry into the four stages of the "supramundane path," where nibbana itself becomes the object of meditation. This "stream entry," as it is known, is possible only when the meditator has developed the seven factors of enlightenment to a heightened degree. These factors are: mindfulness, wisdom, energy, rapture, calm, concentration, and equanimity. These seven factors are artfully balanced to speed the meditator's mind toward nibbana (Goldstein, 1976, p. 147):

> These are the seven qualities of enlightenment that have to be brought to maturity in our practice. Three of them are arousing factors, and three are tranquilizing ones. Wisdom, energy and rapture all arouse the mind; they make it wakeful and alert. Calm, concentration and equanimity tranquilize the mind and make it still. They all have to be in harmony: if there is too much arousal, the mind becomes restless; if too much tranquility it goes to sleep. The factor of mindfulness is so powerful because it not only serves to awaken and strengthen all the other factors, but it also keeps them in their proper balance.

In Abhidhamma, nibbana is said to bring radical and lasting alteration of one's mental states. The significance for personality of nibbana is in its aftereffect. Unlike jhana, which has a short-lived effect on the meditator's personality, a person's post-nibbana personality is said to be irrevocably altered. A person's first experience of nibbana initiates a progression of changes which can finally lead to the point where unhealthy factors no longer occur. Not only are there no unhealthy factors in his states, but he has also eradicated any and all latent tendencies that could potentially lead to an unhealthy factor arising in his mind.

This transformation of consciousness is gradual. Though the experience of nibbana is always the same, as the meditator's insight strengthens he can attain nibbana at increasingly profound depths. At each successive level, groups of the unhealthy factors become totally inhibited. Finally, not a single unhealthy factor will appear in any of the person's mental states. A meditator who reaches this point is called an arahat, literally, "one worthy of praise." He still, however, retains vestiges of his unique personality traits, as is evident from the vast range of personal styles in stories of enlightened beings.

Arahat: Ideal Type of the Healthy Personality

The arahat embodies the essence of mental health in Abhidhamma. His personality traits are permanently altered; all his motives, perception, and actions that he formerly engaged in under the influence of unhealthy factors will have vanished. Rune Johansson, in *The Psychology of Nirvana* (1970), has culled Abhidhamma sources for the personality attributes of the arahat. His list includes:

1. *absence of:* greed for sense desires; anxiety, resentments, or fears of any sort; dogmatisms such as the belief that this or that is "the truth"; aversion to conditions such as loss, disgrace, pain, or blame; feelings of lust or anger; experiences of mental suffering; need for approval, pleasure, or praise; desire for anything for oneself beyond essential and necessary items; and

2. *prevalence of:* impartiality toward others and equanimity in all circumstances; ongoing alertness and calm delight in experience no matter how ordinary or even seemingly boring; strong feelings of compassion and loving-kindness; quick and accurate perception; composure and skill in taking action; openness to others and responsivity to their needs.

While the arahat may seem virtuous beyond belief from the perspective of other personality theories, he embodies characteristics common to the ideal type in most every Asian psychology. The arahat is the prototypic saint, a prototype notable in the main by its absence in Western personality theory. Such a radical transformation of personality overreaches the goals and hopes of our psychotherapies. From the perspective of most modern personality theories the arahat must seem too good to exist; he lacks many characteristics which they assume intrinsic to human nature. However, the arahat is an ideal type, the end point in a gradual transformation which anyone can undertake, and in which anyone can succeed to whatever small measure. Thus the monk or lay meditator may not become a saint overnight, but he may well experience himself changing so that he has a greater proportion of healthy mental states.

Eastern versus Western Models of Mental Well-being

The models of contemporary psychology foreclose the acknowledgment or investigation of a mode of being which is the central premise and summum bonum of virtually every Eastern psychospiritual system. Called variously arahatship, enlightenment, Buddhahood, liberation, the awakened state, and so on, there is simply no fully equivalent category in contemporary psychology. The paradigms of traditional Asian psychologies, however, are capable of encompassing the major categories of contemporary psychology as well as this mode of supreme well-being.

The Tibetan Wheel of Life, for example, depicts pictorially six realms of existence, each a metaphor for a different psychological state. One realm, that of the "stupid beast," stands for the level of behavior which is totally conditioned, and corresponds to a world in which habit and simple stimulus response are the principle determinants of action and thought. The hell realms represent aggression and anxiety states, and are emblematic of all anxiety-based behavior; this is the realm of psychopathology as mapped by contemporary psychologists like Freud, Sullivan, and Laing. The realm of the *pretas,* or hungry ghosts, corresponds to insatiable appetite or needfulness—what Maslow has characterized as "deficiency motivation." The realm of heaven depicts godlike beings who represent sensual bliss and gratification of the highest order; the "peak experience" would be subsumed by this category as would many of the experiences which have emerged from humanistic psychology. Shown at war with the gods of the heaven realm are the "jealous gods" who represent an attitude shaped not by needfulness, but by envy; these reflect a motivational state of overweening competitiveness and self-aggrandizement—a state of mind studied widely within Western social science. The sixth realm is that of human beings, and denotes the potential for insight into the human condition; this insight is very similar to the understanding formulated in Freud's tragic vision: that suffering is inescapable.

The Buddhist psychologist, in stating the same insight as the "First Noble Truth," offers an alternative: alter the processes of ordinary consciousness and thereby end suffering. The state of consciousness which transcends all the ordinary realms of being is the "Buddha realm," portrayed on the Wheel of Life as outside and above the circle of conditioned existence containing the six ordinary realms. Like arahatship, Buddhahood is attained by transforming ordinary consciousness, principally through meditation, and once attained is characterized by the extinction of all those states (e.g., anxiety, needfulness, pride) which mark the ordinary realms of existence.

This state of well-being seems to be a higher-order integration than any suggested by the developmental schema of contemporary psychology. For example, the key attributes of "ego integrity," Erickson's (1960) final psychosocial stage in the epigenesis of the life cycle, include: an acceptance of one's own life history, an appreciation of dignity and love, a readiness to defend the unique life-style which has been the source of one's own integrity, and an emotional integration which allows one to participate by following as well as leading. The failure to integrate successfully at this stage is marked by despair, fear of death, and self-contempt which is expressed as contempt directed toward others. This enumeration of characteristics stands in contrast to the attributes of an arahat, enumerated above. There is some overlap between Erikson's final stage and the arahat's personality, mainly in terms of the theme of acceptance of one's life circumstances, lack of resentment, and absence of fear (for Erikson, specifically fear of death). Divergences between the schema are most obvious in terms of defending one's life-style; while this is a hallmark of ego integrity, such behavior would be unlikely for an arahat because of the extinction of ego identity itself. Indeed, the arahat is said to have no sense of a separate self at all. Another trait of the arahat uncharacteristic of ego integrity is the prevalence of actions which are guided by consideration of the good of others rather than one's own desires, a by-product of the falling away of identity in the sense of self-interest; this is a step beyond Erikson's final stage in ego development, as is the notion that this final integration can occur via a transformation of consciousness. What is particularly intriguing about the Buddhist developmental schema is that it not only expands the constructs of contemporary psychology's view of what is possible for men, but also gives details of the means whereby such a change can occur.

Many of the psychological principles implied by the Buddhist path to well-being were tentatively anticipated in the West in the thought of William James (1910): he recognized the existence of states of consciousness other than the ordinary, he suggested the possibility of retraining neural "habits," and he saw the importance of attentional processes. He did not, however, develop the same theoretical interrelationships between these phenomena as have Buddhist psychologists, namely, that via meditation—an attentional manipulation—one can enter an altered state, and that through systematic retraining of attentional habits one can alter consciousness as a trait of being.

Many contemporary therapies begin from an understanding of the human condition similar in certain respects to that of the Abhidhamma. Freud, for example, saw the "universal neurosis in man"; Buddha saw that "all world-ings are deranged." While the insight was similar, the response differed. Freud sought through analysis to help his patients face, understand, and reconcile themselves to this "tragic" condition of life. Buddha sought through meditation to eradicate the source of suffering in a radical reorientation of consciousness.

Psychodynamic therapy since Freud has worked within the constraints of the fundamental processes of consciousness to alter the impact of the contents of one's past as it effects the present. Asian psychologies have largely ignored psychologically loaded contents of awareness, including psychodynamics, while seeking to alter the context in which they—and all other information—are registered in awareness. Conventional psychotherapies assume as givens the mechanisms underlying perceptual, cognitive, and affective processes, while seeking to alter them at the level of socially conditioned patterns. Asian systems disregard these same socially conditioned patterns, while aiming at the control and self-regulation of the underlying mechanisms themselves. Therapies break the hold of past conditioning on present behavior; meditation aims to alter the process of conditioning per se so that it will no longer be a prime determinant of future acts. In the Asian approach, behavioral and personality change is secondary, an epiphenomenon of changes, through the voluntary self-regulation of mental states, in the basic processes which define our reality.

Consciousness is the medium which carries the messages that compose experience. Psychotherapies are concerned with these messages and their meanings; meditation instead directs itself to the nature of the medium, consciousness. These two approaches are by no means mutually exclusive, but rather complementary. A therapy of the future may integrate techniques from both approaches, possibly producing a change in the whole person more thoroughgoing and more potent than either in isolation.

REFERENCES

Anguttara-Nikaya T. Nyanaponika, translator. Kandy, Ceylon: Buddhist Publication Society, 1975.

Aung, Z. V. *Compendium of Philosophy*. London: Pali Text Society, 1972.

Erikson, E. *Childhood and Society*. New York: W. Norton, 1960.

Goldstein, Joseph. *The Experience of Insight*. Santa Cruz: Unity Press, 1976.

James, W. *Psychology: Briefer Course*. New York: Harper (First edition, 1910), 1962.

Johansson, R. *The Psychology of Nirvana*. New York: Anchor, 1970.

Ledi, S. *The Requisites of Enlightenment*. Kandy, Ceylon: Buddhist Publication Society, 1971.

Nyanaponika, T. *Abhidhamma Studies*. Colombo, Ceylon: Frewin, 1949.

Nyanaponika, T. *The Heart of Buddhist Meditation*. London: Rider, 1962.

Nyanaponika, T. *Five Hindrances*. Kandy, Ceylon: Buddhist Publication Society, 1963.

Nyantiloka. *Path to Deliverance*. Colombo, Ceylon: Buddha Sahitya Sabha, 1952.

Samyutta-Nikaya (I.B. Horner, translator). London: Pali Text Society, 1958.

Visuddhimagga (B. Nyanamoli, translator). Berkeley: Shambhala, 1975.

The Zen masters all proclaim that there is no enlightenment whatever which you can claim to have attained. If you say you have attained something this is the surest proof that you have gone astray. Therefore, not to have is to have; silence is thunder; ignorance is enlightenment.

D. T. Suzuki

This chapter presents Zen Buddhism's vision of enlightenment. At one level, it attempts to present the vision with the simplicity and quiet humor that the vision deserves and which is true to the form of Zen.[1] Therefore, the fact that the chapter represents a belief system, that there are blinders within the belief system, and an analysis of the strengths and weaknesses of the vision are discussed elsewhere.[2,3]

Of all the branches of Buddhism, Zen is perhaps the most challenging to Western intellectual assumptions. Indeed, the master may refuse to even begin intellectual discussion about Zen; may deny there is any such thing as Zen, enlightenment, or illusion; may respond to apparently reasonable queries with apparently irrelevant nonsense; or may pile paradox on paradox until the inquirer either leaves in disgust or begins to intuit that the nature of Zen is to be sought through experience rather than through the intellect.

On those occasions when they do talk about Zen and enlightenment, one of their most frequent metaphors is a mirror. Mirrors have qualities of reflecting reality without distortion, judgment, or attachment—qualities which Zen believes are characteristic of the clear mind. Mirrors and mirrorlike minds are thus the subject of this chapter by Deane Shapiro.

Besides being interested in mirrors, the author of this chapter is also an avid detective fan. Combining these interests, he is quite attached to, and wants to recommend to readers, the works of Janwillem van de Wetering. Van de Wetering wrote The Empty Mirror[4] *(from which this chapter title is borrowed), a first-person account of his experiences of studying Zen while in Japan, and also writes Zen detective stories, in which the essential mirrorlike Buddha nature of policemen and criminals is in evidence.*

As editor of this introduction, I am reminded of the parable of Ungan:

When Ungan was making tea, Dago asked, "To whom are you serving tea?"
Ungan: "There is one who wants it."
Dago: "Why don't you make him serve himself?"
Ungan: "Fortunately, I am here."[5]

In Zen, in the timeless moment, subject/object dichotomies disappear. The editor now introduces the author.

10

Zen and the Art of Enlightenment: Reflections on an Empty Mirror

Deane H. Shapiro, Jr., Ph.D.

Zen may be seen as a dewdrop, reflecting the world. It has variously been called philosophy[6] and non(anti)-philosophy, a religion and a non-religion,[7] and a psychology with no content to teach. Zen has been compared with existentialism,[7,8] Sullivanean interpersonal theory,[9] psychoanalysis,[10,11] behavior therapy,[3] humanistic psychology,[12,13] and transpersonal psychology,[3,14]

Historically, Zen came to China through Bodhidharma who was traditionally thought of as the twenty-eighth patriarch of Buddhism, counting from the Buddha himself.[15] The Indian idea of *Dhyana,* a system of religious practices centering around quiet meditation and quiet contemplation, came into contact with both Confucianism and Taoism. It was this intermingling, called Chan Buddhism, which later found its roots in Japan as Zen.[16]

Alan Watts has warned, however, that we need to distinguish among square Zen, a formal, rigid Zen dogma; beat Zen, which is the "anything goes" Zen of the Kerouac generation of the 1950s; and the actual "spirit" of Zen.[17]

The teaching, such as it be, is that experience is more important than words and intellect. As D. T. Suzuki said,

> A special transmission outside the scriptures. No reliance on words and intellect.[18]

There is a story about Suzuki Roshi, the late Zen Master who founded the Zen Center in San Francisco, which illustrates this need to teach by experience. According to the story, he gave a one-hour lecture at Stanford University. He began by saying that in Zen, one must experience directly, and that meditation is a vehicle to develop that direct understanding. In meditation, he said, one sits with legs crossed in a half or full lotus (which he then did). One puts one's hands in a mudra* position in one's lap (which he did); one sits with one's back erect, but not tight, focuses the eyes a few feet ahead, and breathes gently and with awareness (which he did for the next hour). He then got up, bowed, and left. He was, so the story goes, never invited back!

How would we react to such a teaching? In truth, normally we are used to speech and words as teaching tools. Even a book of this nature, which talks of extreme visions of health, is filled with lots of words. Yet, much of what the spiritual traditions in general, and Zen in particular, emphasize are the qualities of emptiness, nonanalysis, and ceasing the word play of the mind. Yet again I ask how we would react to this. To a blank page in a book? Would it have meaning for us, or would we think the printer, editor, or writer left something out or made a mistake?

How can we understand this emptiness as fullness? As in the Zen *koan*,* what does the "sound of one hand clapping" mean? Or what is the sound of a stringless harp, as in the following *mondo*?†

A monk came to Shuzan and asked him to play a tune on the stringless harp. The master was quiet for some while, and then said, "Do you hear it?"
Monk: "No, I do not hear it."
Master: "Why did you not ask me to play louder?"[5]

How, then, are we to proceed? What is the best way to understand the sound of the stringless harp? Certainly, words, though they may be necessary, do not seem to be sufficient.

Pupil: Whenever appeal is made to words, Master, there is a taint. What is the truth of the highest order?
Master: Whenever appeal is made to words, there is a taint.[5]

Again, how can we be guided in our efforts to conceptualize and understand the Zen "true self," particularly when Zen suggests that we are already

---

*Thumbs touching together, with one palm holding the back of the other hand.
* A koan is an intellectual riddle of the Rinzai school of Zen, which has no intellectual answer.
† Mondos are discourses between masters and monks, used as teaching tools.

whole and enlightened, and the very task of *searching* for understanding is illusory and unnecessary?

> Pupil: Where is the one solitary road to being oneself?
> Master: Why trouble yourself to ask about it?[5]

In this brief article we are going to use the concept of a "mirror" to help us understand this Zen view more fully. Many authors and traditions in this book make reference to the mirror analogy. For example, Smith talks about the sacred unconscious as being like a mirror, the Tibetans talk of a "crystal" mirror, Deikman suggests Sufi stories can help us attain enlightenment by providing a mirror for us, and both Walsh and Wilber also use mirror analogies.

How does the concept of the mirror help us? To clarify this, we will use four tools: (1) a parable to set the stage, (2) a more refined discussion of the mirror as an analogy, (3) an experience, and (4) additional reflections on the empty mirror.

1. A Parable

Strivata stood in front of the oak panel door, waiting for Naciketas to come with the key. Strivata waited anxiously at first, looking quickly over both shoulders for Naciketas' arrival. Several minutes passed, and still there was no sign of Naciketas. Realizing the anxiety within, Strivata decided to sit at the base of the door, wait patiently, and meditate on the intricate carvings which extended in coiled fashion from the upper right-hand corner. Naciketas approached from behind, and his shadow climbed over Strivata's and ascended the door.

"I am glad you have come," said Strivata. "There is no way for me to enter without the key." Naciketas laughed. "Do not laugh," Strivata responded angrily. "The sun is setting, I am becoming cold, and I have waited long for you."

"I thought you would return before me, so I left the door unlatched," Naciketas replied. Strivata entered the unlocked door. The sun went down, casting all in dark shadows. Yet, even before the fire was built, Strivata saw more clearly.

There are several points worth noticing in this parable. For example, notice that the door (symbolizing the barriers to Strivata's true self) was unlocked and that Strivata could have opened it without help; the "key" (to enter the door, to enter the self) was within all the time. However, although Strivata needed no teacher to open the door—to find his "real self"—it seemed that a teacher was, in fact, needed, if only to point out that no teacher was needed. Once Strivata realized this lesson, even though the room was becoming dark, he "saw more clearly."

2. The Mirror Analogy: A Refinement

Historically, the mirror as a teaching tool has been quite important in Zen. In fact, it determined the successor to Hung-jen, the fifth Zen patriarch. To determine who would be his successor, Hung-jen had each contender submit a poem. The leading contender Shen-hsiu's poem went as follows:

Let the body be a Bodhi tree,
Let the mind be a looking glass;
Take care to keep it always clean,
Lest it attract the dust.[19]

This view is an expression of the gradual enlightenment approach (what becomes known as the Northern school or Northern Zen in China).

Hui-neng, on the other hand, submitted the following verse:

There was never a Bodhi tree,
Nor was the bright mirror on its stand.
There was never anything,
Whence then should the dust come?[19]

Hui-neng's poem suggests an altered state of consciousness which maintains a holistic, nondichotomous view. There is no good and bad, no opposites, and Shen-hsiu's distinction between a "dirty mirror" and a "clean mirror" is a relativistic mistake. The enlightened mind does not make such distinctions between dust and nondust. Thus, Hui-neng became the sixth patriarch and his school is referred to as the school of sudden enlightenment.

It can be seen that both teachers taught of the empty mirror. One said that we gradually uncovered our true Buddha nature, and the other said that we need to enter directly into our Buddha nature.

The mirror can be understood as part of Zen's "real me" or Buddha nature, based on four qualities (or wisdoms). These are the qualities of emptiness, acceptance, accurate discrimination, and nonattachment.*

Quality of Emptiness. When a mirror is clean and free from dust, dirt, and stains, it reflects clearly, accurately, and without distortion. It is then

*The author wishes to express his thanks and appreciation to Nishimura Roshi for his lecture, comments, and discussion about this.

said to be empty. In psychological terms, when our "minds" are empty (that is, free of verbal statements and images), there is an absence of preconceptions, strivings, and thoughts. Since, as many authors in this book have pointed out, preconceptions influence the way we interpret reality, the "emptiness" of the mind allows us to see "what is" without the ordinary cognitive chatter and constructs.

According to the Zen way, we are born with this wisdom of emptiness, and are therefore able to interact fully and "clearly" with whatever is around. Thus, in the words of the *Prajna Paramita Sutra,* "the emptiness [of the mirror] is actually [its] fullness." However, our mirrorlike nature subsequently becomes "stained" by words, labels, desires, and aversions, and reality soon becomes distorted to meet one's preconceptions of it. Therefore, one aspect of finding the "real me" is to return to a state of emptiness by wiping the preconceptions from the face of the mirror.

Quality of Acceptance. The second quality of a mirror might be referred to as acceptance or nonevaluation. The mirror accepts everything into itself without evaluations or judgments (wisdom of equalness). Any object put in front of the mirror—a big ball, a red cat, a poor person, a rich person—is reflected with equal accuracy. The mirror does not comment on whatever is around it; it merely accepts it into itself.

In psychological terms, the mirror reflects in a manner that Carl Rogers would call *nonjudgmental*—what social learning theorists would call *without evaluation.* A person who has this "mirror nature" would be able, in Paul Tillich's words, to "accept that you are accepted."

Naranjo and Ornstein have elaborated on the concept of consciousness as a mirror as follows:

> The mirror allows every input to enter equally, reflects each equally, and cannot be tuned to receive a special kind of input. It does not add anything to the input and does not turn off receptivity to stimuli. It does not focus on any particular aspect of input and retune back and forth but continuously admits all inputs equally. . . .[20]

Quality of Accurate Discrimination. The third quality of a clean mirror is that it is able to differentiate and discriminate, for example, large from small, green from red, a happy face from a sad face. This has been referred to as the *wisdom of accurate reflection.* Thus, at the same time the mirror accepts everything into itself (quality of nonevaluation), it is also able to tell the difference between the objects that it is reflecting (quality of discrimination). In other words, our true selves, according to Zen, are both able to see and able to accept everything into themselves equally and fully, while at the same time making discriminations about different objects.

Quality of Nonattachment.   Finally, the clean mirror may be characterized by the wisdom of nonclinging or nonattachment. As we saw above, the mirror reflects instantly and without distortion. Further, as soon as the object is taken away, the mirror is able to immediately "yield," or let it and its reflection go. Thus, the "real me," according to Zen, fully and completely interacts with whatever is in front of it, and yet does so in a nonpossessive, nonclinging manner.

Thus, we see that our true nature, according to Zen belief, is like the empty mirror: it interacts fully with the environment, accepts all into itself without evaluation, is able to discriminate, and is yielding and nonpossessive. As Chuang-Tzu noted, "The perfect man employs his mind as a mirror: it grasps nothing, it receives, but does not keep."

3. An Experience

Publisher's Note: To clarify any misconception, it should be noted that the blank page represents the experience.

4. Reflections on and Implications of the Empty Mirror

What is the experience of emptiness like? According to the Zen view, once we remove our preconceptions, we will see our true self, and this "real me" is positive, unifying, and innately good. In D. T. Suzuki's words, every human being is "so constituted by nature that he can become an artist of life," and "Zen, in its essence, is the art of seeing into the nature of one's being—giving free play to all the creative and benevolent impulses inherently lying in our heart."[5] This basic, good, and real self is quite different from Freud's warring, aggressive id. Rather, it is similar in certain ways to the Jungian integrated, *individuated self*, to Buckes' *cosmic consciousness*, and to Rogers', Maslow's, and Goldstein's *self-actualizing ego*.

However, within the Zen framework, if we conceptualize these potentials in terms of positive traits, we are distorting reality. Traits, even positive traits, are but *descriptions* of reality, and not reality itself. Thus, in Zen, the "real me" is often referred to as "no-self" or "egolessness" or the Tao: that which is beyond words.

The Zen tradition includes many of the qualities associated with the humanistic tradition (e.g., developing inner directedness and a strong sense of oneself), but it also has qualities representative of the transpersonal.[21] Maslow,[22] for example, referred to the goal of therapy as not only learning how to build a strong sense of ego, but learning how to surrender the ego. Eventually, the individual is taught how not to identify with his or her thoughts, including the thoughts of "self." As Goleman noted, "The phenomena contemplated are distinct from the mind contemplating them: the goal of therapy is to develop a high degree of perceptual clarity about one's thought patterns, habits, behaviors without accompanying affect: a mindfulness of each moment.''[23]

Thus, in Zen the goal is to help the person to develop a nonintellectual understanding of the world and of oneself. This nonintellectual understanding—satori, enlightenment, nirvana—is an experience of oneness or wholeness which goes beyond ego boundaries and teaches one a sense of harmony both with oneself and with the world around. This "self-nature" is represented by three characters in the Chinese language. The first character is the one for "sun," and the second is for "rising." Those two characters—"sun rising"—mean "sound." The third character refers to heart, so self-nature is the sound of one's heart or hearing the sun rise in one's heart. By allowing the silence of emptiness, the fullness of one's "Self" can be heard.

Some Implications. Zen posits that the mirrorlike nature of our *self* is innately good and positive. Further, this real self is within all of us now, if only we are willing to see it. There are three important implications of this view of personality. First, the individual who is searching for the "real me" is able to *trust him/herself* in the very act of searching. Believing that our inner nature is good, we are "content to let behavior bring out a self which cannot be fully conceptualized. One trusts this self enough to suspend conscious reflective control over it."[13] This allows us not only to trust ourselves more, but also to be more willing and able to see the spark of goodness within others.

Secondly, this Zen view of the self implies a possible causal relationship between the individual's self-perception and his/her behavior. That is, if we believe in ourselves, we may be more likely to act skillfully and fulfillingly. We might, for example, trust ourselves enough to take more risks, try new paths, let ourselves be free to act creatively, and listen to and trust our body signals regarding physical and emotional health and healing.

Finally, this Zen view of the person has important implications for the therapist and educator. If these professionals believe and trust in the innate ability and goodness of the individual, they will be more likely to allow their students/clients room for personal exploration and latitude for acting creatively. For example, within the therapy practiced by Carl Rogers, the client is treated as a person competent to direct his/her own actions and healing process. Likewise, a physician "healer" of psychosomatic complaints who believes in innate abilities will be more likely to encourage the patient to take an active role in healing him/herself.

Thus, the relationship between mind and body, between our view of ourself and our subsequent behavior, and between the educator/therapist's view of the individual and his/her subsequent style of healing and teaching are all areas that may be affected by the Zen view of the "real me."

Summary

Analogies, parables, personal anecdotes, and even blank pages are tools to help us understand and experience the essence of the "empty mirror." For some, they may provide helpful guideposts. However, guideposts must be thought of in Zen terms as:

A finger pointing to the moon: once the moon has been seen, the finger is no longer necessary.[5]

The mirror can be a useful metaphor, or finger pointing to enlightenment. However, as Huston Smith noted, if there is this sacred unconscious layer and it's like a mirror, then we can't really call it ours. "Even if it were there, in what sense could we call it ours? For when we look toward it we see simply—world."[24]

We can see liberation and enlightenment as qualities of the empty mirror in the following passage from Walsh and Vaughan:

Finally, states of consciousness may emerge in which identification of awareness with some objects to the exclusion of others is permanently dismantled. Shorn of dualism and exclusivity, awareness now experiences itself as transcendent to both time and space, as pure consciousness and yet one with the universe, transcendent to the limitations and suffering which seem so real, absolute, and inescapable from its former perspective.[25]

Ultimate enlightenment is being and experiencing in the here and now. It is both detached observation (nonattachment) and feeling the sorrow and pain. It is reflected in Huston Smith's story of the Zen master who cries at life's suffering, while also observing it, and maintaining the "yes" experience of the East.

Finally, as Wilber notes,[26] Brahman hurls himself back into the formless void to take on another life game, knowing that mirror and reflections are one and the same. Or, in the words of the birthday present from my wife several years ago:

The puddle reflects
Rain drops dissolving
In the image it contains.

REFERENCES

1. Hyers, C. Zen and the comic spirit. Philadelphia: The Westminster Press, 1973.
2. Shapiro, D. A content analysis of traditional and new age, Eastern and Western therapies. This book.
3. Shapiro, D. Precision Nirvana. Englewood Cliffs, N.J.: Prentice Hall, 1978.
4. van de Wetering, J. The empty mirror: Experiences in a Japanese Zen monastery. New York: Pocket Books, 1973.
5. This mondo and all mondos in this chapter are taken from Suzuki, D.T. *Introduction to Zen*. London: John Murray Limited, 1949.
6. Izutsu, T. *Toward a Philosophy of Zen Buddhism*. Tehran: Imperial Iranian Academy of Philosophy, 1977.
7. Suzuki, D.T. *Zen Buddhism* (W. Barrett, Ed.). New York: Doubleday Books, 1956.
8. Hora, T. Tao, Zen, and existential psychotherapy, *Psychologia*, 1959, *2*, 236–242.
9. Stunkard, A. Interpersonal aspects of an oriental religion. *Psychiatry*, 1951, *14*, 419–31.
10. Fromm, E. Zen and psychoanalysis. *Psychologia*, 1959, *2*, 79–99.
11. Haimes, N. Zen Buddhism and psychoanalysis. *Psychologia*, 1972, *15*, 22–30.
12. Keefe, T. Meditation and the psychotherapist. *American Journal of Orthopsychiatry*, 1975, *45*(3), 484–489.
13. Lesh, T. Zen meditation and the development of empathy in counselors. *Journal of Humanistic Psychology*, 1970, *10*(1), 39–74.
14. Owens, C. Zen Buddhism. In *Transpersonal Psychologies* (C. Tart, Ed.). New York: Harper & Row, 1976.
15. Conze, E. *Buddhist Meditation*. New York: Harper & Row, 1969.
16. Harai, T. *Zen Meditation Therapy*. Tokyo: Japan Publications Inc., 1975.
17. Watts, A. Beat Zen, square Zen, and Zen. In *This Is It*. San Francisco: City Lights Bookstore, 1959.
18. Cited in Suzuki, D. T. In *Zen Buddhism* (W. Barrett, Ed.). New York: Doubleday, 1956, p. 9. Original author unknown. Quote is often attributed to Bodhi-dharma.
19. Awakawa Y. *Zen Painting*. Tokyo: Kodensha International Ltd., 1971, pp. 14–15.
20. Naranjo, C. and Ornstein, R. *The Psychology of Meditation*. New York: Viking, 1971, p. 194.
21. Tart, C. (Ed.). *Transpersonal Psychologies*. New York: Harper & Row, 1976.
22. Maslow, A. *Toward a Psychology of Being*. Princeton: Van Nostrand, 1968.
23. Goleman, D. Meditation and metatherapy: Hypotheses toward a proposed fifth state of consciousness. *Journal of Transpersonal Psychology*, 1971, *3*(1), 1–25.
24. Smith, H. The sacred unconscious. This book.
25. Walsh, R. N. and Vaughan, F. Toward an integrative psychology of well-being. This book.
26. Wilber, K. The evolution of consciousness. This book.

The greatest things which are done on earth are done within.
St. Louis de Montfort

The difficulty of describing the highest good has been a notorious problem for both psychology and philosophy. In "The Sacred Unconscious," Huston Smith points to the ways in which people have attempted to circumvent this difficulty and then goes on to describe the nature of a jivanmukti, or fully realized person. Such a person, he suggests, is one "whose doors of perception have been cleansed," leaving clear perception of both the world and the deepest (sacred) levels of the unconscious uncontaminated by greed, aversion, or ignorance. From this perspective he or she is able to open fully to the entire spectrum of human experience though all the while both aware of the numinous and continuing to do whatever is required in the world.

Huston Smith is Professor of Religion and Adjunct Professor of Philosophy at Syracuse University. Born of missionary parents in Soochow, his childhood and youth in China provided an appropriate background for his ensuing work in comparative philosophies and religions. His book on The Religions of Man *has sold over two million copies; his documentary films on Tibetan Buddhism, Sufism, and Hinduism have won international film festival awards; and his phonograph record, "The Music of Tibet," which embodies his discovery of the capacity of certain lamas to sing multi-tones simultaneously, was acclaimed by* The Journal of Ethnomusicology *as "an important landmark in the study of extra-European musics, and in fact of music itself."*

Dr. Smith is a holder of six honorary degrees, and his books include The Purposes of Higher Education *(Harper & Row, 1955),* The Religions of Man *(1958),* The Search for America *(Prentice-Hall, 1958),* Condemned to Meaning *(Harper & Row, 1964),* Forgotten Truth: The Primordial Tradition *(Harper & Row, 1976), and* Beyond the Post-Modern Mind *(1982).*

11

The Sacred Unconscious

Huston Smith

In *The Next Million Years,* a book published around the time of Darwin's Centennial, his grandson, Charles Galton Darwin, considered the prospects for genetic engineering. Writing as a geneticist, he concluded that the difficulties were formidable but solvable. What was not solvable, he thought, was the goal of such engineering—agreement as to the kind of person we would like it to produce. Nietzsche and van Gogh were geniuses but went mad—would we want their genes in our gene pool? It's a good question. It makes us see the nerve of a book—the present one—that tries to define the highest good for man.

As a philosopher and historian of religions, let me venture my perception of this "human best" as follows: if Marx unmasked our social unconscious and Freud our personal unconscious, both piercing through superstructures, or rather substructures, that hide true causes and motives, the supreme human opportunity is to strike deeper still and become aware of the "sacred unconscious" that forms the bottom line of our selfhood.

I shall not go into reasons for assuming that this final unconscious exists; I have discussed some of them in my book *Forgotten Truth: The Primordial Tradition* (Harper & Row, 1976) where I use the word "spirit" for what I am here calling the sacred unconscious. Nor will I here map our human consciousness to show the relation of this deepest level to ones that are more proximate; that I attempted in the chapter on "The Levels of Selfhood" in the book just mentioned. Instead I shall try to surmise what our lives would be like if our deepest unconscious were directly available to us. What would a supremely realized human being, human here conceived as one who is consciously aware of his or her sacred unconscious, be like? How would such beings look to others and feel to themselves?

It is easier to say what such a person would *not* be like than to picture him or her positively, as the "tragic flaw" theory of art reminds us. No writer would dream of trying to create a perfect hero; he would sense instinctively that such a figure would seem completely fictitious—a cardboard cutout. However, let the author endow an otherwise strong character with a tragic weakness—Hamlet's indecision is the standard example—and our imaginations will correct that weakness on their own; convincingly, moreover, for we graft the missing virtue onto a character whose imperfection makes him believable. The same principles apply when we try (as here) to describe human wholeness not concretely as the artist does, but abstractly: we are on firmest ground when we state the case negatively. To cite a historical instance, the Buddha's characterization of enlightenment as the absence of hatred, greed, and ignorance draws its force from being solidly anchored in real life: its key terms refer to traits we live with all the time. Yet if we try to restate his formula in positive terms and say that to be enlightened is to be filled with love, wisdom, and an impartial acceptance of everything, our description becomes abstract. Obviously we have some acquaintance with these virtues, but acquaintance is not what is at stake. The goal is to be *suffused* with these virtues: to be filled by them completely. That we have only the faintest notion of what these positive terms mean when they are raised to their maximum goes without saying.

So we now have two wise caveats before us: Darwin's, that we don't know what the summum bonum is; and Buddha's, that we do best to approach it negatively. In keeping with what I take to be the presumptuous spirit of this book as a whole, I propose to throw these warnings to the wind and attempt a positive depiction of a *jivanmukta,* as the Indians would refer to a fully realized person: a *jiva* (soul) that is *mukti* (liberated, enlightened) in this very life. The project must fail, of course, but that doesn't keep it from being interesting. Perhaps, in keeping with the tragic flaw theory I just alluded to, its very failure may induce the reader to round out in his own imaging the picture which words can never adequately portray.

An enlightened being, I am proposing, is one who is in touch with his deepest unconscious, an unconscious which (for reasons I shall be introducing) deserves to be considered sacred. Our century has acquainted us with regions of our minds that are hidden from us and the powerful ways they control our perceptions. My thesis is that underlying these proximate layers of our unconscious minds is a final substrate that opens mysteriously onto the world as it actually is. To have access to this final substrate is to be objective in the best sense of the word and to possess the virtues and benefits that go with this objectivity.

Normally we are not in touch with this objective component of ourselves—which paradoxically is also our deepest subjective component—because intermediate layers of our unconscious screen it from us, while at the same time screening the bulk of the *world* from us. Our interests, drives and concerns, their roots largely hidden from our gaze, cause us to see what we *want* to see and *need* to see; most of the rest of reality simply passes us by. The Tibetans make this point by saying that when a pickpocket meets a saint, what he sees are his pockets. Moreover, the things we *do* see, we see through lenses that are "prescription ground," so to speak: our interests and conditionings distort the way they appear to us. When poor children are asked to draw a penny, they draw it larger than do children for whom pennies are commonplace; it looms larger in their mind's eye. In many such ways, what we take to be objective facts are largely psychological constructs, as the Latin *factum,* "that which is made," reminds us.

This much is now psychological truism. We enter more interesting terrain when we note that at a deeper level the thoughts and feelings that control what we see are themselves shaped by what the Buddha called the Three Poisons: desire (lust, greed, grasping), aversion (fear, hatred, anger), and ignorance*—and the greatest of these is ignorance. For it is ignorance—most pointedly ignorance concerning our true identity, who we really are—that causes us to divide the world into what we like and dislike. Thinking that we are separate selves,[1] we seek what augments these selves and shun what threatens them. What we call our "self" is the amalgam of desires and aversions that we have wrapped tightly, like the elastic of a golf ball, around the core of separate identity that is its center.

This tight, constricted, golf-ball self is inevitably in for hard knocks, but what concerns us here is that on the average it doesn't feel very good. Anxiety hovers round its edges. It can feel victimized and grow embittered. It is easily disappointed and can become unstrung. To others, it often seems no prettier than it feels to itself: petty, self-centered, drab, and bored.

I am deliberately putting down this golf-ball self—hurling it to the ground, as it were—because we want to see how high our total self can bounce: how far toward heaven it can rise. In order *to* rise, it must break out of the hard rubber strings that are normally stretched so tightly around it, encasing it in what Alan Watts called "the skin-encapsulated ego." If we

---

*I could get where I want to go through any of the great traditions, but having started with a Buddhist allusion several paragraphs back, I shall continue mainly with Buddhism where historical pointers seem helpful. This also makes sense because the primary orientation of this book is psychological, and of the great traditions it is Buddhism that puts its message most psychologically.

change our image from rubber to glass and picture the Three Poisons as a lens that refracts light waves in keeping with our private, importunate demands, then release from such egocentric distortions will come through progressively decreasing our lens' curve—reducing its bulge. The logical terminus of this would then be clear glass. Through this glass we would be able to see things objectively, as they are in themselves in their own right.

This clear glass, which for purposes of vision is equivalent to no glass at all, is our sacred unconscious. It is helpful to think of it as an absence because, like window glass, it functions best when it calls no attention to itself. Yet it is precisely its absence that makes the world available to us: "the less there is of self, the more there is of Self," as Eckhart put the matter. From clear glass we have moved to no glass—the removal of everything that might separate subject from object, self from world. Zen uses the image of the Great Round Mirror. When the Three Poisons are removed from it, it reflects the world just as it is.

To claim that human consciousness can move permanently into this condition may be going too far, but advances along the asymptotic curve that slopes in its direction are clearly perceptible. When our aversion lens is powerful, bulging toward the limits of a semicircle, we like very little that comes our way. The same holds, of course, for our desire lens which is only the convex side of our aversion's concave: the more these bend our evaluations toward our own self-interests, the less we are able to appreciate things in their own right. Blake's formulation of the alternative to this self-centered outlook has become classic: "If the doors of perception were cleansed every thing would appear to man as it is, infinite."

The fully realized human being is one whose doors of perception have been cleansed. These doors, which up to this point I have referred to as windows, I am here envisioning as successive layers of our unconscious minds.[2] Those that are near the surface vary from person to person, for they are deposited by our idiosyncratic childhood experiences. At some level, though, we encounter the Three Poisons (once again, desire, aversion, and ignorance) that are common to mankind and perhaps in some degree essential for our human functioning. However, the deepest layer, we have seen, is really a no-layer, for being a glass door ajar or a mirror that discloses other things rather than itself, it isn't there. Even if it were there, in what sense could we call it ours? For when we look toward it we see simply—world.

This opening out onto the world's infinity is one good reason for calling this deepest stratum of the human unconscious sacred, for surely holiness has something to do with the Whole, but the concreteness of Blake's formulation is instructive. He doesn't tell us that a cleansed perception discloses the infinite per se. It finds it in the things at hand, in keeping with those Buddhist stories which tell that the most sacred scriptures are its unwritten pages—an old pine tree gnarled by wind and weather, or a skein of geese flying across the autumn sky.

Thus far I have defined a jivanmukta; it remains to describe him or her. What does life feel like to such a person, and how does he appear to others.

Basically he lives in the unvarying presence of the numinous. This does not mean that such a person is excited or "hyped"; his or her condition has nothing to do with adrenaline flow, or with manic states that call for depressive ones to balance the emotional account. It's more like what Kipling had in mind when he said of one of his characters, "He believed that all things were one big miracle, and when a man knows that much he knows something to go upon." The opposite of the sense of the sacred is not serenity or sobriety. It is drabness, taken-for-grantedness, lack of interest, the humdrum and prosaic.

All other attributes of a jivanmukta must be relativized against this one absolute: a honed sense of the astounding mystery of everything.[3] All else we say of such a person must have a yes/no quality. Is he or she always happy? Well, yes and no. On one level he emphatically is not; if he were he couldn't "weep with those who mourn"—he would be an unfeeling monster, a callous brute. If anything, a realized soul is more in touch with the grief and sorrow that is part and parcel of the human condition, knowing that it too needs to be accepted and lived as all life needs to be lived. To reject the shadow side of life, to pass it by with averted eyes—refusing our share of common sorrow while expecting our share of common joy—would cause the unlived, rejected shadows to deepen in us as fear, including the fear of death. A story that is told of the recent Zen master Shaku Soen points up the dialectical stance of the realized soul toward happiness that we have been noting. When he was able to do so he liked to take an evening stroll through a nearby village. One evening he heard wailing in a house he was passing and, on entering quietly, found that the householder had died and his family and neighbors were crying. Immediately he sat down and began crying too. An elderly gentleman, shaken by this display of emotion in a famous master, remarked, "I would have thought that you at least were beyond such things." "But it is this which puts me beyond it," the master replied through his sobs.[4]

The master's tears we can understand; the sense in which he was "beyond" them is more difficult to fathom, like the peace that passeth understanding. The peace that comes when a man is hungry and finds food, is sick and recovers, or is lonely and finds a friend—peace of this sort is readily intelligible; but the peace that *passeth* understanding comes when the pain of life is not relieved. It shimmers on the crest of a wave of pain; it is the spear of frustration transformed into a shaft of light. The master's sobs were real, yet paradoxically they did not erode the yes-experience of the East's "it is as it should be" and the West's "Thy will be done."

In our efforts to conceive the human best, everything turns on an affirmation that steers between cynicism on the one hand and sentimentality on the other. A realized self isn't incessantly, and thereby oppresively, cheerful—oppressively, not only because we suspect some pretense in an unvarying smile, but also because it underscores our moodiness by contrast. Not every room a jivanmukta enters floods with sunlight; he can flash indignation and upset money changers' tables. Not invariance but appropriateness is his hallmark, an appropriateness that has the whole repertoire of emotions at its command. The Catholic church is right in linking radiance with sanctity, but the paradoxical, "in spite of" charcter of this radiance must again be stressed. Along with being a gift to be received, life is a task to be performed. The adept performs it: whatever his hand finds to do, he does with all his might. Even if it proves his lot to walk stretches of life as a dessert waste, he walks it rather than pining for an alternative. Happiness enters as by-product. What matters focally, as the Zen master Dogen never tired of noting, is resolve.

If a jivanmukta isn't forever radiating sweetness and light, neither does he constantly emit blasts of energy. He can be forceful when need be; we find it restoring rather than draining to be in his presence, and he has reserves to draw on, as when Socrates stood all night in a trance and outpaced the militia with bare feet on ice. In general, though, we sense him as relaxed and composed rather than charged—the model of the dynamic and magnetic personality tends to have a lot of ego in it; it demands attention. Remember, everything save the adept's access to inner vistas, the realms of gold I am calling the sacred unconscious, must be relativized. If leadership is called for, the adept steps forward; otherwise, he is just as happy to follow. He isn't debarred from being a guru, but equally he does not need to be one—he doesn't need disciples to prop up his ego. Focus or periphery, limelight or shadow—it doesn't really matter. Both have their opportunities; both, their limitations.

All these relativities I have mentioned—happiness, energy, prominence, impact—pertain to the jivamukti's finite self which he progressively pushes aside as he makes his way toward his final, sacred unconscious. As his goal is an impersonal, impartial one, his identification with it involves a dying to his finite selfhood. That part of his being is engaged in a vanishing act, as Coomaraswamy suggested when he wrote, "Blessed is the man on whose tomb can be written, *'Hic jacet nemo,'*" here lies no one.[5]

However, having insisted above that there is only one absolute or constant in the journey toward this self-naughting, namely, the sense of the sacred, that luminous mystery in which all things are bathed, I must now admit that there is another: the realization of how far we all are from the goal that beckons, how many ranges of hills remain to be crossed. "Why callest thou me good ... ?" As human beings we are made to surpass ourselves and are truly ourselves only when transcending ourselves. Only the slightest of barriers separates us from our sacred unconscious; it is infinitely close to us. Yet we are infinitely far from it, so for us the barrier looms as a mountain that we must remove with our own hands. We scrape away at the earth, but in vain; the mountain remains. Still we go on digging at the mountain, in the name of God or whatever. Of the final truth, we for the most part only hear; very rarely do we actually see it. The mountain isn't there. It never was there.

REFERENCES

1. One of the most interesting and original recent analyses of this most universal (yet ultimately questionable) assumption is to be found in Comfort, A. *I and That.* New York: Crown Publishers, 1979. Many studies now approach this subject in terms of both Asian and Western thought, but few also draw recent science as ably into the discussion as does this one.
2. Daniel Brown has uncovered something here that is interesting and probably important—I am indebted to Kendra Smith for pointing this out to me as well as for other helpful suggestions in this chapter. Writing in the *International Journal of Clinical and Experimental Hypnosis* (October 1977, *24, 4*), he notes that the steps in Tantric Buddhist meditation reverse the stages of perceptive and cognitive development as these have been discovered by the constructivist school in child psychology: Piaget, Gesell, Kagan, Lois Murphy, Brunner, et al. Whereas the infant successively acquires (constructs), first a sense of self around which to organize his experience and then structures for organizing his perceptions and after that his thoughts, Tantric meditation throws this process into reverse. After an initial stage that trains the lama to introspect intently, a second state disrupts his thought structures, regressing him to the world of pure perception. Step three takes over from there and disrupts the perception-patterning processes he developed in infancy. The fourth and final stage breaks through the organizing mechanisms that constructed the infant's sense of ego and enables the lama to experience a world in which there is no obstructing sense of self. In the vocabulary we are using here, such meditation peels back intermediate layers of our unconscious minds and allows us to be in direct touch with our sacred unconscious.
3. Isaac Newton provides a lovely instance of the quality I am thinking of. What could be more everyday or obvious than gravity, enabling and ruling (as it does) our every action. Yet Newton pierced through our habituation with the force to see that it is incomprehensible. "That one body may act upon another at a distance through a vacuum without the mediation of anything else," he wrote to a friend, "is to me so great an absurdity that . . . no man who has in philosophic matters a competent faculty of thinking could ever fall into it." Quoted in Zukav, G. *The Dancing Wu Li Masters.* New York: Morrow, 1979, p. 49.
4. Schloegl, I. *The Wisdom of the Zen Masters.* New York: New Directions, 1975, p. 21.
5. *Hinduism and Buddhism.* Westport, Conn.: Greenwood Press, 1943, p. 30.

Certainly it seems more and more clear that what we call 'normal' in psychology is really a psychopathology of the average, so undramatic and so widely spread that we don't even notice it.

Abraham Maslow

In this chapter, "Sufism and The Mental Health Sciences," Arthur Deikman argues that one of the major tasks confronting health care professionals and their patients is the developemnt of a sense of meaning and purpose in the world. The questions Why am I? Who am I? and How do I fit into the world? are among the most fundamental questions that people have to address, and yet often little attention is paid to them by traditional Western psychotherapies. He says that this need for new goals within psychiatry in particular, and the mental health professions in general, is critical and calls for the learning of intuition as expressed in the science of Sufism. Deikman knows the Eastern disciplines well and points out some potential dangers which may occur when Westerners try to graft them onto Western thought. This chapter provides an excellent mix of clear Western logic and ancient Sufi stories.

Arthur J. Deikman received his A.B. and M.D. degrees from Harvard University and his psychiatric residency training at Yale University and at the Austen Riggs Center. He has investigated the effects of meditation on consciousness and developed a theoretical approach to the mystical experience based on developmental and cognitive psychology. He has been on the faculty at the University of Colorado Medical Center and is an Associate Clinical Professor at the University of California, San Francisco (Langley Porter Institute). He also maintains a private practice in San Francisco and Mill Valley. In addition to publishing several research articles he has written Personal Freedom *(Grossmam-Viking, 1976), and* The Observing Self-Mysticism and Psychotherapy *(Beacon, 1982).*

12

Sufism and The Mental Health Sciences

Arthur J. Deikman, M.D.

I think it not improbable that man, like the grub that prepares a chamber for the winged thing it never has seen but is to be—that man may have cosmic destinies that he does not understand.

Justice Oliver Wendell Holmes[1]

Psychiatry can be defined as the science of reducing mental suffering and enhancing mental health. To date, the field has been primarily concerned with the first part of the definition. For example, in the Index to the *Standard Edition of the Complete Psychological Works of Sigmund Freud,*[2] the word "neurosis" has over 400 references. In contrast, "health" is not even listed. The imbalance tends to be true of contemporary texts, as well. This situation is understandable because psychiatry originated to deal with disordered function. The question, What is the function of a healthy person? which requires the further question, What is the purpose of human life? is not usually asked because it is assumed to be answered by simple observation of the everyday activities of the general population.*

Underlying all of our activities are purposes that give meaning and direc-

---

* In fairness to Freud it should be noted that in his later, philosophical writings, he did consider that question, and when he did his answer was more in keeping with mystical literature than with modern psychology. "I may now add that civilization is a process in the service of Eros, whose purpose is to combine single human individuals, and after that families, then races, peoples and nations, into one great unity, the unity of mankind."[3]

tion to our efforts. One might go to college to become a lawyer, save money to buy a car, or vote to elect an official—all these actions are vitalized by purpose and if the purpose is removed, the activities may cease. That being the case, what is the purpose of human life itself? What answer do we have to the question, Why am I? A direct answer is not usually attempted in our culture, but an indirect answer is there, implicit in scientific publications and in the world view that permeates from scientific authority to the public-at-large. We are told either that the question lies outside the scope of science or that the question is false because the human race has developed by chance in a random universe. The physicist Erwin Schrödinger commented on this problem:

> Most painful is the absolute silence of all our scientific investigations towards our questions concerning the meaning and scope of the whole display. The more attentively we watch it, the more aimless and foolish it appears to be. The show that is going-on obviously acquires a meaning only with regard to the mind that contemplates it. But what science tells us about this relationship is patently absurd: as if the mind had only been produced by that very display that it is now watching and would pass away with it when the sun finally cools down and the earth has been turned into a desert of ice and snow.[4]

We pay a price for the nonanswer of science. Psychiatry has recognized the existence of "anomie"—the "illness" of meaninglessness, of alienation or estrangement from one's fellow men. Anomie stems from the absence of a deeply felt purpose. Our contemporary scientific culture also has had little to say about meaning, itself, except to suggest and assume that man imposes meaning; he does not discover it. That this assumption may be incorrect and productive of pathology is a possibility that needs to be considered. It may be that the greatest problem confronting psychiatry is that it lacks a theoretical framework adequate to provide meaning for its patients, many of whom are badly handicapped in their struggle to overcome neurotic problems because the conceptual context within which they view themselves provides neither meaning, direction, nor hope. That context derives from the modern, scientific world view of an orderly, mechanical, indifferent universe in which human beings exist as an interesting biochemical phenomenon—barren of purpose. Survival is a purpose, but not enough. Working for the survival of others and alleviating suffering is a purpose, but it loses its meaning against a picture of the human race with no place to go, endlessly repeating the same patterns, or worse.

The issue of meaning increases in importance as one's own death becomes less theoretical and more probable. Life goals of acquisition become utterly futile, for no achievements of money, fame, sex, power, and security are able to stop the relentless slide towards extinction. Our bodies age and our minds grow increasingly restless seeking a solution to death. As former goals lose their significance, life can easily appear to be a random cycle of trivial events, and the search may end in the most profound despair or a dull resignation. The widespread use of sedatives, alcohol, and narcotics is related to the wish to suppress despair and substitute sensation for meaning.

Such "existential" despair is so culturally accepted that it is often defined as healthy. Consider the following extract from *The American Handbook of Psychiatry:*

> To those who have obtained some wisdom in the process of reaching old age, death often assumes meaning as the proper outcome of life. It is nature's way of assuring much life and constant renewal. Time and customs change but the elderly tire of changing; it is time for others to take over, and the elderly person is willing to pass quietly from the scene.[5]

So we should end, according to the voice of reason, not with a bang or a whimper, but in a coma of increasing psychological fatigue.

The problem is illustrated concretely and poignantly by the dilemma of many psychiatrists themselves. A recent article in the *American Journal of Psychiatry* concerned a number of professional therapists, ages 35 to 45, mostly of a psychoanalytic background, who formed a group which at first provided peer supervision and later attempted to function as a leaderless therapy group for its members who, as it turned out, were in a crisis:

> The original members of the group we have described were remarkably homogenous in their purposes in joining. The conscious reason was to obtain help in mastering a phase in their own development, the mid-life crisis. We refer to that stage of life in which the individual is aware that half of his time has been used up and the general pattern or trajectory of his work and personal life is clear. At this time, one must give up the normal manic defenses of early life—infinite faith in one's abilities and the belief that anything is possible. The future becomes finite, childhood fantasies have been fulfilled or unrealized, and there is no longer a sense of having enough time for anything. One becomes aware that one's energy and physical and mental abilities will be declining. The individual must think of prolonging and conserving rather than expanding. The reality of one's limited life span comes into sharp focus, and the work of mourning the passing of life begins in earnest.[6]

The "healthy" attitude recommended here would seem to be a stoical and courageous facing of a reality defined by certain assumptions prevalent in our culture: limited human capacity and limited meaning to life. From this point of view, it can be maintained that the second half of life should be used to adjust oneself to the final termination of individual consciousness. The grimness of such a goal may have resonated in the author's minds for they go on to brighten up the picture:

> In Erikson's terms, the individual must at this time struggle to achieve intimacy and creativity and avoid isolation and stagnation. If the work of mourning one's lost youth is carried through and the realities of the human situation are fully accepted, the ensuing years can be a period of increased productivity and gratification.[7]

"Increased productivity" and "gratification" are envoked to suggest that something good is still possible after 40, but the possibilities still would seem to call more for resignation than for vitality and continued growth. This ultimately circumscribed view of human life is widely held by psychiatrists. Even in the relatively affirmative writings of Erikson, the Eight Stages of Man has some of the flavor of a survival manual.[8]

In contrast to our scientific culture and its psychology, Eastern introspective (mystical) disciplines have focused on meaning and purpose but have employed a strategy in which the use of intellect and reason is neither central nor basic to the process of investigation. Procedures such as meditation, fasting, chanting, and other unusual practices have been employed as part of an integrated strategy whose exact pattern and content depended on the nature and circumstances of the individual and of the culture in which the teaching was taking place.

Unfortunately, the literature of Eastern psychological disciplines has not been of much practical use for contemporary Western readers. Academic study of such texts does not seem to develop wisdom or improve personality functioning, and exotic practices themselves have proven to be elusive and tricky instruments. For example, procedures such as meditation that were once part of a unique and individually prescribed pattern of development are now extracted from their original context and offered for consumption as if they were a kind of vitamin that was good for everyone, ridiculously cheap, and devoid of side effects. Those who use these components of a specialized technology may obtain increased calmness, enjoyment, and improvement of efficiency—but usually without noticeable gain in wisdom. They answer the question, Who am I? by recitation, not realization, and for all the "bliss" that may be displayed the person's essential knowledge appears unchanged. For those who fare less well with meditation, schizoid withdrawal, grandiosity, vanity, and dependency flourish under the disguise of spiritual practice. Perhaps the worst effect of indiscriminate and unintegrated use of these techniques is that people come to believe that the effects they experience are the measure of Eastern esoteric science. The end result is that they confirm and strengthen their customary conceptual prison from which they desperately need to escape.

The crux of the problem is that modern Westerners need technical means specific to their time and culture. Although such a statement makes perfect sense to most people when the subject concerns the training of physicians or physicists, training in the "spiritual" is believed to be a different matter. Programs and techniques 2000 years old are assumed to be adequate to the task: indeed, it seems that the older and more alien they are, the better they are received.

Fortunately, some traditional materials have recently been made available in a form suitable for contemporary needs; they offer practical benefits of interest to psychiatry as well as to the general public. These materials address themselves to the question, Who am I? but they do so in a unique manner:

WHY WE ARE HERE[9]*

Walking one evening along a deserted road, Mulla Nasrudin saw a troop of horsemen coming towards him.

His imagination started to work; he saw himself captured and sold as a slave, or impressed into the army.

Nasrudin bolted, climbed a wall into a graveyard, and lay down in an open tomb.

Puzzled at his strange behavior, the men—honest travelers—followed him.

They found him stretched out, tense and quivering.

"What are you doing in that grave? We saw you run away. Can we help you?"

"Just because you can ask a question does not mean there is a straightforward answer to it," said the Mulla, who now realized what had happened. "It all depends upon your viewpoint. If you must know, however: *I* am here because of *you,* and *you* are here because of *me.*"

"Why We Are Here" is a teaching story adapted from the classical literature of Sufism. Teaching stories, in a form appropriate to the modern reader, are the means now being made available to prepare Western intellects for learning what they need to know. The stories, such as "Why We Are Here," are built of patterns, depth upon depth, offering resonance at the

---

* All the stories quoted in this article are copyrighted by Idries Shah and are reproduced by his permission.

readers's level, whatever that may be. Teaching stories have more than one function. They provide the means for people to become aware of their patterns of behavior and thinking so as to accomplish a refinement of their perception and the development of an attitude conducive to learning. Some stories are also designed to communicate with what is conceived to be the innermost part of the human being. Speaking metaphorically, Sufis say the stories make contact with a nascent "organ" of superior perception, supplying a type of "nutrition" that assists its development. It is this latter function that is of particular importance to understand; it is the key to the importance of Sufism in helping to diagnose and cure, eventually, the basic illness afflicting psychiatrists as well as their patients.

Sufism is usually thought of as a Middle Eastern mystical religion. According to Idries Shah,* that description is misleading. Referring to copious Sufi classics, he states that Sufism is the method of developing the higher, perceptual capacity inherent in human beings and vital to their happiness.

This method is referred to by classical Sufi authorities as a "science" in the sense that it is a specific body of knowledge, applied according to the principles known by a Teacher, to achieve a specific and predictable result. That result is the capacity to *know* directly (not through the senses or the usual intellectual functions) the meaning of human life and the inner significance of ordinary events. The development of this channel of knowing adds a new dimension to ordinary consciousness, and the change that results is regarded as the next step in the evolution of the human race, a step that we must take or perish.

Ordinarily, we do not consider that the zone of normal perception may be so limited as to preclude the experience of this aspect of reality, the special "sight" with which mystical disciplines were ordinarily concerned. According to the Sufis, meaning is just such a perceptual problem.

An illustration of this issue at the level of biology, has been described by C. F. Pantin, former Chairman of Trustees of the British Museum:

A danger in this sort of behavior analysis—one which I fell into myself - is that it looks so complete that if you are not careful, you may start to imagine that you can explain the whole behavior of the sea anemone by very simple reflexes—like the effect of a coin in a slot machine. But quite by accident, I discovered that apart from reflexes, there was a whole mass of purposive behavior connected with the spontaneous activity of the

*Idries Shah has written many books on Sufism, and his position as spokesman for contemporary Sufism has been accepted by a large number of authorities (see *Sufi Studies: East and West).*[10]

anemone about which we simply know nothing. (Actually, this behavior was too slow to be noticed; it was outside our sensory spectrum for the time being.)[11]

Similarly, the purpose of human life may be outside the perceptual spectrum of the ordinary person. To widen that spectrum, to provide the necessary capacity to "see," is the goal of Sufism.

The Sufis claim that mankind is psychologically "ill" because people do not perceive who they really are and what their situation is. Thus, they are "blind" or "asleep" because their latent, higher capacity is under-developed—partly because they are too caught up in the exercise of intellect and emotion for purposes of vanity, greed, and fear. The development of the necessary perception is called "awakening," and the perception itself is called "knowledge." It is often said that the science of awakening mankind has been present for many thousands of years but, because of the special nature of the process and of the knowledge that it brings, the dissemination of the science has fluctuated throughout history and has never taken place on a large scale, partly because of the resistance this idea provokes.[12]

The resistance is a result of several factors. To begin with, "the seeming completeness of the world" (Rumi) seems to contradict the idea of an unseen reality. "Where is it?" the intellect and senses ask. Futhermore, the wish for control and the anxiety of helplessness lead us to overestimate what we know and to balk at the idea that we may be as undeveloped as children. Missing from our culture are the bases whereby the concept of virtue can be seen to have a functional, rather than a moral, significance. Establishing such a basis in the culture at large will be necessary before mystical science can be utilized by large numbers of people. This issue is illustrated by the arrogance of Western civilization, particularly the mental health sciences' attitude towards mysticism. For example, consider the fact that humility is the fundamental requirement for participation in the mystical traditions. "This is so, not because humility is a virtue, something that earns one credit in a heavenly bank account, but because humility is instrumental—it is the attitude required for learning. Humility is the acceptance of the possibility that someone else or something else has something to teach you which you do not already know. Western scientists view the mystical tradition with the arrogance of British Colonials who could live for years in India without bothering to learn the language of the country because it was considered inferior. Perhaps science's long battle to free itself from religious control, from demonology and divine authority, has left us with an automatic and costly reaction against anything that bears the outward signs of religion. Actually, mystics outside the Western tradition tend to share our suspicion and describe their disciplines as a science of development—not a religion, as ordinarily understood."*

Thus, the attempt to transmit mystical science to the modern Western citizen has proved to be a slow and laborious task, even though the essential concepts are not difficult to understand and are not magical, at all.

RADIOS[13]

I was once in a certain country where the local people had never heard the sounds emitted from a radio receiver. A transistorized set was being brought to me; and while waiting for it to arrive I tried to describe it to them. The general effect was that the description fascinated some and infuriated others. A minority became irrationally hostile about radios.

When I finally demonstrated the set, the people could not tell the difference between the voice from the loudspeaker and someone nearby. Finally, like us, they managed to develop the necessary discrimination of each, such as we have.

And, when I questioned from afterwards, all swore that what they had imagined from descriptions of radios, however painstaking, did not correspond with the reality.

If, instead of talking of a radio receiver, the term "intuition" is used, the meaning of the analogy might be more clear. Ordinary intuition, however, is considered by the Sufis to be a lower-level imitation of the superior form of intuition with which Sufism is concerned. For the moment, however, some consideration of the place of ordinary intuition in the activity of the scientist may be hlepful in illustrating the practical reality of the Sufic position.

Although the scientific method is taught as if data plus logic equal discovery, those who have studied how discoveries are actually made come to quite different conclusions. Eugene Wigner, a Nobel prize winning physicist, comments:

The discovery of the laws of nature requires first and foremost intuition, conceiving of picture and a great many subconscious processes. The use and also the confirmation of these laws is another matter . . . . logic comes after intuition.[14]

An extensive, detailed study of the process of scientific discovery was made by Michael Polanyi, formerly Professor of Physical Chemistry at the University of Manchester and now Senior Research Fellow at Merton College, Oxford.[15] Polanyi studied scientists' descriptions of how they arrived at

*Deikman, A. Comments on the GAP report on mysticism. *Journal of Nervous and Mental Disease,* 1977, *165*(5), 217.

their "breakthroughs" to a new view of reality. He found, like Wigner, that logic, data, and reasoning came last—another channel of knowing was in use. There was no word for that channel in ordinary vocabularly so he used an analogy to convey its nature:

And we know that the scientist produces problems, has hunches, and, elated by these anticipations, pursues the quest that should fulfill these anticipations. This quest is guided throughout by feelings of a deepening coherence and these feelings have a fair chance of proving right. We may recognize here the powers of a dynamic intuition. The mechanism of this power can be illuminated by an analogy. Physics speaks of potential energy that is released when a weight slides down a slope. Our search for deeper coherence is guided by a potentiality. We feel the slope toward deeper insight as we feel the direction in which a heavy weight is pulled along a steep incline. It is this dynamic intuition which guides the pursuit of discovery.[16]

The Sufis contend not only that man needs more than intellect and emotion to guide him, but that those two "servants," in the absence of the "master," have taken over the house and forgotten their proper function:

THE SERVANTS AND THE HOUSE[17]

At one time there was a wise and kindly man, who owned a large house. In the course of his life he often had to go away for long periods. When he did this, he left the house in charge of his servants.

One of the characteristics of these people was that they were very forgetful. They forgot, from time to time, why they were in the house; so they carried out their tasks repetitiously. At other times they thought that they should be doing things in a different way from the way in which their duties had been assigned to them. This was because they had lost track of their functions.

Once, when the master was away for a long time, a new generation of servants arose, who thought that they actually owned the house. Since they were limited by their immediate world, however, they thought that they were in a pardoxical situation. For instance, sometimes they wanted to sell the house, and could find no buyers, because they did not know how to go about it. At other times, people came inquiring about buying the house and asking to see the title-deeds, but since they did not know anything about deeds the servants thought that these people were mad and not genuine buyers at all.

Paradox was also evidenced by the fact that supplies for the house kept "mysteriously" appearing, and this provision did not fit in with the assumption that the inmates were responsible for the whole house.

Instructions for running the house had been left, for purposes of refreshing the memory, in the master's apartments. But after the first generation, so sacrosanct had these apartments become that nobody was allowed to enter them, and they became considered to be an impenetrable mystery. Some, indeed, held that there was no such apartment at all, although they could see its doors. These doors, however, they explained as something else: a part of the decoration of the walls.

Such was the condition of the staff of a house, which neither took over the house nor stayed faithful to their original commitment.

The Sufis specify that the development of man's superior capacity has its own rigorous requirements: adequate preparation of suitable students, the correct learning situation, and the activity of a Teacher—one who has reached the goal and by means of that special knowledge is equipped to teach according to the needs of the particular culture, the particular time, the particular historical period, and the particular person. Because of these requirements, there is no set dogma or technique that is utilized in a standard fashion: the form is only a vehicle and is constantly changing.

All religious presentations are varieties of one truth, more or less distorted. This truth manifests itself in various peoples, who become jealous of it, not realizing that its manifestation accords with their needs. It cannot be passed on in the same form because of the difference in the minds of different communities. It cannot be reinterpreted, because it must grow afresh. (Khwaja Salahudin of Bokhara [18])

Thus, Sufis differentiate their science from traditional religions, whether Christian, Judaic, Buddhist, Moslem, or Hindu, because such religions have solidified around set rituals, forms, exercises, and dogmas that tend to be handed out to everyone regardless of the context and individual differences. According to Idries Shah, even organizations designated as Sufi Orders may undergo this " . . . crystallization into priesthood and traditionalism. In the originally Sufic groupings where this fossilization has indeed taken place, their fixation upon a repetitious usage of Sufi materials provides a warning for the would-be Sufi that such an organization has 'joined the world.'" [19]

We have examples of this problem within the field of psychiatry, itself. In Freud's time, for example, the Vienna Circle was open to all who had sufficient interest and capacity to participate, regardless of what formal degrees or titles they possessed. Today, the American Psychoanalytic Institute will not accord full membership to anyone not possessing an M.D., even though the functional relevance of a medical degree for the theory and practice of psychoanalysis can scarcely be discerned. A similar stiffening, sclerosing process seems to invade every human organization. With this in mind, we can understand the Sufic contention that religions were intially based on the development of a higher form of perception, but inevitably, they became ossified, lost their capacity to function in that way, and now persist as archaic structures, hollow shells good only for fulfilling social and emotional needs. Furthermore, most "mystical experiences" are regarded by the Sufis as being primarily emotional and having little practical importance—except for the deleterious effect of causing people to believe they are being "spiritual" when they are not. Self-deception is at work in such cases and blocks progress towards the development of higher perceptions.

STRANGE AGITATION[20]

Sahl Abdullah once went into a state of violent agitation, with physical manifestations, during a religious meeting.

Ibn Salim said: "What is this state?"

Sahl said: "This was not, as you imagine, power entering me. It was, on the contrary, due to my own weakness."

Others present remarked: "If that was weakness, what is power?"

"Power," said Sahl, "is when something like this enters, and the mind and body manifest nothing at all."

The ordinary man is said to suffer from confusion or "sleep" because of his tendency to use his *customary* thought patterns and perception to try to understand the meaning of his life and reach fulfillment. Consequently, his experience of reality is constricted, and dangerously so, because he tends to be unaware of it. Sufis assert that the awakening of man's latent perceptual capacity is not only crucial for his happiness but is the principal goal of his current phase of existence—it is man's evolutionary task. Rumi, the great Sufi poet, stated this explicitly:

THIS TASK[21]

You have a duty to perform. Do anything else, do any number of things, occupy your time fully, and yet, if you do not do this task, all your time will have been wasted.

HOW FAR YOU HAVE COME![22]

Originally, you were clay. From being mineral, you became vegetable. From vegetable, you became animal, and from animal, man. During these periods man did not know where he was going, but he was being taken on a long journey nonetheless. And you have to go through a hundred different worlds yet.

According to the Sufis, only with the knowledge that perceptual development brings can human beings know the meaning of human life, both in terms of the particular events of a person's life and the destiny of the human race.

CITY OF STORMS[23]

Once upon a time there was a city. It was very much like any other city, except it was almost permanently enveloped in storms.

The people who lived in it loved their city. They had, of course, adjusted to its climate. Living amid storms meant that they did not notice thunder, lightning and rain most of the time.

If anyone pointed out the climate they thought he was being rude or boring. After all, having storms was what life was like, wasn't it? Life went on like this for many centuries.

This would have been all very well, but for one thing: the people had not made a complete adaptation to a storm-climate. The result was that they were afraid, unsettled and frequently agitated.

Since they had never seen any other kind of place in living memory, cities or countries without some storms belonged to folklore or the babbling of lunatics.

There were two tried recipes which caused them to forget, for a time, their tensions: to make changes and to obsess themselves with what they had. At any given moment in their history, some sections of the population would have their attention fixed on change, and others on possessions of some kind. The unhappy ones would only then be those who were doing neither.

Rain poured down, but nobody did anything about it because it was not a recognized problem. Wetness was a problem, but nobody connected it with rain. Lightning started fires, which were a problem, but these were regarded as individual events without a consistent cause.

You may think it remarkable that so many people knew so little for so long.

But then we tend to forget that, compared to present-day information, most people in history have known almost nothing about anything—and even contemporary knowledge is daily being modified—and even wrong.

Most psychotherapy focuses on uncovering the fantasies that shape neurotic action and on clarifying and resolving the conflicts of wishes and fears that lead individuals to the repetitive, self-defeating behaviors for which they usually seek therapy. These functions of psychotherapy are necessary and important. However, the resolution of neurotic problems, while it may be a necessary first step for an individual, is the measure neither of health nor of human potentiality. Freud's model of man as an organism seeking relief from tension, forced to negotiate a compromise between instinct, reason, and society, leaves even the most successful negotiator in a position of impoverishment as pathological, in its own way, as any illness listed in the diagnostic manual. This is because the usual psychiatric concept of health is both barren and narrow. Even the most "humanistic" of current psychologies that offer, in principle, equal attention to such dimensions of human experience as the playful, the creative, and "the spiritual," have no clear concept of the nature of the problem and little to suggest for its solution. "Self-realization" is advocated, but just what the self is that is to be realized and what that realization might be is not made explicit.

All these therapies and theories are in the same boat because they share the fundamental limiting assumptions about man that are basic to our culture. Unwittingly, they help maintain the lack of perception that is the basic dysfunction of the human race and hinders the development of the higher capacities that are needed. In this sense, psychiatry, whether of the neurochemical or psychoanalytic variety or a combination of both, perpetuates the endemic illness of meaninglessness and arrested human development—it has no remedy for the cultural affliction that cripples normal people. Thus, we arrive at the dilemma of the group of psychiatrists in mid-life crisis described above. They illustrate the point. Their science is caught within the same closed room in which they find themselves; indeed, it helps to bar the door. Psychoanalytic theory, the masterpiece of a genius, is so powerful and encompassing a schema that all phenomena seem to be contained within its walls; its proponents have come to love their city—storms notwithstanding, and they are almost never forced to reappraise their world.

However, existentialism has helped some psychiatrists look to the underpinnings of their profession. Rychlak, writing in the *American Handbook of Psychiatry,* summarizes: "Building on the theme of alienation first introduced by Hegel, and then popularized in the writings of Kierkegaard, the existentialists argue that man has been alienated from his true [phenomenal] nature by science's penchant for objective measurement, control, and stilted, non-teleological description."[24] Through existentialism, purpose and meaning have come to have advocates such as the psychoanalyst Avery Weisman: "*The existential core of psychoanalysis is whatever nucleus of meaning and being there is that can confront both life and death.* Unless he accepts this as his indispensable reality, the psychoanalyst is like a man wandering at night in a strange city."[25] Yet how can he find that nucleus of meaning, let alone accept it? The group of psychiatrists in mid-life crisis, described earlier, are missing that center because it is missing from the very discipline they practice and teach. Psychiatry cannot address the issue of meaning because of the limited nature of its concept of man and because of its ignorance of the means needed to develop the capacity to perceive it.

In contrast, Sufism regards its task as the development of the higher perceptual capacity of man, his "conscious evolution." According to Sufi authorities, the knowledge of how to do this has always existed. It had a flowering in Islam during the Middle Ages, during which the term "Sufis" came into use, but it had other names, centuries before. The Sufis regard Moses, Christ, and Muhammad as Teachers of the same basic process—their external forms and the means they employed were different, but the inner activity was the same. The traditional forms that we see around us in current times are said to be the residue of a science whose origins extend back to the beginnings of man's history. The problem is that our thinking has been conditioned to associate "awakening" with vegetarian diets, chanting, chastity, whirling dances, meditation on chakras, koans, and mantras, beards, robes, and solemn faces—because all these features of once vital systems have been preserved and venerated as if they were still useful for achieving the same goal. The parts, or a collection of them, are mistaken for the whole. It is as if a car door, lying on the ground, were labeled "automobile" and hopeful travelers diligently opened and closed its window, waiting expectantly for it to transport them to a distant city.

Meditation, asceticism, special diets, and the like should be regarded as technical devices that sometimes had a specific place in a coherent system prescribed for the individual. When used properly by a Teacher, they formed a time-limited container for a content that was timeless. Now, many old and empty containers labeled "spiritual" litter the landscape. The importation and wide use of these unintegrated forms attest to the immortality of institutions and customs, rather than to the present usefulness of the activities.

The Surfis maintain that, nevertheless, amidst all this confusion, the science of "conscious evolution" continues in a contemporary form, invisibile to those expecting the traditional. "Speak to everyone in accordance with his degree of understanding" was a saying of Muhammad. Idries Shah states that he is one of those speaking now to contemporary man, Eastern as well as Western, in a way appropriate to the task of educating people who do not realize how much they have to learn. R. L. Thompson, writing in *The Brook Postgraduate Gazette,* agrees: "The problems of approaching the Sufis' work are such that Idries Shah's basic efforts do seem necessary. Little help is to be found in the academic approach based on linguistics and history."[26] Most of Idries Shah's writings consist of carefully selected and translated groups of such teaching stories, including the ones I have quoted. His translations are exceptionally clear and digestible to a modern reader.

The stories provide templates to which we can match our own behavior. We accept them because they are so deceptively impersonal—the situations are presented as the history of someone else. The story slides past our vigilant defenses and is stored in our minds until the moment comes when our own thinking or situation matches the template—then it suddenly arises in awareness and we "see," as in a mirror, the shape and meaning of what we are actually doing. The analogical form can evade the categorizing of our rational thought and reach other sectors of the mind.

THE DESIGN[27]

A Sufi on the Order of the Naqshbandis was asked:

"Your Order's name means, literally, 'The Designers.' What do you design, and what use is it?"

He said:

"We do a great deal of designing, and it is most useful. Here is a parable of one such form.

"Unjustly imprisoned, a tinsmith was allowed to receive a rug woven by his wife. He prostrated himself upon the rug day after day to say his prayers, and after some time he said to his jailers:

"'I am poor and without hope, and you are wretchedly paid. But I am a tinsmith. Bring my tin and tools and I shall make small artefacts which you can sell in the market, and we will both benefit.'

"The guards agreed to this, and presently the tinsmith and they were both making a profit, from which they bought food and comfort for themselves.

"Then, one day, when the guards went to the cell, the door was open, and he was gone.

"Many years later, when this man's innocence had been established, the man who had imprisoned him asked him how he had escaped, what magic he had used. He said:

"'It is a matter of design, and design within design. My wife is a weaver. She found the man who had made the locks of the cell door, and got the design from him. This she wove into the carpet, at the spot where my head touched in prayer five times a day. I am a metal-worker, and this design looked to me like the inside of a lock. I designed the plan of the artefacts to obtain the materials to make the key—and I escaped.'

"That," said the Naqshbandi Sufi, "Is one of the ways man may make his escape from the tyranny of his captivity."

Teaching stories, such as the above, are tools that depend on the motivation of the user and his or her capacity or level of skill. As understanding increases, the tools can be used for finer and deeper work. The more one experiences and uses them, the more remarkable they seem to be. They lend credence to Idries Shah's claim that Sufism is a science whose boundaries contain modern psychology but go beyond it. He states, "Sufism is itself a far more advanced psychological system than any which is yet developed in the West. Neither is this psychology Eastern in essence, but human."[28]

According to Shah, the initial step needed to be taken by most human beings is to become aware of *automatic pattern-thinking,* the conditioned associations and indoctrinated values that limit human perception and receptivity. The teaching story is used for this purpose, illustrating at one step removed, the egocentric thinking of which we are usually oblivious.

THAT'S WHY THEY BUNGED IT UP[29]

Nasrudin was very thirsty and was happy when he saw by the roadside a water-pipe whose outlet was bunged with a piece of wood.

Putting his open mouth near the stopper, he pulled. There was such a rush of water that he was knocked over.

"Oho!" roared the Mulla. "That's why they blocked you up, is it? And you have not yet learned any sense!"

PERSONAL WISDOM[30]

"I don't want to be a man," said a snake.

"If I were a man, who would hoard nuts for me?" asked the squirrel.

"People," said the rat, "have such weak teeth that they can hardly do any gnawing!"

"And as for speed . . . ," said the donkey, "they can't run at all, in comparison to me."

Teaching stories such as these have clarified patterns of my own thought, permitting me to notice similar patterns in my patients and to make appropriate interventions. One such story whose content is explicit, is the following:

VANITY[31]

A Sufi sage once asked his disciples to tell him what their vanities had been before they began to study with him.

The first said:

"I imagined that I was the most handsome man in the world."

The second said:

"I believed that, since I was religious, I was one of the elect."

The third said:

"I believed I could teach."

And the fourth said:

"My vanity was greater than all these; for I believed that I could learn."
The sage remarked:
"And the fourth disciple's vanity remains the greatest, for his vanity is
to show that he once had the greatest vanity."

Having read this story, I later observed myself doing the same thing as the
fourth disciple. In my case, I was berating myself for a personal failing. The
context was different from the specific situation of the story *but the pattern
was the same.* The story came to my mind like a mirror and I understood the
role of my vanity in what I was doing. That understanding provoked a wry
smile and ended my self-flagellation. Later, hearing a patient present feelings in a similar pattern, I could recognize it and repond by eliciting and
pointing out the concealed intent. A young male patient with whom I was
working had been castigating himself for having made such a "mess" out of
his opportunities, particularly as there was general recognition that he was
highly intelligent and likable. After listening to him for awhile, I offered an
alternative view: "I think you're doing yourself an injustice. You're not a
good guy who's making a mess of things—you're a mess who is doing a good
job."
He stopped in his tracks—wide-eyed—then threw back his head and
roared with laughter. We both laughed until our sides hurt. The next session,
he reported that he felt much better. The self-recriminations were noticeably
reduced.
My recognition of his concealed vanity, followed by an appropriate interpretation, was matched by the patient, who then responded with laughter,
relaxation, and the disappearance of the behavioral symptom. Would it be
equally correct to say, from the point of view of behavior modification, that
I had applied an aversive stimulus and therefore had extinguished his
response—a case of instrumental conditioning? Judging by my own experience, the "stimulus" does not feel aversive at all, it feels like relief, it is
recognition. Distress is suddenly clarified and disappears, leaving a
delightful sense of new freedom.
Let me give another example of what I am talking about. A woman whom
I had been seeing in once-a-week psychotherapy entered my office almost
frantic with distress, proclaiming anxiously that she was about to "go to
pieces." Ordinarily, I would have listened, drawn out some explanation of
the precipitating circumstances, and worked to clarify her irrational fears
and bring into awareness the emotions or ideas that presumably were being
repressed and were now increasing in intensity so as to produce her current
symptoms. That would most likely have been helpful, to a greater or lesser
extent. What actually happened was that, despite myself, I began to smile,
feeling amused. The woman's distress was genuine by all the criteria

customarily used in such situations. She was not prone to having crises and her statements were not hysterically exaggerated. Yet, I found myself smiling. The situation seemed funny to me because I perceived her as being in no actual danger but completely caught up in her imagination—her observing self was not part of all that commotion but, instead, was reporting it.

The woman suddenly becoming aware of my facial expression, stopped, and indignantly demanded the reason for my "unfeeling" smile in response to her desperation. Her question stimulated me to smile even more broadly and I actually began to laugh. She stared at me in disbelief and a look of outrage took possession of her face. However, in the midst of her rising anger, despite herself, she started to smile, also. "Damn you!" she exclaimed and began to laugh. We laughed together for a long while. The desperate air of crisis, the emergency, the impending breakdown vanished in that laughter like fog evaporating in the sun. The "going to pieces" never happened. The woman's psychotherapeutic progress took a leap forward in succeeding sessions.

This is not an example of a brilliant new therapy. Explanations can be constructed for the incident, using standard theory. However, as far as I can tell, I responded the way I did because of the stories that I had been reading that communicated a particular way of viewing the human situation.

The point of view and the learning principles presented in the teaching stories are tough-minded and emphasize the responsibility of each person for his or her own conduct and fulfillment. Such an attitude is not unfamiliar to psychiatry. However, developing a correct attitude is only the first step in Sufic science, a step called "learning how to learn." Responsibility, sincerity, humility, patience, generosity—these are not ends in themselves but are tools that must be acquired before a person can proceed further. It is what comes after this first step that sharply distinguishes Sufism from all the psychotherapeutic and "growth-oriented" disciplines with which we are familiar. The Sufis regard their system as being far in advance of ours because it extends beyond the conceptual and technical limits of psychology and embodies a method for assisting man to develop the special perception upon which his welfare, and that of the human race, depend. When asked to prove their assertion, Sufis insist on the necessity for undertaking preparatory training and then *experiencing* the domain in question. Such claims and requirements often provoke a haughty dismissal:

THREE EPOCHS[32]

1. *Conversation in the Fifth Century:*

   "It is said that silk is spun by insects, and does not grow on trees."

   "And diamonds are hatched from eggs, I suppose? Pay no attention to such an obvious lie."

"But there are surely many wonders in remote islands?"

"It is this very craving for the abnormal which produces fantastic invention."

"Yes, I suppose it is obvious when you think about it—that such things are all very well for the East, but could never take root in our logical and civilized society."

2. *In the Sixth Century:*

"A man has come from the East, bringing some small live grubs."

"Undoubtedly a charlatan of some kind. I suppose he says that they can cure toothache?"

"No, rather more amusing. He says that they can 'spin silk.' He has 'brought them with terrible sufferings, from one Court to another, having obtained them at the risk of his very life.'"

"This fellow has merely decided to exploit a superstition which was old in my great-grandfather's time."

"What shall we do with him, my Lord?"

"Throw his infernal grubs into the fire, and beat him for his pains until he recants. These fellows are wondrously bold. They need showing that we're not all ignorant peasants here, willing to listen to any wanderer from the East."

3. *In the Twentieth Century:*

"You say that there is something in the East which we have not yet discovered here in the West? Everyone has been saying that for thousands of years. But in this century we'll try anything: our minds are not closed. Now give me a demonstration. You have fifteen minutes before my next appointment. If you prefer to write it down, here's a half-sheet of paper."

If history has any value as a guide, it indicates that we should pay attention to the information now being provided to us by contemporary Sufism and not pass this opportunity without investigating it. Robert E. Ornstein, in his textbook *The Psychology of Consciousness,* concludes: "A new synthesis is in process within modern psychology. This synthesis combines the concerns of the esoteric traditions with the research methods and technology of modern science. In complement to this process, and feeding it, a truly contemporary approach to the problems of consciousness is arising from the esoteric traditions themselves."[33]

Psychiatrists need to recognize that their patients' psychological distress stems from three levels: (1) from conflicts of wishes, fears, and fantasies, (2) from an absence of perceived meaning, and (3) from a frustration of the need to progress in an evolutionary sense, as individuals and as a race. The first level is the domain in which psychiatry functions. The second and third levels require a science appropriate to the task. The special knowledge of the Sufis may enable us to put together materials already at hand—our present knowledge of psychodynamics, our system of universal education, our technology, our resources, and our free society—to create the conditions that will permit the development of man's full capacities, as yet unrealized.

REFERENCES

1. Oliver Wendell Holmes, cited in Murphy, G. *Human Potentialities*. New York: Basic Books, 1958.
2. Strachey, J. (Ed.). *The Standard Edition of the Complete Psychological Works of Sigmund Freud*. London: Hogarth, 1974, XXIV.
3. Strachey, J. (Ed.). *The Standard Edition of the Complete Psychological Works of Sigmund Freud*. London: Hogarth, 1961, XXI, p. 122.
4. Schrödinger, E. *What is Life? Mind and Matter*. Cambridge: Cambridge University Press, 1969, p. 149.
5. Lidz, T. On the life cycle. In *The American Handbook of Psychiatry*. New York: Basic Books, 1974, p. 125.
6. Hunt, W. and Issacharoff, A. History and analysis of a leaderless group of professional therapists. *American Journal of Psychiatry*, 1975, *132*(11), 1166.
7. Ibid., p. 1166.
8. Erikson, E. *Childhood and Society*. New York: W. W. Norton, 1950, pp. 219–234.
9. Shah, I. *The Exploits of the Incomparable Mulla Nasrudin*. New York: E. P. Dutton, 1972, p. 16.
10. Williams, L. F. R. (Ed.). *Sufi Studies: East and West*. New York: E. P. Dutton, 1974.
11. Greene, M. (Ed.). Toward a unity of knowledge. *Psychological Issues,* 1969, *6*(2), 60.
12. Shah, I. *The Sufis*. Garden City, N. Y.: Doubleday, Anchor Books, 1971, p. 28.
13. Shah, I. *The Magic Monastery,* New York: E. P. Dutton, 1972, pp. 13–15.
14. Greene, M. (Ed.). Toward a unity of knowledge. *Psychological Issues, 22,* 45.
15. Polanyi, M. *Personal Knowledge*. Chicago: University of Chicago Press, 1958.
16. Greene, M. (Ed.). Toward a unity of knowledge. *Psychological Issues,* 6(2), 60.
17. Shah, I. *Tales of the Dervishes*. New York: E. P. Dutton, 1970, pp. 211–212.
18. Shah, I. *The Way of the Sufi*. New York: E. P. Dutton, 1970, p. 264.
19. Ibid., p. 259.
20. Ibid., p. 182.
21. Ibid., p. 110.
22. Ibid., p. 102.
23. Shah, I. *The Magic Monastery*. New York: E. P. Dutton, 1972, pp. 140–141.
24. Rychlak, J. F. *American Handbook of Psychiatry*. New York: Basic Books, 1974, p. 162.
25. Weisman, A. *The Existential Core of Psychoanalysis*. Boston: Little, Brown, 1965, p. 242.
26. Thomson, R. L. Psychology and science from the ancient east. *The Brook Postgraduate Gazette,* 1973, *2*(1), 7–9.
27. Shah, I. *Thinkers of the East*. Baltimore: Penguin Books, 1972, p. 176.
28. Shah, I. *The Sufis*. Garden City, N. Y.: Doubleday, Anchor Books, 1971, p. 59.
29. Shah, I. *The Pleasantries of the Incredible Mulla Nasrudin*. New York: E. P. Dutton, 1971, p. 48.
30. Shah, I. *The Magic Monastery*. New York: E. P. Dutton, 1972, p. 157.
31. Ibid., p. 47.
32. Ibid., p. 25.
33. Ornstein, R. E. *The Psychology of Consciousness*. San Francisco: W. H. Freeman, 1972.

I believe there is no source of deception in the investigation of nature which can compare with a fixed belief that certain kinds of phenomena are impossible.

William James

Beginning in the late 1960s the reports of a young anthropologist claiming to describe his experiences and training at the hands of a Yaqui indian "man of knowledge" caught the attention of an extraordinarily large audience and became runaway best sellers. Some of the experiences clearly lay well outside the realm of what we usually consider possible, and controversy has raged over their authenticity. However, whether they are factual or fictional, there has been wide agreement that these books represent exceptional teaching tools for the popular introduction of some of the components of a life-style committed to the cultivation of authenticity, impeccability, and wisdom. Because of their clarity and popularity, it seemed appropriate to include a discussion of them in this volume.

Unlike other traditions described in this book the approach presented here is the path of the warrior, the commitment to view everything in life as a challenge or battle to be met with impeccability and unyielding will. Under guidance of a teacher the apprentice must act with increasing impeccability to build personal power by prolonged practice of such skills as adopting responsibility for one's situation, consciously disrupting automatic routines, reducing the significance of one's past, maintaining awareness of the shortness and uncertainty of life, and stopping the internal dialogue—all the while avoiding the traps which await anyone who is less than impeccable. The final result of unyielding pursuit is "the man of knowledge," a person who recognizes the total insignificance and mystery of his life yet lives it fully, joyfully, lightly, and with perfect control.

Both Maria and Gordon Globus have studied the Castaneda books intensely. Maria is a nurse therapist who works primarily with children but with the birth of twins has recently been working primarily on the home front.

Gordon Globus is Professor of Psychiatry at the University of California at Irvine. His main academic interest is the interface between psychiatry and philosophy. In his writings on the consciousness-brain problem, the self, and paradoxes of self-reference, he has made extensive use of the mystical tradition while remaining within a formal framework. He is the author of numerous articles on psychophysiology, consciousness, and philosophy, and is coeditor of Consciousness and the Brain: A Scientific and Philosophical Inquiry, *Plenum Press, 1976.*

13

The Man of Knowledge

Maria Globus
and
Gordon Globus

A man goes to knowledge as he goes to war, wide awake, with fear, with respect, and with absolute assurance.

don Juan to Carlitos*

We consider the "man of knowledge" presented in the works of Carlos Castaneda to illustrate an exceptional case of well-being. Our aim here is to describe the man of knowledge and some of the skills required for achieving this state. We shall not discuss similarities and dissimilarities to other teachings, which is a topic in its own right; in any case, to the extent that we present these teachings clearly, the reader familiar with other esoteric traditions should have no difficulty in making comparisons. For those who are unfamiliar with Castaneda's writings, we have provided an Appendix to this chapter which briefly describes the five volumes published to date.

There is controversy among people who have read Castaneda's books con-

*This quotation is from Carlos Castaneda's *The Teachings of Don Juan: A Yaqui Way of Knowledge,* p. 43 (referred to as T.D.J.). A description of, and references for, Castaneda's books are provided in the Appendix at the end of this chapter. Other abbreviations used are: S.R., *Separate Reality;* J.T.I., *Journey to Ixtlan;* and T.P., *Tales of Power.* All page numbers are from the paperback editions.

cerning how "real" his teacher, don Juan, is and thus how "truthful" the stories are. There is a tendency to discount the teachings because events surrounding them seem so improbable to our intellectual judgments; indeed, some say Castaneda fabricated the character. Others maintain it is essentially reportage, that Castaneda is a kind of mystical Tom Wolfe.

Our position is that these writings have had instructional value for us; we have found deep meaning and challenge in them. It is, as don Juan says, the "bent of our natures," our "personal predilection," to take them at face value. To "choose to believe" in this way has been an enjoyable and worthwhile path for us, and has enhanced our sense of well-being. In conveying some of the notable features of don Juan's teachings here, we shall utilize Castaneda's own language, which has a compelling flair, poignancy, and uniqueness, rather than translating to the dry framework of behavioral science or the murky framework of phenomenology and existentialism.

It may appear that the accomplishments and physical feats discussed are suitable only for men since, following Castaneda, we frequently use the term "he." However, both men and women may undertake this path. Indeed, women are said to be "better equipped" for gaining entrance into the world of sorcery and knowledge, while men are "more resilient." Acquiring this special knowledge, then, is an achievement of persons.

BACKGROUND

To recall the story briefly, Castaneda's apprenticeship to the sorcerer and man of knowledge, don Juan, begins while Castaneda is a graduate student in anthropology intent on obtaining data on the use of psychotropic plants for his doctoral dissertation. His association with don Juan extends over a 12-year period. It is, by Castaneda's account, a strenuous and frightening, awesome and wonderful, world-collapsing and world-expanding journey.

Initially, attempting to use this eccentric yet somehow remarkable old man as his informant, Castaneda's frustration mounts as his goal is constantly thwarted by don Juan's compelling maneuvers. He obstinately persists in his struggle to control the outcome of their meetings, only to be outdone by don Juan's greater skill and "personal power." Gradually, his reasons for coming to see this astounding man begin to change. Castaneda is literally tricked into abandoning his original quest and instead becomes an apprentice intent on learning the art of sorcery.

Throughout his association with don Juan, Castaneda takes detailed notes of their actions and interactions, his feelings, and his experiences. These he later sifts and reformulates to comprise the corpus of his writings (see Appendix).

THE WORLD OF SORCERY

The term "sorcery" has a variety of connotations. Popular associations might be to witchcraft and black magic. The *Random House Dictionary* defines it as "the art, practices or spells of a person who is supposed to exercise supernatural powers through the aid of evil spirits; black magic; witchery." Castaneda elaborates an alternative description of sorcery that focuses not on evil, but on developing power and skill through rigorous practice of unusual tasks and altering personal habits under the careful guidance of a sorcerer-teacher.

The powers of the sorcerer are limited in certain ways, and Castaneda is urged not to make this his final quest. As the story unfolds, sorcery is utilized as the means to another and even more exceptional goal—becoming a man of knowledge.

To achieve this goal, the apprentice must learn to "see." Seeing is put forth to the apprentice in an attractive and cryptic form to heighten his interest and give him a long-range goal for which to aim. He is cautioned that his actions must be impeccable to master this skill.

Don Juan's sorcery has a certain unique flavor which affronts our *tacit images* of the path to knowledge derived from Eastern traditions. In the latter, we think of the quiet peace of the ashram filled with loving devotees. In don Juan's community, however, apprentices struggle for power in potentially murderous ways. The bodhisattva's compassion and love for all sentient beings is a far cry from don Genaro's poignant discovery on his lonely "journey to Ixtlan" that human beings are all apparitions. Further, there is a sovereign quality to the sorceric man of knowledge. He is a "solitary bird" that "flies to the highest point. . . does not suffer for company . . . aims its beak to the skies . . . does not have a definite color . . . [and] sings very softly."

THE APPRENTICE AND THE TEACHER

The sorceric apprenticeship does not come about simply because a person decides he wants to begin one. One who is qualified to learn about the sorcerer's world must be pointed out to the teacher by "power" through special signs or omens. The teacher "seizes his cubic centimeter of chance" and "hooks" the attention of his apprentice-to-be. The relationship between teacher and student thus initiated develops into an enduring one based on trust, commitment, and the skills of the teacher. The course of instruction always proceeds according to signs and omens which the teacher must use as his guides. Goals for the apprenticeship include the development of harmonious and impeccable action and a true silencing of the mind. The intended outcome is major psychological reorganization: for example, profound differences in the student's way of perceiving, feeling, thinking, and acting. It is the awesome nature of "power" in the sorcerer's world, facilitated by the encompassing guidance of the teacher, that triggers these psychological changes.

POWER AND SEEING

Despite its central importance to don Juan's teachings, power eludes precise definition. It must be witnessed to be appreciated.

Power is viewed as existing all around us, though largely unnoticed. Through learning to "trap" and "store" power within his own person, the apprentice gains the stamina to proceed on his journey. ("Personal power" should not be thought of as the power to control others.)

Power is considered to have extraordinary and awesome effects. The person experiences it in his body like a feeling. Power is deliberately sought by sorcerers as a means for gaining knowledge unavailable to ordinary men. At first it seems an incredibly far-fetched affair, but eventually the apprentice is made increasingly aware of an inexplicable force around him that seems to have direction and volition.

> Next power is manifested as something uncontrollable that comes to oneself. . . . It is nothing and yet it makes marvels appear before your very eyes. (J.T.I., p. 97)

Where before the apprentice could not conceive of such a phenomenon as power, he now becomes fascinated by its presence and frightened by its awesomeness.

> And finally power is something in oneself, something that controls one's acts and yet obeys one's commands. (J.T.I., p. 97)

This last achievement comes solely after the apprentice has succeeded in bringing harmony and impeccability into his life and actions. Only under the condition of exceptional well-being can the forces of power be sustained.

Seeing is a special skill which is the profound accomplishment of a man of knowledge. It is mastered with the aid of the teacher and another equally skilled master, known as the benefactor. Seeing allows one to perceive the "essence" of things. "Seeing is contrary to sorcery; it makes one realize the unimportance of it all." It demonstrates that "nothing is pending in the world . . . nothing is finished, yet nothing is unresolved," that all victories and defeats are equal.

Seeing is a "direct knowing."

Upon learning to see a man becomes everything by becoming nothing. He, so to speak, vanishes and yet he is there. (S.R., p. 153)

Seeing enables the person to detach himself from all that is familiar so that "everything is new. Everything has never happened before. The world is incredible." In this perceptual state, people are distinguished as "luminous beings" composed of iridescent fibers. The world is seen as composed of an infinitude of lines emanating from all things and connecting with all other things. Sorcerers say that to *see* allows a person to reach the "totality of himself" well before death overtakes him. For most of us, the moment of our death is the only time we are said to witness this totality of our being.

THE WARRIOR'S WAY

Only a warrior can withstand the path of knowledge. . . . A warrior cannot complain or regret. . . . His life is an endless challange. (T.P., p. 105)

The force of power can defeat a person if he abandons himself to it. It becomes the apprentice's task to measure his steps carefully and faithfully at all times. He must remain humble and alert. To act impeccably requires that he be in full control of himself and, at the same time, light and fluid. Don Juan refers to this condition as that of a "warrior." A major portion of the teachings are an outline of the precise qualities of the warrior. The teacher clearly demonstrates this way of being through his own impeccability.

Teaching the warrior's way includes lessons and exercises designed to help the apprentice gather and store his own power. In the beginning, he is given power directly from his teacher's own personal store. He recognizes his teacher's greater effectiveness and freedom, his command over himself, and his ability to detach himself from the ordinary, endless stream of obligations, anxieties, and routines in life so familiar to the apprentice.

Learning the lessons is neither easy nor predictable, requiring the student to vigorously oppose his ordinary habits with new tasks without becoming impatient. The "familiar" is tenacious and a power in and of itself, having been effectively sustained for years. So the apprentice is helped to see that he must commit himself with "unbending intent" no matter how difficult it seems. He is assured that if he does so he will eventually win because "power convinces the body."

The body likes the changes; it feels the strength and clarity of action even before the rational mind will let the apprentice believe that this is so. Until the suggestions and tasks begin to make sense to him, he proceeds as if blindfolded. His task is to act in spite of what he thinks, *as if* he believed.

The warrior aims to reach a state of exceptional well-being. Don Juan insists, over Castaneda's protestations, that Castaneda doesn't really know what well-being is, because he has never experienced it. Well-being is a condition that must be "groomed" so that one becomes fully acquainted with it. It is an achievement which must be deliberately sought.

The trick is in what one emphasizes.... We either make ourselves miserable, or we make ourselves strong. The amount of work is the same. (J.T.I., p. 184)

The Art of the Warrior: To Act Is What Counts

The basic difference between an ordinary man and a warrior is . . . a warrior takes everything as a challenge . . . an ordinary man takes everything . . . as a blessing or as a curse. (T.P., p. 106)

Learning to live like a warrior is an accomplishment which takes years. The teacher, benefactor, and other warriors are of great importance in convincing the apprentice to want to change his ways. Countless tasks and problems are artfully put forth by the teacher so that the student's fumbling inferior ways of responding can become clear to him. By way of contrast he witnesses the calm, precise actions of his teacher and attunes himself to the teacher's suggestions. "To act is what counts."

Thinking and talking are our familiar form of communication with others and our chief means of understanding. Thus they are considered appropriate tools for the apprentice in his training. Discussion and reflection are essential to allow the rational mind to accept the unfamiliar teachings. Thinking, talking, and understanding, however, are considered part of one's ordinary and routine world rather than the sorceric world for which they are inappropriate.

. . . a sorcerer seeks to act rather than talk and to this effect he gets a new description of the world . . . where talking is not that important . . . where new acts have new reflections. (T.P., p. 24)

In practicing his art, the warrior aims to make his ordinary life trim and efficient. He trains himself to eliminate unsuitable actions—those which are unnecessary or draining. To act inappropriately could mean his death in the sorceric world. Thus, he must endeavor to act with awareness, deliberateness, and simplicity; he must be fluid and shift with the world around him. The rewards of such a path are that the person become clear, powerful, and free of convention. The "warrior's way" becomes his unique "path with heart" which nourishes and fulfills him as he develops patience and diminishes his wants.

> A warrior is in the hands of power and his only freedom is to choose an impeccable life. There is no way to fake triumph or defeat. (T.P., p. 55)

SOME STEPS ON THE PATH TO KNOWLEDGE

> We must follow certain steps, because it is in the steps where man finds strength. Without them we are nothing. (T.D.J., p. 164)

The steps discussed here are by no means an exhaustive study of all that is required to bring about consummate change. Other steps, such as "dreaming" and the use of the "double," are complex and we did not choose to go into them here.

"Erasing Personal History": To Cast a Fog Around Oneself

Sorcerers say that personal history serves only to fix one in definite ways in one's own mind as well as in the minds of others. Yet most of us believe that to have a personal history is unavoidable, necessary, and at times, something of which we can be justly proud. (Witness the recent upsurge of interest in family roots.) To cast doubt on the value of personal history calls into serious question the importance of culture and tradition; at first glance, such a position seems ridiculous.

A warrior is not concerned with culture or tradition and regards personal history as confining and a hindrance. In his apprenticeship he learns that as long as he keeps telling people about himself, e.g., what he's done and where he's been, he is a virtual slave to these statements. In the wish to appear consistent and credible in his mind and the minds of his friends, he will conform to the image he projects. Accordingly, he and everyone who knows him must have no doubt about who he is and what he can do, and the fluid quality of the warrior is lost.

A warrior's purpose is such that he cannot afford to be so fixed, so predictable, or so bored. His task is to "erase himself" so that nobody, including himself, knows for sure who he is or what he does. He is told to begin by not telling people all about himself. He sees less and less of the people who know him best. His goal is to blot out his definiteness; to "create a fog around himself."

As he proceeds with this intent, little by little, he is no longer taken for granted. Though it is a struggle at first, and frightening, eventually the apprentice begins to feel lighter and less "for sure" in his own mind. His life becomes less complicated for he no longer cares about appearing consistent. What others think of him loses its importance. His teacher knows, though, that taken alone, to "erase oneself" has its dangers and can even lead to emotional collapse. Therefore, other steps must be taken in conjunction to provide balance and tone to his endeavors.

"Losing Self-importance": Opening to an Awesome World

Feeling important makes one heavy, clumsy, and vain. To be a man of knowledge one needs to be light and fluid. (S.R., pp. 7–8)

Generally a person's self-identity looms majestically and demandingly in his own thoughts. His attention is taken up with protecting and defending his self-sense to such a degree that he is blinded to the marvels of the world around him. If he goes for a walk he spends most of it involved in his own thoughts about his own plans, judgments, and memories rather than in what surrounds him. Indeed, his surroundings always appear the same and not very interesting on the whole.

For the sorcerer, the surroundings contain unpredictable, powerful forces capable of aiding a man only if he can be aware of them. When self-importance is great, such awareness is impossible. The world for sorcerers is fascinating, awesome, mysterious, and unfathomable. The teacher makes dramatically clear that self-importance is worthless and must be dropped.

The apprentice then directs himself to the task of being aware of all his habits of self-indulgence which reflect how important he feels. Examples include self-pity, defensiveness, irritability when challenged, or an unwillingness to view oneself as equal to everyone and everything else in the world. He earnestly practices seeing himself in balance with the world and waits patiently for this new view to take hold. A warrior begins with "the certainty that his spirit is off balance." He then lives "in full control and awareness . . . without hurry or compulsion," in an effort to gain balance.

The apprentice learns to proceed strategically with the task of losing self-importance, as with all other tasks. His strategy is to want to accomplish the changes yet never to become obsessed with the exercise. He is taught that too much wanting and needing makes for unhappiness and loss of well-being. Part of his strategy then is to reduce his wants to nothing so that whatever comes his way is a true gift.

The power to reduce our wants is all we have to oppose the forces of our lives . . . without it we are dust in the wind. (S.R., p. 142)

"Assuming Responsibility": Ceasing to Regret

Since acting is what counts, there is no room in the warrior's way for doubts or confusion once the decision to act is made. To regret one's own action or cast blame on others for its outcome is also impossible for a warrior.

It is common in our day-to-day living to project responsibility onto others for our own activities or whereabouts: "I'm here because of my boss," or "I'm doing this because of my wife (husband, son, daughter)." There is no recognition of irresponsibility in having adopted these views. Nor does it seem to matter that these views are inefficient and time wasting. After all, it is assumed, one really has plenty of time to think anyway one wants.

The apprentice is shown that irresponsibility is wasteful and progressively debilitating. Taking full and complete responsibility for his actions and decisions is the only way he can prepare himself to act deliberately. To be impeccable means he cannot afford to waste time by being unaware of his own purposes. It is incumbent upon him to assess carefully the conditions around him and within him *before* choosing to act. Once his decision is made, all doubts must vanish. The warrior is obliged to be

> master of his choices. He must fully understand that his choice is his responsibility and once he makes it there is no longer time for regrets or recrimination. (S.R., p. 151)

"Believing without Believing": Following a "Path with Heart"

As the apprentice learns to take all that comes to him as a gift and recognizes his own responsibility for the taking, his appreciation for what is possible in the world is enhanced. He lives by his own choice and that choice need not be limited by narrow vision. His daily world is his challenge and, like all challenges, requires his full attention.

To act requires purpose adopted with conviction. The apprentice is taught to be purposeful and, at the same time, fluid in his actions. To remain in perfect balance, he must "believe without believing" in whatever he is doing. To believe in particular ways is his choice, and he recognizes its usefulness as a force applied to his actions. Once an action is completed, the belief is no longer relevant.

At the same time, he does not tie himself to any one belief to the exclusion of others. He uses the power of believing while remaining free of any belief. His attention is given equally to all that comes to him in the world. Acting impeccably means that he is aware of everything, and from that immensity, he chooses to believe. His choice reflects his "innermost predilection": it is his expression of harmony and grace. He follows his "path with heart" fully commited to the end, yet knowing that the path is arbitrary. For example, rather than wanting life to be easy, the warrior *chooses* to take life as a continual struggle and a challenge. He chooses to believe that the world is unpredictable and mysterious. Thus, he strives to be impeccable at all times in order to fully exploit his fortune as a man.

"Taking Death as an Advisor": As an Advisor, Self-pity Is Nothing Compared to Death

Sorcerers say that to remain unaware of one's death allows one to be timid, self-pitying, and to look for countless excuses to explain away one's problems. By leading the person to conclude he has plenty of time, such a position encourages self-importance, pettiness, and other forms of indulgence. To wait until one is sick or dying to become acquainted with death is too late. Moreover, to shroud death with fear prohibits its effectiveness and leads a person into obsession.

Recognizing the fact of his own inevitable death is of powerful significance for the apprentice.

> A man who follows the path of sorcery is confronted with imminent annihilation every turn of the way, and unavoidably he becomes keenly aware of his death. (S.R., p. 150)

This awareness, at first so alarming and difficult to maintain, is to be used as an aid to him in all his decisions and actions. He is shown that the knowledge of impending death will support him in his refusal to waste time in habits that leave him weak and vulnerable. He learns to regard death as a force that waits patiently, just as he waits, and one that will ultimately overtake him. Nevertheless, death and the warrior are friends.

An immense amount of pettiness can be dropped by consulting one's death, which counsels that the only thing which really matters is that one is still alive. The awareness of death is essential for developing the strength and conviction to act swiftly, lightly, and precisely.

> There is a strange consuming happiness in acting with the full knowledge that whatever one is doing may very well be one's last act on earth. (J.T.I., p. 83)

The apprentice must first make death familiar rather than an enemy or an unknown. He endeavors to recall the fact of his death often. It is regarded as a definite presence that is always there. When he acts, death is there; when he sits, death sits beside him; when he sleeps, death waits.

The apprentice seeks to disengage himself from any notion that death is to be feared or avoided.

> . . . to be concerned with death would force any one of us to focus on the self and that would be debilitating. So the next thing one needs to be a warrior is detachment. (S.R., p. 150)

He must accept that death is not hidden or ominous or overwhelming, but is real and separate from himself. His purpose is to acknowledge his inevitable end without concern, simply as an undeniable fact that will give him power; for without full awareness of death,

> everything is ordinary, trivial. It is only because death is stalking us that the world is an unfathomable mystery. (T.P., p. 114)

"Disrupting Routines": Stalking Personal Habits

One of don Juan's early maneuvers, designed to catch his apprentice's attention, was to engage him in the art of hunting, a favorate pastime for Castaneda as a child. Don Juan then points out that the strategy a successful hunter uses to catch his prey is the same a warrior uses to hunt power.

The hunter carefully observes and studies the habits of his prey until he is thoroughly familiar with its routines, for it is through these routines that the prey succumbs. He builds his traps for efficiency and precision. He leaves very little to chance, calculating his own internal condition, the weather, the direction of the wind, the proper time of day, and the best trap to use as part of his preparation. To succeed he knows he must outsmart and swiftly overtake his prey. He is alert not to leave any scent trail or be in any other way noticeable. He treats the animals he hunts and the natural surroundings with consideration. When he kills an animal for his food, he gives thanks for the gift received and recognizes that his death will also be a gift to someone or something else someday. He apologizes to the plants he injures to make his traps and thanks them for their help.

A warrior hunting power follows a similar pattern. He stalks his own routines, while remaining respectful, unhurried, alert, and confident in his pursuit. When a gift of power is found and he is capable of taking it, he never leaves the spot without acknowledging his gift. To hunt power, the apprentice learns to free himself of his routines, considered to be all his habitual ways of thinking, acting, and feeling, so that he himself is never a prey. Very early in his apprenticeship, he is told not to eat at the same time every day, to take different routes when he walks or drives, to walk instead of driving. His body begins to feel the refreshing effects of these practices, while the teacher provides increasingly greater opportunities for the changes to extend further into his daily life.

"Being Inaccessible": A Passage Which Leaves No Trace of Disturbance

Along with disrupting routines, the apprentice is made aware of the importance of being available to others or to the forces in the world only when he chooses to be. Not to set himself in this way would leave him extremely vulnerable—"a leaf at the mercy of the wind." Being inaccessible entails that

> you touch the world around you sparingly. . . . You don't expose yourself to power unless it is mandatory. You don't use and squeeze people until they have shrivelled to nothing. . . . (J.T.I., p. 69)

The warrior's proper style is to make light contact with the world around him, staying just for a while and then moving on, without leaving a trace. His aim is to avoid draining himself and others and to use his world sparingly and tenderly.

"The Mood of the Warrior": Perfect Control Followed by Complete Abandon

The warrior always acts in the proper mood, and this he learns to create. Whereas an ordinary person's moods seem to be related directly to the people and events around him, the warrior is taught to arrive at and maintain a specific mood independent of people and events.

Two attitudes are required for the proper mood, and they are to be held simultaneously. The first is control over himself and the second is abandon. He must have total command of himself and at the same time be free to let himself go without caring about the outcome. To learn this is a complicated affair. The teacher adroitly leads him into predicaments from which he cannot escape without putting into practice these two elements of the proper mood. Achieving this mood and maintaining it are said to be very difficult, requiring years of practice.

Sorcerers say that when the apprentice recognizes that death is stalking him, when his body is finely tuned and his mind is completely clear, acting in the proper mood is the warrior's only possible course, To act in any other way would drain him or kill him, and a warrior would never abandon himself to death. He cannot be pushed to do anything harmful to himself or against his better judgment since he is tuned to survive in the best of all fashions.

"Controlled Folly": What One Does Is Ultimately Unimportant

... everything I do in regard to myself and my fellow men is folly, because nothing matters. (S.R., p. 85)

Don Juan termed the life he led *controlled folly*. He tells Castaneda that once he developed his capacity to see, his way of living as a man in the world changed. Where previously he cared about what people thought and did, wanted his actions to produce specific outcomes, and felt angry if these did not result, after *seeing* it was no longer the same for him. Once a man is able to *see,*

he realizes that he can no longer think about the things he looks at, and if he cannot think about what he looks at everything becomes unimportant. (S.R., p. 86)

It seems impossible to consider that the life one leads is unimportant when one has been taught the opposite. To consider one's acts ultimately as folly appears at first glance to undermine one's efforts. That response occurs, don Juan counsels, because one is thinking about one's acts and relying solely on what one has learned.

For don Juan, taking life as folly is to be lighthearted, equal to everything else in the world, and without heaviness, clumsiness, or seriousness. A warrior is not trapped by any set of beliefs or by any way of going about things. He is fluid. He has no need to have his acts lead to a certain outcome. His only intent is to act impeccably, and "when he fulfills his acts he retreats in peace."

The mark of a warrior is that his folly is carefully controlled. He lives strategically, measures his course sensitively, is always alert and confident. The paths he chooses to tread are always selected in accordance with what his heart tells him—his innermost predilection. He likes, he enjoys, but he does not care. He takes what comes to him as a challenge, neither good nor bad.

For me there is no victory or defeat or emptiness. Everything is filled to the brim and everything is equal and my struggle was worth my while. (S.R., p. 94)

"Not-Doing": Collapsing the Ordinary World

Not-doing is considered the key to the world of sorcery, essential to *seeing* and becoming a man of knowledge. When the apprentice becomes proficient in the technique of not-doing, then he is able to "stop the world."

Sorcerers say that what a person knows is taught to him by others, leading him to a socially agreed upon description of the world. This description is accepted by the person totally and undeniably as reality. It is repeated in thought and serves to select all that one attends to in the world. One's eyes look only at what one's mind knows, and so the world is maintained in a steady and reasonable state.

One's mind, in its thoughtful selectivity, is upholding a description—it is "doing." To *stop the world,* where world signifies the total way one ordinarily views oneself, everyone, and everything, one must stop "doing," i.e., practice *not-doing.*

Doing encompasses all one's thoughts, actions and habits. (It is what phenomenologists term "intentionality.") Whatever one does is part of doing. Doing holds one in a familiar world and acts as a shield against disruption. Doing upholds the world in the sense that every person within a culture learns to agree to similar ways of thinking, acting, and perceiving.

Not-doing is the undoing of the familiar world. It constitutes the warrior's first deliberate step to storing personal power. An important aspect of this undoing is learning to stop the "internal dialogue."

One activity we all do is talk to ourselves. Usually we go about our day mentally engaged in a continuous stream of talk within the privacy of our minds. Don Juan calls this the "internal dialogue." This flow of thoughts serves to maintain an order we know as the world. When we stop thought, the world changes.

Whenever the dialogue stops, the world collapses and extraordinary facets of ourselves surface, as though they have been kept heavily guarded by our words. (T.P., p. 33)

The apprentice is urged to spend periods in which this talk is totally silenced. He may begin by "listening to the sounds of the world" rather than always looking with his eyes. Other modes include walking in unfamiliar surroundings and sitting quietly attending to clouds, shadows, fog, stars, or plants. His skill at stopping the internal dialogue increases gradually when he is intent and practices for long periods. The night is said to be a particularly good time to train because the environment is transformed to something quite unusual. This uncommon condition forces greater attention to the task of getting around, and less is available for talking to oneself. These practices afford beneficial effects in the forms of increased vigor and deep relaxation.

Not-doing is designed to alter one's ordinary perceptions. The exercises introduced to the apprentice make constant use of the natural surroundings apart from his usual living space. Don Juan takes Castaneda on long journeys into the desert to places that offer particular advantages for practicing, because of certain rock formations, the position of cliffs in relation to the sun, or other configurations of natural forces. These he calls "places of power." Here Castaneda is instructed to observe shadows rather than objects, to practice visually joining objects (rocks, sticks, plants) commonly seen as separate, and to make large what is ordinarily seen as small (pebble, flower, or insect).

Other exercises concern the way the eyes are focused. The eyes are taught to gaze without focusing or, at other times, to be crossed so that two images are seen instead of one. By changing the way in which the eyes usually focus, the world is dramatically altered. Gradually, with practice, the apprentice begins to "Feel" the world with his eyes rather than merely looking at it.

> The most difficult part of the warrior's way is to realize that the world is a feeling. (J.T.I., p. 193)

When the person can maintain this altered perception without becoming anxious or lost in the revelation, his ordinary world collapses and he is said to have *stopped the world*.

For the warrior, not-doing is the foundation for an entirely new realm of perception and capability. Having fully mastered the technique, it then becomes possible for him to contact two regions of perception: one being the common world or the world of reason where doing, thinking, and talking prevail; the other being the sorcerer's world, called the world of will, or the world of not-doing. The world of doing is shared with all human beings, while the world of not-doing, full of mystery and magic and maintained through one's *will,* is shared with only a small number. Not-doing is the way the warrior enters the indescribable void.

This concludes our discussion of some of the steps taken by the apprentice on his path to becoming a warrior. To be a warrior is to reach for an exceptional state of well-being. The warrior is

> joyful because he feels humbled by his great fortune, confident that his spirit is impeccable, and above all, fully aware of his efficiency.... (T.P., p. 289)

His joyful spirit results from

> having accepted his fate, and from having truthfully assessed what lies ahead of him. (T.P., p. 289)

We next focus on the culmination of the path and the sorcerer's "secret." These considerations require further presentation of don Juan's framework including the notions of *will, tonal,* and *nagual.* We then consider the four enemies which a warrior must challenge and defeat to become a man of knowledge. Finally, we describe how the warrior meets his death.

THE WILL

In the sorceric view we are all born with eight points through which we can function. These eight points include: *reason, talking, will, feeling, seeing, dreaming,* the *tonal,* and the *nagual.* We all know reason and talking, and to a lesser degree we know feeling. Through sorcery, the warrior is introduced to the other five.

Reason and will are both points of concentration. Reason is directly connected with talking and indirectly connected with feeling. Will, considered to be the larger center, is directly connected with seeing, feeling, and dreaming. The *tonal* and the *nagual,* discussed below, are in a somewhat different domain.

Like much within the sorceric framework, the will is difficult to define. It is said to be a power or a force which the warrior patiently waits for. No one knows how, or when, but at a certain moment will simply occurs in a warrior's life as long as his body is in a state of perfection. Its manifestation emanates from a specific physical location on the body—a point just below the navel—known as the "gap." Will is something that "has direction and can be focused on anything." The point where will emerges from the body is considered the most sensitive part of a man, the place where death enters.

Will is conceived of not as an idea, an object, or a wish, but as a true force that connects a man to the world. It is

> something very clear and powerful which can direct one's acts. Will is something a man uses to win a battle which he, by all calculations, should lose. (S.R., p. 146)

For a man who *sees,* will is perceived as a sturdy luminous fiber that can actually grab onto rocks, trees, and other physical objects. Will, however, is not observable by those who can only look with their eyes.

Our reason and our senses tell us that the world around us is real, full of objects, and outside of us. The sorcerer regards this world as a description affording us convenient passage on earth. The commonplace world is comprised of fleshy, solid people like ourselves who are grounded or earthbound and generally predictable.

The sorcerer has his reason and his senses like an ordinary man, but he also uses his will to perceive the world. The sorcerer knows that he can actually touch anything he wants with a feeling that comes out of his body from a spot right below or above his naval. That feeling is the will. (S.R., p. 152)

Indeed, it is the sorcerer's will which is said to keep him alive every time he bids for power. For the man of knowledge who *sees* and knows that nothing in the world matters, that nothing is important, his life is maintained by his will rather than plans or hopes or wishes.

THE *TONAL* AND THE *NAGUAL*

If power makes *will* available to the warrior, he must then tune and perfect it. He does this by engaging with power, and if he becomes a man of knowledge, through *seeing*. The inconceivable world which a man of knowledge *sees* is termed, by don Juan, the *nagual*. The world he looks at, the one in which he thinks and acts, is termed the *tonal*. The *nagual* is the exclusive realm of a man of knowledge and is beyond sorcery. To arrive at the awareness of these two points or worlds equally means that the warrior has reached the "totality of himself."

The *tonal* comprises everything we are or know. Our ability to reason, to organize thoughts and actions, to sense—that is, our total daily commonsensical perspective—is the work of the *tonal*. While the *tonal* is intended to be the protective guardian of our being, it generally turns into a jealous, narrow-minded, indomitable guard. Our daily view becomes trivial and constant.

There are two parts to the *tonal*. The outer part is like the surface of an island. It is associated with action and considered to be the most rugged aspect. The inner part is more fragile, delicate, and complex. Here, decision making and judgment take place.

Ordinarily, we are all *tonal* and have no awareness of our other side, the vastness called the *nagual*. Therefore, we belong solely to our island of reason, thinking, and familiar habits of person. On our islands, we "judge, assess, and witness the world" according to the rules of the *tonal*. The *tonal* has formed the rules by which we apprehend the world, and we are usually quite content to stay forever on this island of the familiar. Our islands are usually laden with personal history and self-importance, crowded with habits, and earthbound.

An important feature of the *tonal* is its delicacy. It begins at birth and ends with death; if the *tonal* is destroyed, then so is the man. Thus it must be protected at all costs. This is the teacher's underlying objective throughout the entire instruction, "to prepare the *tonal* not to crap out."

The island of the *tonal* has to be swept clean and maintained clean. . . . A clean island offers no resistance; it is as if nothing is there. (T.P., p. 174)

The warrior's way acts as a vital shield for the *tonal*, giving a man durable options as he struggles to bring the totality of himself into balance. The mark of the warrior's spirit is that he treats his *tonal* in a very special way. He seeks a proper *tonal* that is balanced and harmonious and aware of everything that occurs on his island. "A warrior doesn't ever leave the island of his *tonal*, he uses it."

The *nagual* surrounds the island and should be the most obvious occurrence; yet it is not. The *tonal* and the *nagual* are said to be a true pair, though the manifestations of the *nagual* are virtually eliminated from view by the clever doings of the *tonal*. For the *nagual* to emerge, the *tonal's* unity must be broken and it must shrink; this is a very dangerous affair.

To attempt to define the *nagual* is virtually impossible. It is presented as "that part of us for which there is no description, no words, no names, no feelings, no knowledge." The teacher indicates that to say anything about the *nagual* forces one to borrow from the *tonal*, thus it is easier to simply detail its effects. This is so because our talking makes sense only when we stay within certain boundaries, and those boundaries "are not applicable to the *nagual*." The *nagual* can only be witnessed; it can be neither understood nor explained.

for the *nagual* there is no land, or air or water . . . the *nagual* glides, or flies, or does whatever it may do in *nagual's* time. (T.P., p. 194)

In order to witness the *nagual*, the warrior must come upon a benefactor who is a man of knowledge and capable of leading the way. The benefactor gives many demonstrations over a period of time, while the teacher aids the warrior in fortifying his *tonal* during the onslaughts. The emergence of the *nagual* is a jolt which is said to terrify the *tonal*, and specific practices are required to soothe the *tonal* so that it can maintain the view of the *nagual*.

In the presence of his masterful benefactor, the apprentice encounters extraordinary occurrences.

. . . I felt completely disoriented . . . I felt unknown to myself. Don Genaro was doing something to me, something which kept me from formulating my thoughts the way I am accustomed. (S.R., p. 257)

The benefactor forces the *nagual* into the apprentice's awareness, and marked physical sensations herald its appearance.

I felt a sensation of vacuity in my lower abdomen. It was a terribly anguishing sensation of falling, not painful, but rather unpleasant and consuming. (S.R., p. 261)

Accompanying these sensations are observations of astounding performances by the benefactor. These are truly awesome and unimaginable feats, and to perceive them (i.e., to perceive the *nagual*) is true *seeing*. For example, Castaneda *sees* don Genaro bound to the top of great trees.

... he glided through the air, catapulted in part by his formidable yell, and pulled by some vague lines emanating from the tree. (T.P., p. 182)

It appeared that "the tree had sipped him through its lines."

The warrior is first placed in the position of witnessing the *nagual* so that his body is "soaked" with memories of it, and then he is invited to enter this indescribable domain in order to learn how to negotiate from within. He is told that it is really impossible to predict what will occur once one is within the *nagual*, except that it will never be like anything he knows. Nevertheless he must enter confidently, trusting his personal power and his warrior's spirit to protect him.

SORCERIC FEATS

The man of knowledge who can use his will and enter the crack between the two worlds of the *tonal* and the *nagual* is able to perform stupendous feats, such as flying through the air. Castaneda is continually amazed at these feats and presses don Juan to divulge whether or not they "really" happened. Some of Castaneda's readers consider don Juan to have supernatural powers, wheras others consider the events related to be nothing but tall tales told to the gullible. However, don Juan repeatedly makes clear that these miraculous occurrences are *feats of perception*. This is the sorcerer's secret, this extraordinary capacity to perceive according to nonordinary descriptions of the world.

It is not difficult to understand intellectually the sorcerer's explanation that we are enclosed, as don Juan says, within a "bubble of perception" from the moment of birth, a bubble in which we see the reflection of our own description. Nor is it difficult to understand intellectually that if freed from social consensus, we could constitute an unconventional "separate reality." Also, we might intellectually agree that we have no objective basis for concluding that ordinary perception is more authentic than extraordinary perception (or vice versa).

Yet this cognitive stance will not sustain sorceric feats. As don Juan relates to Castaneda,

Personal powder decides who can or who cannot profit by a revelation; my experiences with my fellow men have proven to me that . . . very few . . . would be willing to listen. (T.P., p. 231)

Don Juan goes on to say that of those few who would listen, not all would be willing to act

and of those who are willing to act even fewer have enough personal power to profit by their acts. (T.P., p. 231)

We illustrate the perception required by considering events recounted in *Tales of Power* (pp. 256–260), wherein Castaneda had an experience of making astounding leaps into a deep ravine. The setting was a great rock situated above the ravine. Don Juan and don Genaro each whispered synchronously into his ears, and told him that he was surrounded by fibers via which he could leap from the rock to the bottom. For Castaneda, every word had a "unique connotation" and was retained "as if I were a tape recorder." As they urged him to leap to the bottom of the ravine, they gave a precise description of the perception entailed.

They said that I should first feel my fibers, then isolate one that went all the way down to the bottom of the ravine and follow it. (T.P., p. 259)

With amazement he realized that he could experience feelings that paralleled their words exactly. He identified precise sensations that were wholly unique.

I sensed an itching all over me, especially a most peculiar sensation of a "long itching." My body could actually feel the bottom of the ravine. . . . (T.P., p. 259)

Castaneda was coaxed to "slide through the feeling," but he did not know how to break his bubble of ordinary perception and leap. He had not yet unfolded his "wings of perception."

Then don Genaro grabbed or pushed or embraced him (it was unclear which). They plunged together into the abyss, while Castaneda felt physical anguish in his gut, yelled at the top of his lungs, and could not tell whether his eyes were open or closed or where his body was. He again experienced physical anguish, and then had the impression that he had woken up and found himself standing on the rock with don Juan and don Genaro.

However, this confused perceptual achievement was insufficient for the two sorcerers. They said that Castaneda had "goofed again" and that

> ... it was useless to leap if the perception of the leaps was going to be chaotic. (T.P., p. 260)

The experiencing of the *nagual* had to be "tempered" by the *tonal*. He must leap into the abyss willingly and with total awareness.

Castaneda hesitated, and then some strange mood overtook him. "I leaped with all my corporealness." He did not have a sequential perception of falling, but the sensation that he was actually on the ground at the bottom. He was unable to maintain this perception for long, however.

> After a moment I panicked and something pulled me up like a yo-yo. (T.P., p. 260)

He was made to perform the feat over and over again so as to improve his perception. Each time they appealed to him not to hold back, not to refuse the experience but open to it. Don Juan revealed that

> The sorcerer's secret in using the "nagual" was in our perception, that leaping was simply an exercise in perception. (T.P., p. 260)

They said that his jump would only be complete

> after I had succeeded in perceiving, as a perfect "tonal," what was at the bottom of the ravine. (T.P., p. 260)

Finally he achieved an inconceivable sensation.

> I was fully and soberly aware that I was standing on the edge of the rock ... then in the next instant I was looking at the bottom of the ravine. (T.P., p. 260)

The magnitude of such feats should not be discounted by their being "only in imagination," for the man of knowledge fully believes in the authenticity of his own act and relies solely on the personal power he has acquired through impeccable action. For him, such a leap is incorrigibly the case. To "leap" in this manner from a monumental cliff is thus both a feat of perception and a feat of courage.

OBSTACLES ALONG THE PATH TO KNOWLEDGE

The state of being a man of knowledge is a process, a becoming, a challenging dance along a path with heart. It is not a condition lastingly achieved. It is said that most people who begin on this path succumb along the way, giving in to one of the four natural enemies that stalk them mercilessly. Only through "unbending intent" can an individual overcome such formidable opponents.

One's first battle is with *fear,* a notorious adversary that seeks to paralyze its victim. Fear is unfailingly persistent—a constant threat that will reduce a man's vision and force him to abandon his quest unless he is strong and equally persistent. To overcome his fear, he must defy it and continue his learning.

> He must be fully afraid . . . yet he must not stop. . . . A moment will come when his first enemy retreats. . . . (T.D.J., pp. 79–80)

Now his confidence increases, his commitment deepens, and he feels a great surge of triumph and freedom. He is clear about what he wants and how to get it. Learning is no longer such a mystery because he understands his own responses. His vision becomes much sharper and wider.

A brilliant *clarity* envelops him and very soon becomes his second enemy. He feels invulnerable, extremely confident, and willing to take great personal risks. Yet if he fails to realize that this feeling is not true power, he will falter and collapse through impatient action or imprudent misjudgment. To outmaneuver this second threat,

> he must defy clarity. . . . Use it only to see . . . wait patiently and measure carefully before taking new steps: he must think above all, that his clarity is almost a mistake. (T.D.J., p. 81)

If he perseveres, the apprentice will eventually overcome clarity and reach a point of true invincibility that is no mistake. He has acquired *power.* The temptation to give into this beguiling condition is immense. He may decide he has reached his limit, enjoying the feeling of mastery to the exclusion of any further challenge. Though he will remain powerful if he gives up, he will never learn how to handle it. If he chooses to defy power, he then regards it as a marvelous gift which is never, in fact, his. He proceeds knowing that to gain power means he must remain continually fit and ready.

> If he can see that clarity and power, without his control over himself, are worse than mistakes, he will reach a point where everything is held in check. (T.D.J., p. 82)

The warrior, then, free from fear, with his clarity well grounded and his power under his control, faces his fourth and final enemy, *old age*. This is a critical period when the warrior feels a desire to rest that will not yield.

If he gives in totally to his desire to lie down and forget, if he soothes himself in tiredness, he will have lost his last round. . . . (T.D.J., p. 83)

He must resist his tiredness, fend off his desire to retreat, all the while knowing that he will never be able to fully defeat his fourth enemy, but only push it away.

If he is capable of fighting back his fatigue so that he "lives his fate through," he then can be called a "man of knowledge." The man of knowledge knows his death will overtake him in the end. After all, he and his death are friends.

THE WARRIOR'S LAST DANCE

As old age acts upon the warrior and makes him feeble, at some point his death unavoidably taps him. When, finally, he feels this tap he prepares to meet death at his own "place of predilection."

Every warrior has a place to die . . . soaked with unforgettable memories . . . where he has witnessed marvels, where secrets have been revealed to him. (J.T.I., p. 153)

A warrior stores his personal power at his place of predilection. He finds this place long before, with the aid of his teacher, and he cares for it, grooming it throughout his life. This place gives him a feeling of profound wellbeing; it nourishes and restores him. Such a unique capacity is what makes it his special place. So when death taps him, this is where he goes to dance his "last dance." For each warrior there is

a specific form, a specific posture of power, which he develops throughout his life . . . a sort of dance. A movement that he does under the influence of his personal power. (J.T.I., pp. 153–154)

During his life, as the warrior bids for power, he forms his dance—the story of his life which grows as he gains power. His last dance may be long or it may be short; it is the recounting of his tale, in all its greatness and hardship, an expression of his deep respect and of the truths he has learned in his lifetime. His death is his only audience. For the last time, he rejoices in commemorating the power of his life, the final act of a man of knowledge. There remains nothing

> to oppose the silent force of his death, and his life becomes like the lives of all his fellow men, an expanding fog moving beyond its limits. (S.R., p. 198)

★ ★ ★

This concludes our presentation of the man of knowledge. For those who "choose to believe" in it, such a path makes for a joyful journey. It points toward extraordinary achievement, wisdom, and profound well-being through mental, physical, and spiritual training. Yet, "all paths are the same; they lead nowhere." To know which one to take, one must try them out, each as often as necessary. Neither fear nor ambition must direct one's actions and, finally, one must ask oneself the question,

> Does this path have heart? If it does, the path is good; if it doesn't it is of no use.... (T.D.J., p. 106)

Acknowledgment. The authors thank Ellen McGrath and the editors for their comments.

APPENDIX

Castaneda's first book, *The Teachings of Don Juan: A Yaqui Way of Knowledge* (New York, Ballantine Books, 1969), recounts the initial years of his apprenticeship to a Yaqui indian, the sorcerer "don Juan." The setting of the relationship is primarily Mexico. Castaneda, a graduate student in anthropology at the University of California, Los Angeles, is seeking an informant on the indigenous use of psychotropic plants. He is introduced to don Juan on a chance encounter, and finds himself strongly drawn to the man. He takes extensive field notes on his discussions with don Juan as they talk at don Juan's house, roam the chaparral, and meet various people. Castaneda also describes his experiences with psychotropic plants administered under don Juan's supervision. The book includes an appendix that is an anthropological analysis of don Juan's system of knowledge.

In *Separate Reality* (New York, Simon and Schuster, 1971), Castaneda continues his account, with special focus on his experiences induced by naturally occurring hallucinogenic drugs. The doctoral dissertation begins to recede in importance and the apprenticeship becomes more explicit. The compelling figure of don Juan dominates the narrative. Castaneda himself appears to be intellectually a prototypically Western man, but with an unusually adventurous spirit. Drug-induced experiences are both profound and terrifying, indeed shattering, so that Castaneda finally breaks off the apprenticeship.

Castaneda's return to his apprenticeship is described in *Journey to Ixtlan* (New York, Simon and Schuster, 1973). (This book comprises the body of Castaneda's doctoral dissertation.) He reconsiders his entire apprenticeship and reorganizes the material, appreciating that don Juan has been systematically teaching him. The psychological changes entailed in becoming a man of knowledge are focused on, and the drug-induced experiences are no longer central. Castaneda's "benefactor," the sorcerer don Genaro, forcefully demonstrates "power" to Castaneda. The book ends with don Genaro's poignant recounting of his "journey" to Ixtlan, in which he experiences the immense isolation of a man of knowledge from the social community, such that people become only "apparitions" for him.

In *Tales of Power* (New York, Simon and Schuster, 1974), Castaneda's apprenticeship is brought to a close. With the aid of his benefactor, don Genaro, he witnesses extraordinary events without any drug influence. The problems a reasonable person like Castaneda has in grasping such notions are again shown and balanced by don Juan's penetrating instructions about the strategy of the warrior. In the final period of his apprenticeship, don Juan gives Castaneda a sweeping survey of the scope and purposes of the teachings. The last point made to him is the "sorcerer's explanation," which concerns complex feats of perception that Castaneda is induced to perform.

The fifth and, at this writing, last work published by Castaneda is *The Second Ring of Power* (New York, Simon and Schuster, 1978). The apprenticeship has been concluded. Don Juan and don Genaro have disappeared into the *nagual*. Castaneda returns to don Juan's homeland to talk with three men, also former apprentices, who had joined with him during certain later periods of the instruction. He discovers five more former apprentices, all women, some of who try to injure or kill him initially. Each apprentice has something further to teach him. Emphasis is on his relationship with one of the women, La Gorda, who imparts further instruction that don Juan has directed her to give him.

Let us study not cripples, but the closest approach we can get to whole, healthy men. In them we find qualitative differences, a different system of motivation, emotion, value, thinking, and perceiving. In a certain sense only the saints *are* mankind.

Abraham Maslow

What does it feel like to be deeply enlightened? What does it feel like to be a master of Zen, a lama of Tibetan Buddhism, a Christian mystic, or a Christian missionary whose lifetime of selfless service and dedication to the poor has won worldwide recognition?

Myths abound about the experiences which supposedly accompany transcendental insights, enlightenment, or completely selfless service. We tend to think first of intense bliss and joy but there also seem to be suggestions of more—a loss of ego and sense of separation, a cosmic sense in touch with the most profound depths of mind, and a source of deep religious experience from which stream depths of compassion for one's less fortunate fellow beings. These are some of the feelings one gets reading the literature about such people, but it would be nice to have some firsthand accounts.

This is exactly what Jack Kornfield has provided. Searching through diverse sources, he has culled quotations by people who are widely believed to be outstanding masters or saints and who have described the nature of their own experience. From these descriptions he points to the similarities which underlie the experience of people from diverse traditions, cultures, and centuries.

Jack Kornfield is a psychologist and meditation teacher at the Insight Meditation Center in Barre, Massachusetts. He was introduced to meditation and Buddhism while working in the Peace Corps in Southeast Asia. Following the completion of his assignment there, he remained for several years as a Buddhist monk doing very intensive meditation practice. On returning to the United States he completed his doctorate in psychology and was one of the founders of the Insight Meditation Center. From there he travels throughout the United States and Europe, lecturing and teaching meditation courses. In accordance with the Buddhist tradition, he does not charge for these services. He has conducted empirical studies of the effects of meditation, has written widely on Buddhism, meditation, and the integration of Western and non-Western psychologies, and is author of the book Living Buddhist Masters, *Unity Press, 1977.*

14

Higher Consciousness: An Inside View

Jack Kornfield, Ph.D.

In this chapter I wish to present, in the words of some respected masters and their students, a descriptive sense of the awakened mind. Although perhaps not yet measured or tested by our modern psychological science, these expressions point to a greater human possibility of development in wisdom and love. The sense of such capacity within each of us, reminded by the words of these masters, may provide the impetus for the further study, practice, and discipline that would allow us to better understand and incorporate these possibilities into our lives.

The central experience of enlightenment involves a breaking down of a limited personality/body-centered view of oneself. This process was alluded to by Albert Einstein when he said,

A human being is a part of the whole called by us "universe," a part limited in time and space. He experiences himself, his thoughts and feelings, as something separated from the rest—a kind of optical delusion of his consciousness. This delusion is a kind of prison for us, restricting us to our personal desires and to affection for a few persons nearest to us. Our task must be to free ourselves from this prison by widening our circle of understanding and compassion to embrace all living creatures and the whole of nature in its beauty.[1]

The expressions of many enlightened teachers speak directly of this nonidentification with one's ordinary, limited view of oneself. That this is not an intellectual construct, but a dramatically altered way of perceiving oneself and the world, is illustrated in this remarkable dialogue with Sri Nisargadatta Maharaj, an 84-year-old master of Advaita Vedanta. He is asked about his mind state and responds directly to this point:

QUESTION: I see you sitting in your son-in-law's house waiting for lunch to be served. And I wonder whether the content of your consciousness is similar to mine, or partly different, or totally different. Are you hungry and thirsty as I am, waiting rather impatiently for the meal to be served, or are you in an altogether different state of mind?

MAHARAJ: There is not much difference on the surface but very much of it in depth. You know yourself only through the sense and the mind. You take yourself to be what they suggest; having no direct knowledge of yourself, you have mere ideas; all mediate, second-hand, by hearsay. Whatever you think you are you take it to be true; the habit of imagining yourself perceivable and describable is very strong with you.

I see as you see, hear as you hear, taste as you taste, eat as you eat. I also feel thirst and hunger and expect my food to be served on time. When starved or sick, my body and mind go weak. All this I perceive quite clearly, but somehow I am not in it, I feel myself as if floating over it, aloof and detached. Even not aloof and detached. There is aloofness and detachment as there is thirst and hunger; there is also the awareness of it all and a sense of immense distance, as if the body and the mind and all that happens to them were somewhere far out on the horizon. I am like a screen—clear and empty—the pictures pass over it and disappear, leaving it as clear and empty as before. In no way is the screen affected by the pictures, nor are the pictures affected by the screen.

QUESTION: When I ask a question and you answer, what exactly happens?

MAHARAJ: The question and the answer—both appear on the screen. The lips move, the body speaks—and again the screen is clear and empty.

QUESTION: When you say: clear and empty, what do you mean?

MAHARAJ: I mean free of all contents. To myself I am neither perceivable nor conceivable; there is nothing I can point out and say: "this I am." You identify yourself with everything so easily; I find it impossible. The feeling: "I am not this or that, nor is anything mine" is so strong in me that as soon as a thing or a thought appears, there comes at once the sense "this I am not."

QUESTION: Do you mean to say that you spend your time repeating "this I am not, that I am not"?

MAHARAJ: Of course not. I am merely verbalizing for your sake. By the grace of my Guru I have realized once and for good that I am neither object nor subject and I do not need to remind myself all the time.

QUESTION: I find it hard to grasp what exactly you mean by saying that you are neither the object nor the subject. At this very moment, as we talk, am I not the object of your experience, and you the subject?

MAHARAJ: Look, my thumb touches my forefinger. Both touch and are touched. When my attention is on the thumb, the thumb is the feeler and the forefinger—the self. Shift the focus of attention and the relationship is reversed. I find that somehow, by shifting the focus of attention, I become the very thing I look at and experience the kind of consciousness it has; I become the inner witness of the thing. I call this capacity of entering other focal points of consciousness—love; you may give it any name you like. Love says: "I am everything." Wisdom says: "I am nothing." Between the two my life flows. Since at any point of time and space I can be both the subject and the object of experience, I express it by saying that I am both and neither and beyond.[2]

In some few individuals this detachment or nonidentification arises spontaneously or easily. However, in most of the great spiritual traditions (Buddhist, Christian mustic, Hindu, Chasid, etc.), a sustained discipline, a training of awareness, and a cultivation of nonattachment precede such awakening. In the Buddhist practice of insight meditation as taught by the greatest contemporary master Mahasi Sayadaw, one undertakes a systematic training of mindfulness and concentration, practicing the constant noticing of whatever is predominant in one's awareness. After some weeks or months of such sustained cultivation of awareness, there begin to arise spontaneously the inner qualities of an enlightened mind. So the Venerable Sayadaw describes the experience at this level of practice as follows:

When the meditator, in the exercise of noticing, is able to keep exclusively to the present body-and-mind process, without looking back to past processes or ahead to future ones, then, as a result of Insight, [the mental vision of] a *brilliant light* will appear to him. To one it will appear like the light of a lamp, to others like a flash of lightening, or like the radiance of the moon or the sun, and so on. With one it may last for just one moment, with others it may last longer.

There will also arise in him strong *mindfulness* pertaining to Insight. As a result, all the successive arisings of bodily and mental processes will present themselves to the consciousness engaged in noticing, as if coming to it of themselves; and mindfulness too, seems as if alighting on the processes of itself. Therefore the meditator then believes: "There is no body-and-mind process in which mindfulness fails to engage."

His *knowledge* consisting in Insight, here called "noticing," will be likewise keen, strong and lucid. Consequently he will discern clearly and in separate forms all the bodily and mental processes noticed, as if cutting to pieces a bamboo sprout with a well-sharpened knife. Therefore the meditator then believes: "There is no body-and-mind process that cannot be noticed." When examining the characteristics of Impermanence, etc., or other aspects of reality, he understands everything quite clearly and at once, and he believes it to be the knowledge derived from direct experience.

Further, strong *faith* pertaining to Insight, arises in him. Under its influence, the meditator's mind, when engaged in noticing or thinking, is serene and without any disturbance; and when he is engaged in recollecting the virtues of the Buddha, the Dhamma* and the Sangha†, his mind quite easily gives itself over to them. There arises in him: the wish to proclaim the Buddha's Teaching, joyous confidence in the virtues of those engaged in meditation, the desire to advise dear friends and relatives to practice meditation, grateful remembrance of the help received from his meditation master, his spiritual mentor, etc.,—these and many other similar mental processes will occur.

There arises also *rapture* in its five grades, beginning with minor rapture. When Purification of Mind is gained, that rapture begins to appear by causing "goose-flesh," tremor in the limbs, etc.; and now it produces a sublime feeling of happiness and exhilaration, filling the whole body with an exceedingly sweet and subtle thrill. Under its influence, he feels as if the whole body had risen up and remained in the air without touching the ground or as if it were seated on an air cushion, or as if it were floating up and down.

There arises *tranquility* of mind with the characteristic of quietening the disturbances of consciousness and its mental concomitants; and along with it appear mental agility, etc. When walking, standing, sitting or reclining there is, under the influence of these mental qualities, no disturbance of consciousness and its mental concomitants, nor heaviness, rigidity, unwieldiness, sickness or crookedness. Rather his consciousness and its mental concomitants are tranquil through having reached the supreme relief in nonaction. They are agile in always functioning swiftly; they are pliant in being able to attend to any object desired; they are wieldy in being able to attend to an object for any length of time desired; they are quite lucid through their proficiency, that is, through the ease with which Insight penetrates the object; they are also straight through being directed, inclined and turned only towards wholesome activities.

---

* The path, the teaching.
† The people practicing meditation, studying the teaching.

There also arises a very sublime feeling of *happiness* suffusing all his body. Under its influence he, then, becomes exceedingly joyous and he believes; "Now I am happy all the time" or "Now indeed, I have found happiness never felt before," and he wants to tell others of his extraordinary experience.

There arises in him *energy* that is neither too lax nor too tense, but is vigorous and acts evenly. For formerly his energy was sometimes lax, and so he was overpowered by sloth and torpor; hence, he could not notice keenly and continuously the objects as they became evident, and his understanding, too, was not clear. And at other times his energy was too tense, and so he was overpowered by agitation, with the same result of being unable to notice keenly, etc. But not his energy is neither too lax nor too tense, but is vigorous and acts evenly: and so getting over these shortcomings of sloth, torpor and agitation, he is able to notice the objects present keenly and continuously, and his understanding is quite clear, too.

There also arises in him strong *equanimity* associated with Insight, which is neutral towards all formations. Under its influence he regards with neutrality even his examination of the nature of these formations with respect to their being impermanent, etc.; and he is able to notice keenly and continuously the bodily and mental processes arising at the time. Then his activity of noticing is carried on without effort, and proceeds, as it were, of itself.

He cherishes no desire nor hate with regard to any object, desirable or undesirable, that comes into the range of his sense doors, but taking them as just the same in his act of noticing, he understands them (that is to say, it is a pure act of understanding).[3]

This description has been corroborated by modern meditation studies such as "The Phenomenology of Insight Meditation."[4] From this meditative tradition, the qualities of enlightenment are described as arising spontaneously in the mind when two things occur. The first is an ability to stay/be in the present moment, and the other is the ability to do so without grasping or self-identification. This nongrasping presentness allows the spontaneous flow of well-being and creative responsiveness frequently attributed to enlightened persons. Trudy Dixon, close student of the great Zen master Shunryu Suzuki Roshi, describes her teacher thus:

A roshi is a person who has actualized that perfect freedom which is the potentiality for all human beings. He exists freely in the fullness of his whole being. The flow of his consciousness is not the fixed repetitive patterns of our usual self-centered consciousness, but rather arises spontaneously and naturally from the actual circumstances of the present. The results of this in terms of the quality of his life are extraordinary—buoy-

ancy, vigor, straightforwardness, simplicity, humility, serenity, joyous-
ness, uncanny perspicacity and unfathomable compassion. His whole being testifies to what it means to live in the reality of the present. Without
anything said or done, just the impact of meeting a personality so
developed can be enough to change another's whole way of life. But in the
end it is not the extraordinariness of the teacher which perplexes, in-
trigues, and deepens the student, it is the teacher's utter ordinariness.
Because he is just himself, he is a mirror for his students. When we are
with him we feel our own strengths and shortcomings without any sense of
praise or criticism from him. In his presence we see our original face, and
the extraordinariness we see is only our own true nature.[5]

Although many texts on spiritual development emphasize a gradual
elimination of greed, fear, hatred, and dullness, with constant vigilance until
these are uprooted in the mind (Buddhaghosa, Patanjali, St. John of the
Cross, etc.), other masters speak of this occurring spontaneously. Such a
spontaneous arising of unselfishness, joy, and responsiveness to the present
situation comes about through a distinct change in perspective. The new
perspective moves us from a limited, identified self-view to one which
transcends this. Once the limitations of the field of self-identification are
seen clearly and the concepts of I-as-separate lose their hold, there manifests
a holistic perception and an automatic compassion. At this point there is no
longer an effort to maintain or produce purity and awareness, only its spontaneous manifestation. The Tibetan lama, Chogyam Trungpa Rinpoche,
describes this experience in this way:

Q: Is the "awake quality" different from just being in the now?
A: Yes. Enlightenment is being *awake* in the nowness. For instance,
animals live in the present, and, for that matter, an infant child lives in the
present; but that is quite different from being awake or enlightened.
Q: I do not quite understand what you mean by animals and babies living
in the present. What is the difference between living in the present in that
form and being an enlightened person?
A: I think it is a question of the difference between dwelling upon
something and really being in the nowness in terms of "awake." In the
case of an infant or animal, it is being in the nowness but it is dwelling
upon the nowness. They get some kind of feedback from it by dwelling
upon it, although they may not notice it consciously. In the case of an
enlightened being, he is not dwelling upon the idea—"I am an enlightened
being"—because he has completely transcended the idea of "I am." He is
just fully being. The subject-object division has been fully transcended.
Q: If the enlightened being is without ego and feels the sorrows and the
sadness of those around him but does not feel his own necessarily, then

would you call his willingness to help them get over their difficulties "desire"?

A: I don't think so. Desire comes in when you want to see someone happy. When that person is happy, then you feel happy because the activities you have engaged in to make him happy are, in a sense, done for yourself rather than for the other person. *You* would like to see him happy. An enlightened being has no such attitude. Whenever someone requires his help, he just gives it; there is no self-gratification or self-congratulation involved.[6]

For the Nobel prize winning saint, Mother Theresa of Calcutta, this presentness brings an ability to manifest compassion and loving assistance in even the most difficult situations.

I do not agree with the big way of doing things. To us what matters is an individual. To get to love the person we must come in close contact with him. If we wait till we get the numbers, then we will be lost in the numbers. And we will never be able to show that love and respect for the person. I believe in person to person; every person is Christ for me, and since there is only one Jesus, that person is only one person in the world for me at that moment.[7]

Thus she prays:

JESUS MY PATIENT

Dearest Lord, may I see you today and every day in the person of your sick, and, whilst nursing them, minister unto you.

Though you hide yourself behind the unattractive disguise of the irritable, the exacting, the unreasonable, may I still recognize you, and say: "Jesus, my patient, how sweet it is to serve you."

For Mother Theresa the same process of letting go of self-identification described by Einstein and Nisargadatta is expressed through the Christian metaphor:

Let there be no pride or vanity in the work. The work is God's work, the poor are God's poor. Put yourself completely under the influence of Jesus, so that he may think his thoughts in your mind and do his work through your hands.

It is an expanded vision of oneself and the world, of perspective, which allows this seeing of each person as Jesus himself, of letting Jesus think the thoughts in your mind and do the work of your hands. Selfish thoughts and limiting perspectives such as fear and doubt are not seen as qualities which must be actively fought, uprooted, or overcome. Instead, they drop away naturally as the limited identification with body, mind, and smaller parts of the world ceases. The mind becomes simple, spacious, and untouched by the effects of praise and blame, or loss and gain. Thus the Chinese master Chuang Tsu writes:

> The men and women in whom Tao
> Acts without impediment
> Harm no other being
> By their actions
> Yet they do not know themselves
> To be "kind," to be "gentle."

> The men and women in whom Tao
> Acts without impediment
> Do not bother with their own interests
> And do not despise
> Others who do.
> They do not struggle to make money
> And do not make a virtue of poverty.
> They go their way
> Without relying on others
> And do not pride themselves
> On walking alone.

> While they do not follow the crowd
> They won't complain of those who do.
> Rank and reward
> Make no appeal to them.
> Disgrace and shame
> Do not deter them.
> They are not always looking
> For right and wrong
> Always deciding "Yes" or "No."[8]

or the modern Indian saint Meher Baba writes:

> No amount of slander can affect or change me, nor any amount of admiration or praise enhance my divinity. Baba is what he is. I was Baba, I am Baba, and I shall forever remain Baba.[9]

This unchangeability and freedom of mind has come to many masters only as a result of great surrender and arduous mental training. One such master from Tibet, the joyful Milarepa, expressed this freedom through the creation of thousands of songs, the vehicle through which he taught. Yet the songs were produced only after many years of traditional training in the mountain solitude. How fully Milarepa transcended the form of his tradition to touch the universal is expressed in his following song:

Having meditated on love and compassion,
I forgot the difference between myself and others.
Having meditated on my lama,
I forgot those who are influential and powerful.
Having meditated constantly on my yidam,
I forgot the coarse world of the senses.
Having meditated on the instruction of the secret tradition,
I forgot the books of dialectic.
Having maintained pure awareness,
I forgot the illusions of ignorance.
Having meditated on the essential nature of mind as Trikaya,
I forgot my hopes and fears.
Having meditated on this life and the life beyond,
I forgot the fear of birth and death.
Having tasted the joys of solitude,
I forgot the need to please my relatives and friends.
Having assimilated the teaching in the stream of my consciousness,
I forgot to engage in doctrinal polemics.
Having meditated on that which is non-arising, non-ceasing, and non-
    abiding,
I disregarded all conventional forms.
Having meditated on the perception of phenomena as the Dharmakaya,
I forgot all conceptual forms of meditation.
Having dwelt in the unaltered state of naturalness,
I forgot the ways of hypocrisy.
Having lived in humility in body and mind,
I forgot the disdain and arrogance of the great.
Having made a monastery within my body,
I forgot the monastery outside.
Having embraced the spirit rather than the letter,
I forgot how to play with words.[10]

This universality comes from the direct perception that all things are one, not as an idea, but as an experience. Zen master Suzuki Roshi, speaking to students in California, led them to understand in this way:

It will take quite a long time before you find your calm serene mind in your practice. Many sensations come, many thoughts or images arise, but they are just waves of your own mind. Nothing comes from outside your mind. Usually we think of our mind as receiving impressions and experiences from outside, but that is not a true understanding of our mind. The true understanding is that the mind includes everything; when you think something comes from outside it means only that something appears in your mind. Nothing outside yourself can cause any trouble. You yourself make the waves in your mind. If you leave your mind as it is it will become calm. This mind is called big mind. That everything is included within your mind is the essence of mind. To experience this is to have religious feeling. Even though waves arise, the essence of your mind is pure; it is just like clear water with a few waves. Actually, water always has waves. Waves are the practice of the water. To speak of waves apart from water or water apart from waves is a delusion. Water and waves are one. Big mind and small mind are one. When you understand your mind in this way, you have some security in your feeling. . . . A mind with waves in it is not a disturbed mind, but actually an amplified one. Whatever you experience is an expression of big mind.[5]

Here the modern master teacher of awareness, Krishnamurti, describes his own experience of the oneness, of big mind:

Woke up this morning rather early, with a sense of a mind that had penetrated into unknown depths. It was as though the mind itself was going into itself, deeply and widely and the journey seemed to have been without movement. And there was this experience of immensity in abundance and a richness that was incorruptible.

It's strange that though every experience, state, is utterly different, it is still the same movement; though it seems to change, it is still the changeless.[11]

From this level of perception, gain and loss, pleasure and pain, are seen as equal. Thus, Zen master Suzuki Roshi could meet even his painful death of cancer with profound equanimity. In some of his last words to his students he said:

If when I die, the moment I'm dying, if I suffer, that is all right, you know; that is suffering Buddha. No confusion in it. Maybe everyone will struggle because of the physical agony or spiritual agony, too. But that is all right, that is not a problem. We should be very grateful to have a limited body . . . like mine or like yours. If you had a limitless life it would be a real problem for you.[5]

Many generations before, Zen master Rinzai, in whom the same spirit flowed, spoke to his students in this way:

> If you love the sacred and dislike the worldly, you will go on floating and sinking in the ocean of birth and death. The passions arise depending on the heart. If the heart is stilled, where then do you find the passions? Do not tire yourselves by making up discriminations, and quite naturally, of itself, you will find the Way.[12]

From this profoundly altered perspective where pleasure and pain are seen as simply a play of energy, arises true and unchanging love. So Mother Theresa speaks in this way:

> . . . here in the slums, in the broken body, in the children, we see Christ and we touch Him.[7]

From a modern Western woman who has practiced meditation deeply under a famous Indian teacher, we can see the capacity for growth in equanimity and love together. This woman had suffered greatly in prison camps during the Second World War, and writes in a letter to her teacher describing effects that her recently successful meditation training has had on her life:

> A few weeks ago I was sorting out old files with notes, stories, thoughts, etc., which I had written down over the years. Reading through them, before destroying them, I was more amazed than I have ever been in my life . . . so much misery and unhappiness! How is it possible that any human being can live for 55 years through so much unhappiness, fear, despair, morbidity, depression, suffering, pain and devastation, and not be utterly destroyed by it! I must have been stronger than I thought. . . . And when I now look back over the past four years, since the first time I came to you in India, life has just been so simple and serene that it is unbelievable. After reaching the first stage in my mental development, I lost all my depressions, headaches, fears and nightmares. And after reaching the second stage during my second visit to you, I don't even understand any more what all the fuss was about those first 55 years of my life. I now just live life as it is and as it comes and as a whole, in calmness and equanimity; and I am happy and content.
>
> Sometimes I meditate intensely and sometimes I don't meditate at all. But you see, in a way my whole life is one total meditation, because I live every minute of the day in full mindfulness and awareness. And somehow nothing seems to be able to touch me anymore. It is living on two levels:

the outer level will make conversation with people and say the right things at the right time. And under that is the second level, where is a core of untouched and untouchable stillness and quiet attention and peace. Because somehow, life is so simple, uncomplicated, and all those old upheavals were after all just of my own making. You only get upheavals through the way you react to things. And once you react the right, direct, simple way, there are no problems left. And somehow, the right way of reacting is most of the time nonreacting. I hope all this makes sense to you!

I'll tell you a little story which will show you what an enormous success you are as a Teacher: A few months ago the man whom I loved more than any other man in the world and who was for the past 17 years as close to me as any man and woman can be, died rather suddenly. If that had happened before you started to teach me in 1975, I am sure it would have completely destroyed me . . . I would have committed a quick suicide to end it all. But now . . . I just felt a little sad about losing this man's close love for me and I missed his company. But for the rest—no, a stone thrown in the water would have caused more ripples than his death did to me. I accepted his death with complete serenity and detachment. He has just finished this life-trip of his and may already have started another one. I don't know that, but apart from a certain personal loss of his companionship, there is no upset or conflict in me about his death.

Apparently I have always been able to see and understand other people's problems and have been able to help them somehow. But in the old days other people's miseries tore out my heart and gave me stomach ulcers, in my pity and concern for them. But now, when people come to see me in their misery, I can listen to them, help them, have a truly great compassion for them; but when they leave, it is over and done with and they have not torn my guts out in the process. I have been working with an alcoholic this past month or so and for some odd reason my listening seems to help in his struggle to stay away from the alcohol and to find himself again. I think you can be proud of yourself as a teacher and content with me as your pupil! [13]

By examining these reports, we can see phenomenologically that these people experience a growth in love and balance of mind as a result of a radically new vision of the world. For some, this vision change results from arduous practice; for others, from deep faith and surrender. Again in the words of Sri Nisargadatta, we can see clearly that the growth of love comes directly out of this new vision. He says:

As I told you already, my Guru showed me my true nature—and the true nature of the world. Having realized that I am one with and yet beyond the world, I became free from all desire and fear. I did not reason out that I should be free—I found myself free—unexpectedly, without the least effort. This freedom from desire and fear remained with me since then. Another thing I noticed was that I do not need to make an effort; the deed follows the thought without delay and friction. I have also found that thoughts became self-fulfilling; things would fall in place smoothly and rightly. The main change was in the mind; it became motionless and silent, responding quickly but not perpetuating the response. Spontaneity became a way of life, the real became natural and the natural became real. And above all, infinite affection, love, dark and quiet, radiating in all directions, embracing all, making all interesting and beautiful, significant and auspicious.[2]

From the perception of one so awakened, even the idea of the journey of awakening is seen as untrue. Although there are many paths and spiritual practices associated with the masters we have quoted in this chapter, in fact the truth is here right now; things are as they are and nothing need be changed. It is simply a question of awakening to this truth as it exists. One of the greatest Indian saints of this century was Ramana Maharshi. When asked about the attainment of liberation, he said this:

Our real nature is Liberation, but we imagine that we are bound and make strenuous efforts to get free, although all the while we are free. This is understood only when we reach that state. Then we shall be surprised to find that we were frantically striving to attain something that we always were and are. An illustration will make this clear. A man goes to sleep in this hall. He dreams he has gone on a world-tour and is travelling over hill and dale, forest and plain, desert and sea, across various continents, and after many years of weary and strenuous travel, returns to this country, reaches Tiruvannamalai, enters the Ashram and walks into the hall. Just at that moment, he wakes up and finds that he has not moved at all, but has been sleeping where he lay down. He has not returned after great effort to this hall, but was here all the time. It is exactly like that. If it is asked why, being free, we imagine ourselves bound, I answer, "Why, being in the hall, did you imagine you were on a world-tour, crossing hill and dale, desert and sea?" It is all in the mind or maya. . . . In a sense, speaking of Self-realization is a delusion. It is only because people have been under the delusion that the non-Self is the Self and the unreal the Real that they have to be weaned out of it by the other delusion called Self-realization; because actually the Self always is the Self and there is no such thing as realizing it. Who is to realize what, and how, when all that exists is the Self and nothing but the Self?[14]

SUMMARY

We have attempted in this chapter to illustrate commonality of vision of respected masters from many great traditions. The element of nonidentification with a limited self seems to be central to their experience of the world. Out of this expanded or unified experience comes naturally, as described in many ways here, equanimity, contentment, joy, and profound love. This experience may arise in many traditions and circumstances, and cannot be forced through desire but is awakened through awareness or surrender. To taste this we are thus instructed by the great Thai meditation master, Achaan Cha, in this way:

Each person has his own natural pace. Some of you will die at age fifty, some at age sixty-five and some at age ninety. So too, your practice will not all be identical. Don't think or worry about this. Try to be mindful and let things take their natural course. Then your mind will become quieter and quieter in any surroundings. It will become still like a clear forest pool. Then all kinds of wonderful and rare animals will come to drink at the pool. You will see many wonderful and strange things come and go. But you will be still. This is the happiness of the Buddha.[15]

REFERENCES

1. Goldstein, J. *The Experience of Insight.* Santa Cruz, Calif.: Unity Press, 1976.
2. Sri Nisargadatta Maharaj. *I Am That.* Bombay: Chetana Publishers, 1973.
3. Mahasi Sayadaw. *The Progress of Insight.* Kandy: Buddhist Publication Society, 1973.
4. Kornfield, J. Intensive insight meditation: A phenomenological study. *Journal of Transpersonal Psychology,* 1979, *11,* 41–58.
5. Suzuki Roshi. *Zen Mind, Beginner Mind.* New York: Weatherhill, 1970.
6. Chogyam Trungpa. *Cutting Through Spiritual Materialism.* Berkeley: Shambhala, 1973.
7. Muggeridge, M. *Something Beautiful for God.* New York: Harper & Row, 1971.
8. Merton, T. (translator) *Chuang Tsu.* New York: New Directions, 1965.
9. Meher Baba. *Listen Humanity.* New York: Harper & Row, 1967.
10. Lobsang P. Llalungpa. *Life of Milarepa.* New York: E.P. Dutton, 1977.
11. Krishnamurti, J. *Krishnamurti's Notebook.* New York: Harper & Row, 1976.
12. Rinzai. *The Zen Teachings of Rinzai.* Berkeley: Shambhala, 1976.
13. Anagarika Munindra. Personal correspondence, Bodh Gaya, 1978.
14. Osborne, A. *The Teachings of Ramana Maharshi.* New York: Samuel Weiser, 1962.
15. Kornfield, J. *Living Buddhist Masters.* Santa Cruz, Calif.: Unity Press, 1977.

IV
INTEGRATIONS AMONG PERSPECTIVES

We can consider the process of healthy growth to be a never ending series of free choice situations, confronting each individual at every point throughout his life, in which he must choose between the delights of safety and growth, dependence and independence, regression and progression, immaturity and maturity.

Abraham Maslow

In its breadth of integration, "The Evolution of Consciousness" is unparalleled in developmental psychology. Never before has there been a model which spans the entire range of development from infancy to the highest levels of psychological maturation, which integrates Western and Eastern psychologies, or which suggests a pattern of transformation common to all levels.

By integrating among major schools of Western psychology, Ken Wilber traces psychological development from infancy through adulthood. Turning to Eastern schools he then details the stages of further development which they describe beyond usual levels of health and normality. Particularly important is the fact that he is able to suggest that the underlying processes by which maturation occurs display parallels at all levels. The result is a broad-ranging synthesis which pulls together an extraordinary amount of formerly unrelated data.

He next applies this schema to an examination of the unconscious and meditation. Both, he suggests, need to be viewed developmentally. By doing so he abstracts five distinct types or processes of the unconscious and then argues that meditation is a means for heightened development which effects these five types differentially. "The Evolution of Consciousness," and its expansion—The Atman Project—are likely to stimulate developmental psychology for years to come.

15

The Evolution of Consciousness

Ken Wilber

Everywhere we look in nature, said the philosopher Jan Smuts,[1] we see nothing but *wholes*—not just simple wholes, but hierarchical ones. Each whole is a part of a larger whole which is itself a part of a larger whole: fields within fields within fields, stretching through the cosmos, interlacing each and every thing with each and every other.

Further, said Smuts, the universe is not a thoughtlessly static and inert whole—the cosmos is not lazy, but energetically dynamic and even creative. It tends to produce higher- and higher-level wholes, ever more inclusive and organized. This overall cosmic process, as it unfolds in time, is nothing other than *evolution,* and the drive to every-higher unities, Smuts called *holism.*

If we continued this line of thinking, we might say that because the human mind or psyche is an aspect of the cosmos, we would expect to find, in the psyche itself, the same hierarchical arrangement of wholes within wholes, reaching from the simplest and most rudimentary to the most complex and inclusive (cf. Welwood).[2] In general, such is exactly the discovery of modern psychology. As Werner put it, "Wherever development occurs it proceeds from a state of relative globality and lack of differentiation to a state of increasing differentiation, articulation, and hierarchical integration."[3] Jakobson speaks of "those stratified phenomena which modern psychology uncovers in the different areas of the realm of the mind," where each stratified layer is more integrated and more encompassing than its predecessor.[4] Bateson points out that even learning itself is hierarchical, involving several major levels, each of which is "meta-" to its predecessor.[5] As a general approximation, then, we may conclude that the psyche—like the cosmos at large—is many layered (pluridimensional), composed of successively higher-order wholes and unities and integrations.

Now the holistic evolution of nature—which produces everywhere higher and higher wholes—shows up in the human psyche as *development* or *growth*. The same force that produced man from amoebas produces adults from infants. That is, a person's growth, from infancy to adulthood, is simply a miniature version of cosmic evolution. Or, we might say, psychological growth or development in humans is simply a microcosmic reflection of universal growth on the whole, and has the same goal: the unfolding of ever higher-order unities and integrations. This is one of the major reasons that the psyche is, indeed, stratified. Very like the geological formation of the earth, psychological development proceeds stratum by stratum, level by level, stage by stage, with each successive level superimposed upon its predecessor in such a way that it includes but transcends it ("envelopes it," as Werner would say).

Now in psychological development, the *whole* of any level becomes merely a *part* of the whole of the next level, which in turn becomes a part of the next whole, and so on throughout the evolution of consciousness. Take, as but one example, the development of language: the child first learns babbling sounds, then wider vowel and consonant sounds, then simple words, then small phrases, then simple sentences, and then extended sentences. At each stage, simple parts (e.g., words) are integrated into higher wholes (e.g., sentences), and as Jakobson points out, "new additions are superimposed on earlier ones and dissolution begins with the higher strata."[6]

Modern developmental psychology has, on the whole, simply devoted itself to the exploration and explanation of the various levels, stages, and strata of the human constitution—mind, personality, psychosexuality, character, consciousness. The cognitive studies of Piaget and Werner, the works of Loevinger,[7] Arieti,[8] Maslow,[9] and Jakobson, the moral development studies of Kohlberg[10]—all subscribe, in whole or part, to the concept of stratified stages of increasing complexity, integration, and unity.

Having said that much, we are at once entitled to ask, "What, then, is the *highest* stage of unity to which one may aspire?" Or perhaps we should not phrase the question in such ultimate terms, but simply ask instead, "What is the nature of some of the higher and higest stages of development? What forms of unity are disclosed in the most developed souls of the human species?"

We all know what the "lower" stages and levels of the psyche are like (I am speaking in simple, general terms): they are instinctual, impulsive, libidinous, id-ish, animal, apelike. We also know what some of the "middle" stages are like: socially adapted, mentally adjusted, egoically integrated, syntactically organized, conceptually advanced. Yet are there no higher stages? Is an "integrated ego" or "autonomous individual" the highest reach of consciousness in human beings? The individual ego is a marvelously high-order unity, but compared with the unity of the cosmos at large, it is a pitiful slice of holistic reality. Has nature labored these billions of years just to bring forth this egoic mouse?

The problem with that type of question lies in *finding* examples of truly higher-order personalities—and in deciding exactly *what* constitutes a higher-order personality in the first place. My own feeling is that as humanity continues its collective evolution, this will become very easy to decide, because more and more "enlightened" personalities will show up in data populations, and psychologists will be forced, by their statistical analyses, to include higher-order profiles in their developmental stages. In the meantime, one's idea of "higher-order" or "highly developed" remains rather philosophic. Nonetheless, those few gifted souls who have bothered to look at this problem have suggested that the world's great mystics and sages represent some of the very highest, if not the highest, of all stages of human development. Bergson said exactly that—as did Toynbee, Tolstoy, James, Schopenhauer, Nietzsche, and Maslow.

The point is that we *might* have an excellent population of extremely evolved and developed personalities in the form of the world's great mystic-sages (a point which is supported by Maslow's studies). Let us, then, simply *assume* that the authentic mystic-sage represents the very highest stages of human development—as far beyond normal-and-average humanity as it itself is beyond apes. This, in effect, would give us a sample which approximates the "highest state of consciousness." Furthermore, most of the mystic-sages have left rather detailed records of the stages and steps of their own transformations into the upper reaches of consciousness. That is, they tell us not only of the highest level of consciousness, but also of all the intermediate levels leading up to it. If we take these higher stages and add them to the lower and middle stages/levels which have so carefully been described and studied by Western psychology, we would then arrive at a fairly well-balanced and comprehensive model of the spectrum of consciousness. I have attempted this type of synthesis in a series of books: *The Spectrum of Consciousness*,[11] *No-boundary*,[12] *The Atman Project*,[13] and *Up from Eden*.[14] As a very general and simplistic outline, here is what we find:

THE LOWER REALMS

It is generally agreed, by Eastern and Western psychology alike, that the lowest levels of development involve simple biological functions and processes. That is, the lowest levels involve somatic processes, instincts, simple sensations and perceptions, and emotional-sexual impulses. In Piaget's system, these are the sensorimotor realms;[15] Arieti refers to them as instinctual, exoceptual, and protoemotional;[16] Loevinger calls them presocial, symbiotic, and impulsive.[17] To the Vedanta Hindu, this is the realm of the anna- and pranamayakosa, the levels of hunger and emotional sexuality (those are precise translations). The Buddhist calls them the lower five vijnanas, or the realm of the five senses. The chakra psychology refers to them as the lower three chakras: the muladhara, or root material and pleromatic level; svadhisthana, or emotional-sexual level; and manipura, or aggressive-power level. These also constitute the lower three skandhas in the Hinayana Buddhist system of psychology: the physical body, perception, and emotion-impulse, and they are Maslow's lowest two needs, physiological and safety needs. All of this simply goes to point up one of Freud's major ideas: "The ego," he said, "is first and foremost a body-ego."[18]

Now the bodyego or bodyself tends to develop in the following way: It is generally agreed that the infant initially cannot distinguish self from not-self, subject from object, body from environment. That is, the self at this earliest of stages is literally one with the physical world. As Piaget put it, "During the early stages the world and the self are one; neither term is distinguished from the other.... [The] self is still material, so to speak...."[19] In Freud's words, "The ego-feeling we are aware of now is thus only a shrunken vestige of a far more extensive feeling—a feeling which embraced the universe and expressed an inseparable connection of the ego with the external world."

That initial stage of *material oneness,* which Piaget called "protoplasmic," I call *pleromatic* and *uroboric.* Although in its primal oneness it expresses Atman-consciousness as potential, it is in terms of actualization, the lowest of all stages. "Pleromatic" is an old gnostic (and Jungian) term meaning the material universe—the *materia prima* and *virgo mater.* "Uroboros" is a mythological motif of the serpent eating its own tail, and signifies "wholly self-contained" and "not able to recognize an other"—autistic and narcissistic.

It is out of this primordial fusion state (or rather, out of what we will soon introduce as the "ground unconscious") that the separate self emerges, and, as Freud said, the self emerges first and foremost as a body, a bodyself. The infant bites a blanket, and it does not hurt; he bites his thumb, and it hurts. There is a difference, he learns, between the body and the not-body, and he gradually learns to focus his awareness *from* the pleroma *to* the body. Thus, out of primitive material unity emerges the first real self-sense: the bodyego. The infant *identifies* with the newly emergent body, with its sensations and emotions, and gradually learns to differentiate them from the material cosmos at large.

Notice that the bodyego, by differentiating itself from the material environment, actually *transcends* that primitive state of fusion and embeddedness. The bodyego transcends the material environment and thus can perform physical *operations* upon that environment. Towards the end of the sensorimotor period (around age two), the child has differentiated the self and the not-self to such a degree that he has a fairly stable image of "object constancy" and so he can *muscularly* coordinate physical operations *on* these objects. He can coordinate a physical movement of various objects in the environment, something he could not easily do as long as he could not differentiate himself from those objects.

Let us note that triad: by *differentiating* the self from an object, the self *transcends* that object and thus can *operate* upon it (using the tools that constitute the self at that level—at this stage, the sensorimotor body).

At the bodyego stage(s), then, the self no longer is bound to the pleromatic environment—but it *is* bound to, or identified with, the biological body. The self, as bodyego, is dominated by instinctual urges, impulsiveness, the pleasure principle, involuntary urges, and discharges—all the id-like primary processes and drives described so well by Freud et al. For this reason, we also call the bodyego the "typhonic self"—the typhon, in mythology, was half human, half serpent (uroboros). In physiological terms, the reptilian complex and the limbic system dominate the self at this stage.

Eventually, however, true *mental* or conceptual functions begin to emerge out of, and differentiate from, the bodyego. As language develops, the child is ushered into the world of symbols and ideas and concepts, and thus is gradually raised above the fluctuations of the simple, instinctual, immediate, and impulsive bodyego. Among other things, language carries the ability to picture things and events which are *not immediately* present to the body-senses. "Language," as Robert Hall put it, "is the means of dealing with the non-present world."

By the same token, then, language is the means of transcending the simply present world (language, in the higher realms of consciousness, is itself transcended, but one must go from the preverbal to the verbal in order to get to the transverbal; we are here talking about the transcendence of the preverbal by the verbal which, although only half the story, is an extraordinary achievement). Through language, one can anticipate the future, plan for it, and thus gear one's present activities in accordance with tomorrow. That is, one can delay or control one's present bodily desires and activities. This is, as Fenichel explains, "a gradual substituting of actions for mere discharge reactions. This is achieved through the interposing of a time period between stimulus and response." [15] Through language and its symbolic, tensed structures, one can postpone the immediate and impulsive discharges of simple biological drives. One is no longer totally dominated by instinctual demands but can to a certain degree *transcend* them, and this simply means that the self is starting to differentiate from the body and emerge as a *mental* or verbal or syntactical being.

Notice again: as mental-self emerges and differentiates from the body (with the help of language), it *transcends* the body and thus can *operate* upon it using its own mental structures as tools (it can delay the body's immediate discharges and postpone its instinctual gratifications using verbal insertions). At the same time, this allows a sublimation of the body's emotional-sexual energies into more subtle, complex, and evolved activities.

At any rate, a fairly coherent mental-ego eventually emerges (usually between ages four and seven), differentiates itself from the body, transcends the simple biological world, and *therefore* can to a certain degree operate on the biological world (and the earlier physical world) using the tools of simple representational thinking. This whole trend is consolidated with the emergence (usually around age seven) of what Piaget calls "concrete operational thinking"—thinking that can *operate* on the world and the body by use of concepts.

By the time of adolescence, another extraordinary differentiation begins to occur: in essence, the self simply starts to differentiate *from* the representational thought process. And because the self starts to differentiate itself from the representational thought process, it can to a certain degree *transcend* the thought process and therefore *operate* upon it. Piaget calls this—his highest stage—"formal operational," because one can operate on one's own formal thought (i.e., work with linguistic objects as well as physical ones), a detailed operation which, among other things, results in the 16 binary propositions of formal logic. However, the only point I wish to emphasize here is that this can occur because consciousness differentiates itself from syntactical thought, transcends it, and hence can operate upon it (something that it could not do when it *was* it). Actually, this process is just beginning at this stage—it intensifies at the higher stages—but the overall point seems fairly clear: consciousness, or the self, is *starting* to transcend the verbal ego-mind. It is starting to go transverbal.

(To touch bases with other researchers: the verbal ego-mind is known in Mahayana Buddhism as the manovijnana, in Hinduism as the manomaya-kosa, in Hinayana Buddhism as the fourth and fifth skandhas. It is Freud's ego and secondary process, Arieti's language and conceptual levels, Loevinger's conscientious and individualistic stages, Sullivan's syntactic mode, Maslow's self-esteem needs. It is also the fifth chakra, the visuddha chakra or lower verbal-mind, and the lower aspects of the sixth or ajna chakra. These are all very general but very significant correlations.)

Now as consciousness begins to transcend the verbal ego-mind, it can integrate the ego-mind with all the lower levels. That is, because consciousness is no longer identified with any of these elements to the exclusion of any others, all of them can be integrated: the body and mind can be brought into a higher-order holistic integration. This stage is referred to as the "integration of all lower levels" (Sullivan et al.[21]), "integrated" (Loevinger[22]), "self-actualized" (Maslow), "autonomous" (From,[23] Riesman[24]). My favorite descriptive phrase comes from Loevinger's statement of Broughton's work: his highest stage, stage 6, is one wherein "mind and body are both experiences of an integrated self."[25] This integrated self, wherein mind and body are harmoniously one, we call the "centaur"—the great mythological being with animal body and human mind existing in a state of at-one-ment. The centaur, we say, is starting to go transverbal, but it is not yet transpersonal.

As I mentioned, both Eastern and Western psychology are in agreement as to the nature of all these lower levels, from pleroma to body to ego-mind, but the West has contributed a rather exact understanding of a phenomenon that is only vaguely understood in the East: namely, the process of dynamic repression. For what the West discovered is that as higher-order levels of consciousness *emerge* in development, they can *repress* the lower levels, with results that range from mild to catastrophic.

In order to take into account this process of dynamic repression, we simply use the Jungian terms "shadow" and "persona." The shadow is the personal unconscious, a series of "feeling-toned complexes." These complexes are images and concepts which become "contaminated" by the lower levels—in particular, the emotional-sexual—and thus are (erroneously) felt to be threatening to the higher-order structure of the ego-mind. These complexes are thus split off from consciousness (they become shadow), a process which simultaneously distorts the self-concept (the ego), and thus leaves the individual with a false or inaccurate self-image (the persona). If the persona and shadow can be reunited, then the higher-order integration of the total ego can be established. That, in very general terms, is the major aim of orthodox Western psychotherapy.

So far, then, we have these major levels of increasing integration and transcendence: the simple and primitive fusion-unity of the pleroma; the next higher-order unity of the biological bodyself; then the mental-persona, which, if integrated with the shadow, yields the higher-order unity of the total ego; and finally the centaur, which is a higher-order integration of the total ego with all preceding and lower levels—body, persona, and shadow.

THE INTERMEDIATE REALMS

With the exception of transpersonal psychology, the centaur is the highest level of consciousness taken seriously by Western psychology. The existence of levels above and prior to the centaur is thus viewed by Western psychology with a jaundiced eye. Western psychiatrists and psychologists either deny the existence of any sort of higher-order unities or—should they actually confront what seems to be a higher-order level—simply try to pathologize its existence, to explain it by diagnosis. Thus, for indications as to the nature of any higher levels of consciousness beyond the ego and the centaur, we have to turn to the great mystic-sages, Eastern and Western, Hindu and Buddhist, Christian and Islamic. It is somewhat surprising, but absolutely significant, that all of these otherwise divergent schools of thought agree rather unanimously as to the nature of the "farther reaches of human nature." There are indeed, these traditions tell us, higher levels of consciousness—as far above the ego-mind as the ego-mind is above the typhon.

Beginning with (to use the terms of yogic chakra-psychology) the sixth chakra, the ajna chakra, consciousness *starts* to go transpersonal. Consciousness is now going transverbal *and* transpersonal. It begins to enter what is called the "subtle sphere." This process quickens and intensifies as it reaches the highest chakra—the sahasrara—and then goes supra-mental as it enters the seven higher stages of consciousness beyond the sahasrara. The ajna, the sahasrara, and the seven higher levels are, on the whole, referred to as the subtle realm.

For convenience sake, however, we speak of the "low-subtle" and the "high-subtle." The low-subtle is epitomized by the ajna chakra—the "third eye"—which is said to include and dominate both astral and psychic events. That is, the low-subtle is "composed" of the astral and psychic planes of consciousness. Whether one believes in these levels or not, *this* is where they are said to exist.

The astral level includes, basically, out-of-the-body experiences, certain occult knowledge, the auras, true magik, "astral travel," and so on. Although this is the very lowest of the intermediate realms, it has today become something of a fashion to regard this plane as an extraordinarily high state of being.

The psychic plane includes what we would call "psi" phenomena: ESP, precognition, clairvoyance, psychokinesis, and so on. Some individuals seem to occasionally "plug in" to this plane, and evidence random or higher-than-random psychic abilities, but to actually *enter* this plane is to more or less master psychic phenomena, or at least certain of them, such as teleportation or levitation. Patanjali has an entire chapter of his *Yoga Sutras* devoted to this plane and its structures (which are *siddhis,* or paranormal powers). I should also say that many researchers feel that the astral is higher than the psychic, and others feel that they are the same body, but the general points are as outlined above.

The whole point of the low-subtle—the astral-psychic—is that consciousness, by further differentiating itself from the mind and body, is able in some ways to *transcend* the normal capacities of the gross bodymind and therefore *operate* upon the world and the organism in ways that appear, to the ordinary mind, to be quite fantastic and farfetched. For my own part, I find them a natural extension of the transcendent function of consciousness.

The high-subtle begins at the sahasrara and extends into seven more levels of extraordinarily high-order transcendence, differentiation, and integration. This is, on the whole, the realm of high religious intuition and inspiration; of symbolic visions; of blue, gold, and white light; of audible illuminations and brightness upon brightness; it is the realm of higher presences, guides, angelic beings, ishtadevas, and dhyani-buddhas, all of which are simply high archetypal forms of one's own being (although they initially and necessarily appear "other"). It is the realm of Sar Shabd, of Brahma the Controller, of God's archetypes, and of Sat Shabd—and beyond these realms lie three higher and totally indescribable levels of being. Dante sang of it thus:

> Fixing my gaze upon the Eternal Light
> I saw within its depths,
> Bound up with love together in one volume,
> The scattered leaves of all the universe. . . .
> Within the luminous profound subsistence
> Of that Exalted Light saw I three circles
> Of three colors yet of one dimension
> And by the second seemed the first reflected
> As rainbow is by rainbow, and the third
> Seemed fire that equally from both is breathed.

Keep in mind that this is what Dante *saw,* literally, with his eye of contemplation.

The psychiatrist Dean reports this:

> An intellectual illumination occurs that is quite impossible to describe. In an intuitive flash, one has an awareness of the meaning and drift of the universe, an identification and merging with creation, infinity and immortality, a depth beyond depth of revealed meaning—in short, a conception of an over-self, so omnipotent. . . .[26]

In Hinduism, this is the vijnanamayakosa; in Mahayana Buddhism, the manas. Aspects of this subtle realm have been called the "over-self" or "over-mind" or "supra-mind"—as in Aurobindo and Emerson. The point is simply that consciousness, in a rapid ascent, is differentiating itself entirely from the ordinary mind and self, and thus can be called an "over-self," "over-mind," or "supra-mind." It embodies a transcendence of all mental forms, and discloses, at its summit, the intuition of that which is above and prior to mind, self, world, and body—something which, as Aquinas would have said, all men and women would call God.

Yet this is not God as an ontological other, set apart from the cosmos, from humans, and from creation at large. Rather, it is God as an archetypal summit of one's own consciousness. In this way only could St. Clement say that he who knows himself knows God. We could now say, he who knows his over-self knows God. They are one and the same.

THE ULTIMATE REALMS

As the process of transcendence and integration continues, it discloses even higher-order unities, leading, consummately, to Unity itself.

Beyond the high-subtle lies the causal region, known variously as the alayavijnana, the anandamayakosa, pneuma, etc. Again, for convenience, we divide it into the low-causal and the high-causal.

The low-causal, which is revealed in a state of consciousness known as savikalpa samadhi, represents the pinnacle of God-consciousness, the final and highest abode of Ishvara, the Creatrix of all realms. At this point, all the preceeding subtle-realm manifestations begin to actually and literally reduce to modifications of Consciousness itself, so that one begins to become all that previously appeared as objective visions, lights, sounds, colors (this process begins at the high-subtle, but culminates here). In visualization meditation, this is the point at which the dhyani-buddha or yidam, once created and evoked in the subtle realm, becomes one's own self, or rather, one's self dissolves into that god-archetype. John Blofeld quotes Edward Conze on the Vajrayana viewpoint: " 'It is the emptiness of everything which allows the identification to take place—the emptiness which is in us coming together with the emptiness which is the deity.' By visualizing that identification 'we actually do become the deity. The subject is identified with the object of faith. [As is said,] The worship, the worshipper and the worshipped, those three are not separate.' "[27] At its peak, the soul becomes one, literally one, with God, with Ishvara, with Spirit, with the Dhyani-Buddha. One dissolves into Deity, as Deity—that Deity which, from the beginning, has been one's own Self or highest archetype. At this point, all of the archetypal forms of the previous stages (any yidam, ishtadeva, vision, light, etc.)—as well as one's own self—condense and dissolve into God, which is here seen as a subtle audible-light or bija-mantra from which the individual yidams emerged in the first place.

Beyond that point, into the high-causal, all forms are so radically transcended that they no longer need even appear or arise in consciousness.

This is total and utter transcendence into formless consciousness, boundless being. There is here no self, no God, no objects, no subjects, and no thingness, apart from or other than consciousness-as-such. Note the overall progression: in the high-subtle and low-causal, the self dissolves into Deity; here, the Deity-Self dissolves into formlessness. The Deity is reduced to its own prior ground. Blofeld describes this progression from the Vajrayana view: "As the rite progresses, this deity enters the adept's body and sits upon a solar-disc supported by a lunar-disc above a lotus in his heart; presently the adept shrinks in size until he and the deity are coextensive [the subtle realm]; then, merging indistinguishably [the high-subtle], they are absorbed by the seed-syllable from which the deity originally sprang [the low-causal]; this syllable contracts to a single point; the point vanishes and deity and adept in perfect union remain sunk in the samadhi of voidness [the high-causal]. . . ."[28] This is described in much the same way by Lex Hixon,[29] who presents the Hindu view; by Bubba Free John;[30] and by Zen texts on koan study—and it is widely and similarly described by all the traditions that reach this high realm. This state itself is nirvikalpa samadhi, nirodh, jnana samadhi, the high-causal—and the eighth of the ten Zen ox-herding pictures.

Passing through nirvikalpa-samadhi, consciousness totally awakens as its original condition and suchness (tathata), which is, at the same time, the condition and suchness of all that is, gross, subtle, or causal. That which witnesses, and that which is witnessed, are only one and the same. The entire world process then arises, moment to moment, as one's own being—outside of which, and prior to which, nothing exists. That being is totally beyond and prior to anything that arises, and yet no part of that being is other than what arises.

Thus, as the center of the self was shown to be God, and as the center of God was shown to be formlessness, so the center of formlessness is shown to be not other than the entire world of form. "Form is not other than Void, Void is not other than Form," says the Heart Sutra. At that point, the extraordinary and the ordinary, the supernatural and the mundane, are precisely one and the same. This is the tenth Zen ox-herding picture, which reads: "The gate of his cottage is closed and even the wisest cannot find him. He goes his own way, making no attempt to follow the steps of earlier sages. Carrying a gourd, he strolls into the market; leaning on his staff, he returns home."

This is also sahaja samadhi, the Turiya state—the ultimate unity, wherein all things and events, while remaining perfectly separate and discrete, are only one. Therefore, this is not itself a state apart from other states; it is not an altered state;[31] it is not a special state—it is rather the suchness of all states, the water that forms itself in each and every wave of experience, as all experience. It cannot be seen, because it is everything which is seen; it cannot be heard, because it is hearing itself; it cannot be remembered because it only *is.* By the same token, this is the radically perfect integration of all prior levels—gross, subtle, and causal, which, now of themselves so, continue to arise moment to moment in an irridescent play of mutual interpenetration. This is the final differentiation of consciousness from all forms in consciousness, whereupon consciousness-as-such is released in perfect transcendence, which is not a transcendence from the world but a final transcendence into the world. Consciousness henceforth *operates,* not on the world, but only as the entire world process, integrating and interpenetrating all levels, realms, and planes, high or low, sacred or profane.

This, finally, is the ultimate unity towards which all evolution, human as well as cosmic, drives. It might be said that cosmic evolution—that holistic pattern—is completed in and as human evolution, which itself reaches ultimate unity consciousness and so completes that absolute gestalt towards which all manifestation moves. Not only does "phylogeny recapitulate cosmogeny," it completes it.

THE FORM OF DEVELOPMENT

Overall, the process of psychological development—which is the operation, in humans, of cosmic evolution—proceeds in a most articulate fashion. At each stage, a higher-order structure—more complex and therefore more unified—emerges through a differentiation of the preceeding, lower-order level. This higher-order structure is introduced to consciousness, and eventually (it can be almost instantaneous or can take a prolonged time) the self *identifies* with that emergent structure. For example, as the body emerged from its pleromatic fusion with the material world, consciousness became a bodyself: identified with the body. As language emerged in awareness, the self began to shift from a solely biological bodyself to a syntactical ego—the self eventually identified itself with language and operated *as* a syntactical self. Likewise, in advanced evolution, the Deity emerges, is introduced to consciousness directly (in the high-subtle), the self identifies as the Deity, and operates from that identification. The point is that as each higher-order structure emerges, the self eventually identifies with that structure—which is normal, natural, appropriate.

As evolution proceeds, however, each level in turn is differentiated *from* the self-sense, or "peeled off" so to speak. The self, that is, eventually *disidentifies* with that structure (so as to identify with the next higher-order emergent structure), or we might say that the self detaches itself from its *exclusive* identification with that structure. The point is that because the self is differentiated from the lower structure, it *transcends* that structure and thus can *operate* on that lower structure by using the tools of the newly emergent structure (operation *can* become manipulation, but that is a separate issue). As the bodyego was differentiated from the material environment, it could operate on the environment using the tools of the bodyself (muscles). As the ego-mind was differentiated from the body, it could operate on the body and world with its tools (concepts, syntax). As the subtle self was differentiated from the ego-mind, it could operate on mind, body, and world using its structures (psi, siddhi), and so on.

Thus, at each point in psychological growth, we find: (1) a higher-order structure emerges in consciousness; (2) the self identifies its being with that structure; (3) the next higher-order structures then eventually emerges; (4) the self disidentifies with the lower structure and (5) shifts its essential identity to the higher structure; (6) consciousness thereby transcends the lower structure and becomes capable of operating on that lower structure from the higher-order level; (7) all preceding levels can then be integrated in consciousness, and ultimately as consciousness. We noted that each successively higher-order structure is more complex, more organized, and more unified, and evolution continues until there is only unity—ultimate in all directions—whereupon the force of evolution is exhausted, and there is perfect release in radiance as the entire world flux.

A few technical points: using the terms of linguistics, we say that each level of consciousness consists of a *deep structure* and a *surface structure*. The deep structure consists of all the basic limiting principles embedded as that level. The deep structure is the defining *form* of a level, which embodies all of the potentials and limitations of that level. Surface structure is simply a *particular* manifestation of the deep structure. The surface structure is constrained by the form of the deep structure, but within that form it is free to select various contents (e.g., within the form of the subtle deep structure, one may select a particular dhyani-buddha or yidam or ishtadeva as surface structure; what all of these forms of the subtle have in common is the deep structure of the subtle: an ishtadeva is different from a yidam, and each yidam is different from all others, but all of them are equally *forms of* the subtle level).

A deep structure is like a paradigm and contains within it all the basic limiting principles in terms of which all surface structures are realized. To use a simple example, take a ten-story building: each of the floors is a deep structure, whereas the various rooms and objects on each floor are surface structures. All bodyselves are on the second floor; all verbal ego-minds are on the fifth floor; all yidams are on the eighth floor; God is on top, and the building itself is consciousness-as-such. The point is that although all verbal egos are quite different, they are all on the fifth floor: they all share the same deep structure.

Now the movement of surface structures we call *translation;* the movement of deep structures we call *transformation*. Thus, if we move furniture around on the fourth floor, that is a translation; but if we move up to the seventh floor, that is a transformation. Many egos try to think about Buddha, which is merely translation, whereas what is required is a transformation: the fifth floor can't see what's going on on the tenth, and probably shouldn't try.

Two more technical terms: a *sign* is that which points to, represents, or is involved with any element *within* a given level; whereas a *symbol* points to, represents, or is involved with an element of a different level (either higher or lower). Therefore, we say that *translation operates with signs, whereas transformation operates with symbols*. The word "Buddha" is merely a sign if, while on the fifth floor of verbal-ego deep structure, I simply think about "Buddha" or philosophize about what that word might mean, and refuse to identify it with anything higher than my present state of adaptation. "Buddha" is especially a sign if I make the error of identifying it with anything that can be presently seen from the fifth floor. "Buddha" is a symbol when it is understood, by the ego, to represent a transcendent being which cannot be fully understood without transformation to a higher state itself. Finally, "Buddha" visualized as yidam becomes an actual symbol of transformation which discloses that higher realm.

With all of that in mind, we can say that each transformation upward marks the emergence in consciousness of a new and higher level, with a new deep structure, within which new translations or surface structures can unfold and operate. In addition, we say that evolution is a series of such transformations, or changes in deep structure, mediated by symbols or forms in consciousness (the lowest form being the body, the next being the mind, then the subtle, etc.). Most importantly, we say that *all* deep structures are *remembered*, in the precise Platonic sense of *anamnesis*, whereas all surface structures are *learned*, in the sense studied by Western psychologists. A deep structure emerges in consciousness when it is remembered; a surface structure emerges when it is learned. It is generally agreed that one does not learn to become a Buddha, one simply discovers or remembers that one is already Buddha. Just so, no one learns any deep structure, but simply discovers or remembers it prior to (or concomitant with) the course of learning its surface structure. You don't learn to have a body, but you do learn to play baseball with it—you discover deep structures and learn surface structures. Only this view, I have argued in *The Atman Project*,[13] can explain emergence or psychological development.

Every time one remembers a higher-order deep structure, the lower-order structure is subsumed under it. That is, at each point in evolution, what is the whole of one level becomes merely a part of the higher-order whole of the next level. We saw, for example, that the body is, during the earlier stages of growth, the *whole* of the self-sense—that is the bodyego. As the mind emerges and develops, however, the sense of identity shifts to the mind, and the body becomes merely one aspect, one part, of the total self. Similarly, as the subtle level emerges, the mind and body—which together had constituted the whole of the self-system—become merely aspects or parts of the new and more encompassing self.

In precisely the same way, we can say that at each point in evolution or remembrance, a *mode* of self becomes merely a *component* of a higher-order self (e.g., the body was *the* mode of the self before the mind emerged, whereupon it became merely a component of self). This can be put in several different ways, each of which tells us something important about development, evolution, and transcendence: (1) what is *identification* becomes *detachment;* (2) what is *context* becomes *content* (i.e., the context of cognition and experience of one level becomes simply a content of the experience of the next); (3) what is *ground* becomes *figure* (which releases higher-order ground); (4) what is *subjective* becomes *objective* (until both of these terms become meaningless); (5) what is *condition* becomes *element* (e.g., the mind, which is the a priori condition of egoic experience, becomes merely an element of experience in the higher-order realms; as it was put in the *The Spectrum of Consciousness,*[11] one is then looking at these structures and therefore is not using them as something with which to look at, and thus distort, the world).

Each of those points is, in effect, a definition of *transcendence.* Yet each is also a definition of a stage of *development.* It follows that the two are essentially identical and that evolution, as has been said, is actually "self-realization through self-transcendence."

TYPES OF THE UNCONSCIOUS

Although the preceding model is complex, nothing simpler, I believe, is capable of grasping all the facts of the extrordinarily complex phenomenon of consciousness or—what amounts to the same thing—of unconsciousness either. Many accounts of "the unconscious" simply assume that it is there, either as process or as content, from the start, and then proceed to describe its layers, levels, grounds, modes, or contents. However, I believe that approach must be supplemented by developmental or evolutionary concerns on the one hand and dynamic factors on the other.

Let me give a few examples of the problem itself: Transactional Analysis speaks of unconscious (or preconscious) script programming, containing *verbal* injunctions such as "feel guilty" or "collect anxiety." The job of the script analyst is to discover these injuctions, make them explicit and conscious, and thus release the client from their compulsive power. For simplicity's sake, let's call this the "script unconscious."

Let us now note a rather simple point: a preverbal child cannot have a verbal script unconscious. Rather, language itself will have to emerge developmentally, then be loaded with script injunctions which will then have to sink back below the ordinary threshold of consciousness—at which point, and not before, we may speak of the unconscious script. In the same way, a child in the pre-phallic stage cannot have a phallic fixation, the pre-egoic infant doesn't possess unconscious ego character structure, and so on.

Clearly, what exists in "the" unconscious depends in large measure on developmental concerns—*all* of the unconscious, in all its forms, is not just given at the start. Yet, to continue the story, many writers seem to assume that there is a "transpersonal unconscious" that is present but repressed from the beginning, whereas—if it is like verbal programming, character structure, mental capacity, abstract thinking, and higher structures in general—it is not yet repressed because it has not yet developmentally had the chance to emerge. It is not yet repressed from awareness because it has not yet even tentatively emerged in awareness in the first place.

With this developmental and dynamic, as opposed to static and given, viewpoint in mind, I will now outline five basic types of unconscious processes. These are types of unconscious processes, not levels of the unconscious (although we will mention these as well). This outline is meant to be neither exhaustive nor definitive, but only indicative of concerns that I feel transpersonal psychology must address.

The Ground Unconscious

By "ground" I intend an essentially neutral meaning; it is not to be confused with "ground of being" or "open ground" or "primal ground." Although in a certain sense it is "all encompassing," it is basically a developmental concept. The fetus "possesses" the ground unconscious; in essence, it is *all the deep structures existing as potentials ready to emerge, via remembrance, at some future point.* All the deep structures given to a collective humanity—pertaining to every level of consciousness from the body to mind to soul to spirit, gross, subtle, and causal—are enfolded or enwrapped in the ground unconscious. All of these structures are unconscious, but they are *not* repressed because they have not yet entered consciousness. Development—or evolution—consists of a series of hierarchical transformations or *unfoldings* of the deep structures out of the ground unconscious, starting with the lowest (the body) and ending with the highest (God). When—and if—*all* of the ground unconscious has emerged, then there is *only* consciousness: all is conscious *as* the All. As Aristotle put it, when all potential has been actualized, the result is God.

Notice that the ground unconscious is largely (but I don't think we can say totally) devoid of surface structures, for these are basically *learned* during the unfolding (remembrance) of deep structures. This is similar—but only similar—to Jung's idea of the archetypes as "forms devoid of content." As Jung put it, an archetype (deep structure) "is determined as to its content [surface structure] only when it becomes conscious and is therefore filled out with the material of conscious experience."[32] Everyone "inherits" the same basic deep structures, but everybody learns individual surface structures, which can be quite similar or quite dissimilar from those of other individuals (within, of course, the constraints of the deep structures themselves).

Finally, let us note that the closer a deep structure is to emergence, the more profoundly it affects the already-emerged consciousness. This fact turns out to be of the utmost significance.

Now, all of the following four types of the unconscious can be defined *in relation* to the ground unconscious. This gives us a concept of unconscious processes that is at once structural and dynamic, layered and developmental.

The Archaic Unconscious

Freud's initial pioneering efforts in psychoanalysis led him to postulate two basically distinct psychic systems: the system-unconscious, as he called it, and the system-conscious. The unconscious was, he felt, *generated* by repression: certain impulses, because they were dynamically resisted by the system-conscious, were forcefully expelled from awareness. "The unconscious" and "the repressed" were basically one and the same.

Eventually, however, Freud came to speak, not so much of the system-conscious and the system-unconscious, but rather of the ego and the id, and these two formulations did not overlap very clearly. That is, the ego was *not* the same as the system-conscious, and the id was not the same as the system-unconscious. First of all, parts of the ego (the superego, the defenses, and the character structure) were *unconscious,* and parts of the id were unconscious *but not repressed.* In his words, "We recognize that the *Ucs.* does not coincide with the repressed; it is still true that all that is repressed is *Ucs.*, but not all that is *Ucs.* is repressed."[33]

Not all that is unconscious is repressed because, as Freud came to see, some of the unconscious simply finds itself unconscious from the start—it is not first a personal experience which is then repressed, but something that, as it were, *begins* in the unconscious. Freud had once thought that the symbols in dreams and fantasies could be traced back to real life personal experiences, but he came to see that many of the symbols found in dreams and fantasies could not possibly have been generated by personal experience. "Whence comes the necessity for these fantasies, and the material for them?" we hear him ask. "There can be no doubt about the instinctual sources; but how is it to be explained that the same fantasies are always formed with the same content? I have an answer to this which I know will seem to you very daring. I believe that these *primal fantasies* ... are a phylogenetic possession. In them the individual ... stretches out ... to the experiences of past ages."[34] This phylogenetic or "archaic heritage" included, besides instincts, "abbreviated repetitions of the evolution undergone by the whole human race through long-drawn-out periods and from prehistoric ages." Although Freud differed profoundly from Jung on the nature of this archaic heritage, he nevertheless stated that "I fully agree with Jung in recognizing the existence of this phylogenetic heritage."[35]

For Jung, of course, the "phylogenetic heritage" consisted of the instincts and the mental forms or images associated with the instincts, which he eventually termed the "archetypes." For Jung, instinct and archetype were intimately related—almost one. As Frey-Rohn explains it, "The connection between instinct and archetypal image appeared to [Jung] so close that he drew the conclusion that the two were coupled. ... He saw the primordial image [the archetype] as the *self-portrait of the instinct*—in other words, *the instinct's perception of itself*."[36] As for the archic images themselves:

> Man inherits these images from his ancestral past, a past that includes all of his human ancestors as well as his prehuman or animal ancestors. These racial images are not inherited in the sense that a person consciously remembers or has images that his ancestors had. Rather they are predispositions or potentialities for experiencing and responding to the world in the same ways that his ancestors did [they are, that is, archaic deep structures].[37]

Such is the archaic unconscious, which is simply the most primitive and least developed structures of the ground unconscious—the pleroma, the uroboros, and the typhon. They are initially unconscious but unrepressed, and some tend to remain unconscious, never clearly unfolded in awareness except as rudimentary deep structures with little or no surface content. Self-reflexive awareness is out of the question with these structures, so they always retain a heavy mood of unconsciousness, and this with or without repression (which is a significant point). The "prevailing quality of the id," said Freud, "is that of being unconscious,"[38] and that is the nature of the id, not something created by repression. Incidentally, I do not share Jung's enthusiasm over the archaic images; and I do not equate the archetypes, which are highly advanced structures lying in the high-subtle and low-causal, with the archaic images, which are (as Jung himself said) instinctual or typhonic counterparts. The archetypes are exemplary patterns of manifestation, not old images.

At any rate, following both Freud and Jung, we can say in general that the somatic side of the archaic unconscious is the id (instinctual, limbic, typhonic, pranic); the psychic side is the phylogenetic fantasy heritage. On the whole, the archaic unconscious is not the product of personal experience; it is initially unconscious but not repressed; it contains the earliest and the most primitive structures to unfold from the ground unconscious, and even when unfolded, they tend towards unconsciousness. They are preverbal.

Freud himself came to realize the significance of differentiating the personal unconscious (which we will examine in the next section) from the archaic unconscious. In analyzing a client's symptoms, dreams, and fantasies, it is important to distinguish those which are the products of actual past experience or personal fantasy, and those which were *never* personally experienced in this lifetime, but which enter consciousness through the impersonal archaic heritage. My own feeling is that the former are best treated analytically; the latter, mythologically.

The Submergent Unconscious

Once a deep structure has emerged from the ground unconscious and taken on some sort of surface structure, it can for various reasons be returned to a state of unconsciousness. That is, once a structure has emerged, it can be submerged, and the total of such structure we call the submergent unconscious. The submergent unconscious is that which was once conscious in the lifetime of the individual, but is now screened out of awareness.

Now the submergent unconscious can include, in principle, every structure that has emerged, whether collective, personal, archaic, subtle, etc. It can contain collective elements that have clearly and unequivocally emerged and then been suppressed, or it can contain personal elements molded in this lifetime and then suppressed, or it can contain a mixture of both. Jung has written extensively on just that subject and we needn't repeat him here, but we should notice that even Freud was aware of the difference between the archaic unconscious id and the submergent unconscious id, even if it was occasionally hard to perfectly differentiate between them.

In the course of this slow development certain contents of the id were ... taken into the ego; others of its contents remained in the id unchanged, as its scarcely accessible nucleus. During this development, however, the young and feeble ego put back into the unconscious state some of the material it had already taken in, dropped it, and behaved in the same way to some fresh impressions it might have taken in, so that these, having been rejected, could leave a trace only in the id. In consideration of its origin we speak of the this latter portion of the id as *the repressed*.[39]

There is the difference, or rather one of them, between the original archaic unconscious and the repressed or submerged unconscious. However, as Freud says, "It is of little importance that we are not always able to draw a sharp line between these two categories of contents in the id. They coincide approximately with the distinction between what was innately present originally [the archaic unconscious] and what was acquired in the course of the ego's development [the submergent unconscious]."[40] Notice that Freud arrives at these conclusions on the basis of developmental thinking.

The submergent unconscious becomes unconscious for various reasons, and these reasons lie along a *continuum of inattention*. This continuum ranges from simple foregetting through selective forgetting to forceful/dynamic forgetting (the latter alone being repression proper). Of the *personal* submergent unconscious, Jung states:

The personal unconscious . . . includes all those psychic contents which have been forgotten during the course of the individual's life. Traces of them are still preserved in the unconscious, even if all conscious memory of them has been lost. In addition, it contains all subliminal impressions or perceptions which have too little energy to reach consciousness. To these we must add unconscious combinations of ideas that are still too feeble and too indistinct to cross over the threshold. Finally, the personal unconscious contains all psychic contents that are incompatible with the conscious attitude.[41]

Simple forgetting and lack of threshold response constitute the subliminal submergent unconscious. Dynamic or forceful forgetting, however, is repression proper, Freud's great discovery. The repressed submergent unconscious is that aspect of the ground unconscious which, upon emerging and picking up surface structures, is then forcefully repressed or returned to unconsciousness because of an incompatibility with conscious structures (for which, see the next section).

The personal aspect of the repressed submergent unconscious is the *shadow*. Once returned to unconsciousness, the shadow can be strongly influenced by the archaic unconscious (following primary process laws and the pleasure principle, which dominates the typhonic realms), although this is definitely a relative affair. I agree with Jung, for instance, that the shadow *can* be verbal and highly structured (similar in structure and content to the ego). Actually, there seems to be a continuum of structure, ranging from the highly structured verbal components of the unconscious all the way down to the primal chaos of the unstructured *materia prima,* the pleroma base of the archaic unconscious. Needless to say, one of the major reasons for repressing the shadow is that it becomes a vehicle for the archaic unconscious: loaded with instinctual impulses which are felt to be incompatible with the ego.

The Embedded Unconscious

We come now to that aspect of the unconscious which most puzzled Freud, but which is nonetheless one of his greatest discoveries. Recall that Freud abandoned the conscious-unconscious model in favor of the ego-id model because "we recognize that the *Ucs.* does not coincide with the repressed; it is still true that all that is repressed is *Ucs.,* but not all that is *Ucs.* is repressed." Besides the archaic unconscious, which was unconscious but unrepressed, Freud found that "it is certain that much of the ego is itself unconscious." [42] At the same time, he began to locate the origin of repression in the ego, because "we can say that the patient's resistance arises from his ego. . . . " [43]

The point was this: repression *originates* in some part of the ego; it is some aspect of the ego that represses the shadow-id. However, Freud then discovered that part of the ego was itself unconscious, *yet it was not repressed.* He simply put two and two together, and concluded that the *unrepressed* part of the ego was the *repressing* part. This part he called the superego: it was unconscious, unrepressed, but repressing. "We may say that repression is the work of this super-ego and that it is carried out either by itself or by the ego in obedience to its orders . . . portions of the both of them, the ego and the super-ego themselves, are unconscious"; [44] but *not* repressed.

Before we try to make sense of this unrepressed but repressing structure, I must briefly outline the general theory of repression presented in *The Atman Project,* [13] a theory based on the works of Piaget, Freud, Sullivan, Jung, and Loevinger. In essence, we have this: the process of *translation,* by its very nature, tends to screen out all perceptions and experiences which do not conform to the basic limiting principles of the translation itself. This is normal, necessary, and healthy, and forms the basis of "necessary and normal defense mechanisms"—it prevents the self-system from being overwhelmed by its surroundings, internal or external. This is normal "inattention" and—in contrast to a plethora of theories which maintain that "filtering" is reality corrupting—it is absolutely essential for normal equilibration.

Should, however, binds arise in the translation processes of any level, then the individual mistranslates his self and his world (which means that he distorts or deletes, displaces or condenses, aspects of the deep structure that could just as well exist correctly as surface structures). This can occur in any number of ways and for any number of reasons, and it can be expressed in terms of "energy thresholds" or "informational distortion." The essential point is that the individual is now selectively inattentive or forcefully restrictive of his awareness. He no longer simply translates his self and world, he translates *out,* or edits, any aspects of his self and world which are threatening. This mistranslation results in both a symptom and a symbol, and the job of the therapist is to help the individual retranslate ("the interpretation") his symbolic symptoms back into their original forms by suggesting "meanings" for the symptom-symbols ("Your feelings of depression are *really* feelings of masked rage"). Repression is simply a form of mistranslation, but a mistranslation that is not just a mistake but an *intentional* (even if unconscious) editing, a dynamic repression with vested interests. The individual does not just forget: he doesn't want to remember.

We saw that at each level of development, the self-sense *identifies* with the newly emergent structures of that level. When the body emerged from the pleroma, the self identified with it; when the verbal-mind emerged, the self identified with it; and so on. Further, it is the nature of an exclusive identification that one does not and cannot realize that identification without *breaking* that identification. In other words, all exclusive identification is unconscious identification. At the moment the child realizes that he *has* a body, he no longer is *just* the body: he is aware of it; he transcends it; he is looking at it with his mind. At the point the adult realizes he has a mind, he is no longer just a mind—he is actually perceiving it from the subtle regions.

In other words, at each level of development, one cannot totally see the seer. One uses the structures of that level as something with which to perceive and translate the world, but one cannot perceive and translate those structures *themselves,* not totally. That can occur only from a higher level. The point is that each translation process sees but is not seen; it translates, but is not itself translated; *and it can repress, but is not itself repressed.*

The Freudian superego, with the defenses and the character structure, are those aspects of the ego level with which the self is unconsciously *identified,* so much so that they cannot be *objectively* perceived (as can the rest of the ego). They translate without being translated—they are repressing but unrepressed. This fits very well with Freud's own thoughts on the matter, because he himself felt that (1) the superego is created by an *identification,* an unconscious identification ("identifications replace object-choices"), and (2) one of the aims of therapy is to make the superego conscious—to see it as an object and thus cease using it as something through which to see and (mis)translate the world. This is simply an instance of the overall evolution process we earlier described, where one becomes free of a level by disidentifying with it, later to integrate it in a higher-order unity. I should quickly mention that, according to Freud, the superego is frequently severe because it is contaminated by the archaic unconscious.

Anyway, the superego is an instance of what we can call the embedded unconscious: because it is embedded *as* the self, the self cannot totally or accurately see it. It is unconscious, but *not* repressed. It is that aspect of the ground unconscious which, upon emergence, emerges *as* the self-system and so remains essentially unconscious, possessing the power to send other elements to the repressed unconscious. Again, it is unrepressed but repressing. This can occur at any level of consciousness, although the specifics naturally vary considerably, because the tools of resistance are simply the structures of the given level and each level has differrent structures (for example, when the bodyego *was* the embedded unconscious, it used not repression but introjection and projection as the modes of mistranslation, because introjection and projection part of the primary process which dominates the typhonic realms). However, this whole process assumes its most violent, pathological, and characteristic forms with the egoic-mental level and the low-subtle realms. Levels lower than these are not really strong enough to sustain fierce repression (the archaic id is originally unrepressed and unrepressing); levels higher than this become so transcendent and integrated that repression—as we ordinarily think of it—tends to fade out. The higher realms do possess their own forms of resistances, but this is a matter for a separate study.

The Emergent Unconscious

Let us now examine someone who has evolved from the pleroma to the bodyself to the ego-mind. There still remain in the ground unconscious the deep structures of the subtle and causal realms. These structures have not yet emerged; they *cannot,* as a rule, emerge in consciousness until the lower structures have emerged. Since the higher structures encompass the lower ones, the higher have to unfold last. At any rate, it is certainly ridiculous to speak of realizing the transpersonal until the personal has been formed. The transpersonal (the subtle and the causal) realms are not yet repressed—they are not screened out of awareness, they are not filtered out—they have simply not yet had the opportunity to emerge. We do not say of a two-year-old child that he or she is resisting the learning of geometry, because the child's mind has not yet developed and unfolded to the degree that he or she could even begin to learn mathematics. Just as we do not accuse the child of repressing mathematics, we do not accuse him of repressing the transpersonal—not yet, that is.

At any point in the developmental cycle, those deep structures which have not yet emerged from the ground unconscious are referred to as the emergent unconscious. For someone at the ego (or centaur) level, the low-subtle, the high-subtle, the low-causal, and the high-causal are emergent unconscious. They are unconscious, *but not repressed.*

Notice that the subtle-causal emergent unconscious shares several characteristics with the archaic unconscious; namely, they have never (or never yet) been conscious within the lifetime of the individual, and thus are not repressed, and yet find themselves in the unconscious from the start. The difference, other than the fact that one is low and primitive and the other is high and transcendent, is that the archaic unconscious is humanity's past; the emergent unconscious is humanity's future.

However, the unconscious-future is determined only as regards deep structures: the surface structures are not yet fixed. The unconscious-past, on the other hand, contains deep structures as well as surface structures (such as the shadow), because both of these have already emerged and been determined.

Now supposing that development is not arrested at the ego-centaur realm—which is usually the case at this point in history—the subtle will of itself begin to emerge from the ground unconscious. It is not really possible to set timetables for these higher realms and stages, because a collective humanity has only evolved to the ego level, and thus only levels leading up to that have been determined as to emergence. In general, however, the subtle *can* begin to emerge after adolescence, but rarely before. In addition, for all sorts of reasons, the emergence of the subtle can be resisted and even, in a sense, repressed. For the ego is strong enough to repress not only the lower realms but also the higher realms—it can seal off the superconscious as well as the subconscious.

That part of the ground unconscious whose emergence is resisted or repressed we call, naturally enough, the emergent-repressed unconscious. It is that part of the ground unconscious which—*excluding developmental arrest*—remains unconscious *past* the point at which it could just as well become conscious. We are then justified in looking for reasons for this lack of emergence, and we find them in a whole set of defenses, actual defenses, against Deity, transcendence, and bliss. They include rationalization ("Transcendence is impossible or pathological!"); isolation or avoidance of relationship ("My consciousness is supposed to be skin-bounded!"); death terror ("I'm afraid to die to my ego, what would be left?"); desacralizing (Maslow's term for refusing to see transcendent values anywhere); substitution (a lower structure is substituted for the intuited higher structure, with the pretense that the lower *is* the higher); and contraction (into forms of knowledge or experience). Any or all of these simply become part of the ego's translation processes, such that the ego merely continues to translate whereas it should in fact begin transformation.

Because psychoanalysis and orthodox psychology have never truly understood the nature of the emergent unconscious in its higher forms, as soon as the subtle or causal begins to emerge in awareness—perhaps as a peak experience or as subtle lights and bliss—they are all in a dither to explain it as a breakthrough of some archaic material or some past repressed impulses. Since they know not of the emergent unconscious, they try to explain it in terms of the *submergent* unconscious. It is, they say, not a higher structure emerging but a lower one remerging. Thus they trace samadhi back to infantile breast union; they reduce transpersonal unity to prepersonal fusion in the pleroma; God is reduced to a teething nipple and all congratulate themselves on explaining the mystery. This whole enterprise is starting to fall apart of its own weight, because of the ridiculous number of things psychoanalysis has to attribute to the infant's first four months of life in order to account for *everything* that subsequently emerges.

At any rate, with an understanding of these types of the unconscious, as well as of translation/transformation and the stages of development presented in the first part of this paper, we can now turn to a quick study of meditation and the unconscious.

MEDITATION AND THE UNCONSCIOUS

Most of the accounts of meditation and the unconscious suffer from a lack of concern with developmental or evolutionary factors. They tend simply to assume that the unconscious is *only* the submergent unconscious (subliminal, filtered, screened, repressed, or automated), and thus they see meditation as a way to *reverse* a nasty state of affairs: they see it as a way to force entry into the unconscious. Meditation is pictured as a way to lift the repression, halt the filtering, deautomate the automating, or defocalize the focalizing. It is my own opinion that those issues, however significant, are the most secondary aspects of all types of meditation.

Meditation is, if anything, a sustained instrumental path of transcendence, and since—as we saw—transcendence and development are synonymous, it follows that meditation is simply *sustained development* or growth. It is not primarily a way to reverse things but a way to carry them on. It is the natural and orderly unfolding of successively higher-order unities, until there is only Unity, until all potential is actual, until all the ground unconscious is unfolded as consciousness.

Meditation thus occurs in the same way all the other growth/emergences did: one translation winds down and fails to exclusively dominate consciousness, and transformation to a higher-order translation occurs (a higher-order deep structure is remembered, which then underlies and creates new surface structures). There is differentiation, disidentification, transcendence, and integration. Meditation *is* evolution; it *is* transformation—there is nothing really special about it. It seems quite mysterious and convoluted to the ego because it is a development beyond the ego. Meditation is to the ego as the ego is to the thyphon: developmentally more advanced. However, the same process of *growth* and emergence runs through the whole sequence—the way we got *from* the typhon to the ego is the same way we go from the ego to the causal. We grow, we don't dig back.

My first point is that most accounts of meditation assume that the transpersonal realms—the subtle and causal—are parts of the submergent unconscious or repressed submergent unconscious, and that meditation means lifting the repression. I am suggesting that the transpersonal realms are really part of the emergent unconscious and that meditation is just speeding up the emergence.

However, when a person—say a young adult—begins meditation, all sorts of different things begin to happen, some of which are only incidentally related to the actual growth and transcendence process, and this greatly complicates the overall picture of meditation. With that problem in mind, I would like first to discuss the nature of the meditative stance itself, and then its general and complete course.

To begin with, we note that every transformation in development necessitates the surrendering of the particular translation (or rather, the exclusiveness of that translation). For the average person, who has already evolved from the pleroma to the typhon to the ego, transformation into the subtle or causal realms demands that egoic translation wind down and be surrendered (not destroyed). These egoic translations are usually composed of verbal thoughts and concepts (and emotional reactions to those thoughts). Therefore, meditation consists, *in the beginning,* of a way to *break conceptual translating* in order to open the way to subtle transformation.

In essence, this means to *frustrate* the present translation and encourage the new transformation. As explained in *No-boundary,*[12] this frustration/encouragement is brought about by *special conditions*—such as moral precepts, diet regulation, vows, and the more internal conditions of prayer, chanting, and meditation.

Now the heart of the special conditions is an activity which embodies any of the major characteristics of the sought-after higher sphere. That is, the individual is taught to begin translating his reality according to one of the major characteristics of the desired realm. He is therefore using *symbols,* not signs, and thus is open to *transformation* instead of mere translation. For example, the yidam: the individual is shown a symbol of the yidam-deity, a symbol which, precisely because it is a symbol, corresponds to nothing in his present reality. He constructs or translates this symbol into his own consciousness, to the point that the subtle yidam actually *emerges* from the ground unconscious into full awareness. The individual *identifies* (as we explained with *all* development) with this higher structure, which breaks his lower translation as ego and raises him to a higher structure. He then *sees* (translates) reality from the higher viewpoint of Deity: the high-subtle has emerged in his case, because he has evoked it as a process of growth and transcendence from his own ground unconscious.

The Master simply continues to frustrate the old translations, to undermine the old resistances, and to encourage the new transformation by enforcing the special conditions. This is true in *all* forms of meditation—concentrative or receptive, mantric or silent. In concentrative meditation, the special condition has a defined form: in receptive meditation, it is formless—both are enforced special conditions, however, and the individual who drops his formless or defocal awareness is chastised just as severely as the one who drops his koan.

In principle, this is no different than asking a child to put into words something he would rather act out typhonically. We are asking the ego to put into subtle forms that which it would rather think about conceptually. Growth occurs by adopting higher translations until one can actually transform to that higher realm itself. Since major characteristics of the higher realms include timelessness, love, no avoidances, total acceptance, and subject-object unity, these are most often the special conditions of meditation ("Stay in the Now always; recognize your avoidances; be only as love in all conditions; become one with your meditation and your world; accept everything since everything is Buddha"). Our parents helped us move from the first floor to the fifth floor by imposing the special conditions of language and egoic self-control. Just so, the Master helps us from the fifth to the tenth floor by imposing the special conditions of the tenth upon us as practice.

In essence, it does not matter whether the special conditions use a concentrative-absorptive or a receptive-defocal mode of meditation. The former breaks the lower and egoic translation by halting it, the latter by watching it. What they both have in common is what is essential and effective about both: jamming a translation by concentration or watching a translation by defocalizing can only be done from the next highest level. They both accomplish the same goal, the breaking of a lower-order translation. Both are intensely *active* processes. Even "passive receptivity" is, as Benoit said, activity on a higher plane. (This is not to say, however, that the receptive-defocal mode and the concentrative-absorptive mode are identical, or that they produce the same secondary results. This will become obvious when we outline the course of a typical medtation.)

Before discussing what transpires in meditation, however, it is important to realize that not all schools of meditation aim for the same general realm of consciousness. Rather, as explained in *The Atman Project,*[13] they break down into three major classes (cf. Bubba Free John[45]). The first is the Nirmanakaya class, which deals with bodily or typhonic energies and their transmutation into the lower-subtle region. This includes hatha yoga, kundalini yoga, kriya yoga, pranayama, and particularly all forms of tantric yoga. The goal of the Nirmanakaya class is the sahasrara, the crown chakra, and it is exemplified by Patanjali.

The second is the Sambhogakaya class, which deals with the low- and high-subtle regions, and aims for the seven (or ten) inner spheres of bliss and audible realization secreted within and beyond the sahasrara. This includes nada yoga and shabd yoga, and is exemplified by Kirpal Singh.

The third is the Dharmakaya class, which deals with the causal regions. It operates through neither tantric energy manipulation nor subtle light and sound absorption, but rather through inquiry into the causal field of consciousness itself, inquiry into I-ness or the separate-self sense, even in and through the transcendent witness of the causal region, until all forms of subject-object dualism are uprooted. It is exemplified by Sri Ramana Maharshi, Bubba Free John, Zen, etc. At the terminal point of each path, one *can* fall into the prior suchness of all realms, the Svabhavikakaya, although this is both easier and more likely the higher the path one initially adopts.

Let us now assume that a young adult takes up the practice of Zen, in either its concentrative-koan or receptive-shikan-taza form. Both of these are Dharmakaya practices, if employed correctly, and so we will expect to see all sorts of lower-level manifestations in the intermediate stages.

To start with, the meditation practice begins to break the present egoic translation by either halting it (koan) or watching it (shikan). Washburn has given a nice account of some of the specifics of this process.[46] As the present egoic translation begins to loosen, then the individual is first exposed to the subliminal submergent unconscious (the nonrepressed submergent unconscious in general) which includes, among other things, the "innumerable unnoticed aspects of experiences, aspects tuned out due to habit, conditioning, or the exigencies of the situation."[47] All sorts of odd memories float up—screen memories, insignificant memories, memories that are not repressed, merely forgotten or preconscious. Months can be spent "at the movies" watching the subliminal submergent reemerge in awareness and dance before the inward eye.

As meditation progresses, however, the truly resistant aspects of the egoic translation are slowly undermined and dismantled in their exclusiveness. That is, the embedded unconscious is jarred loose from its unconscious identification with the Self and thus tends either to emerge as an actual object of awareness or to at least loose its hold on awareness. Washburn states that psychic immobilization (the halting of the egoic translation) "brings unconscious psychic operations into awareness by interfering with their normal functioning," so that "one can begin to look *at* it, rather than, as hitherto has been the case, merely looking *through* it."[48] I think that is a good point, but I would just add that it applies basically to the embedded unconscious; we don't, for example, bring the causal emergent unconscious into awareness by "interfering with it" but rather by allowing it to emerge in the first place, just as we don't bring mathematics into awareness by interfering with it but by first learning it.

At any rate, the embedded unconscious, by being "interfered with," starts to shake loose its habitual hold. Now recall that the embedded unconscious translations were the unrepressed but repressing aspects of the self-system of a given level. Naturally, then, as the repressor is relaxed, the repressed tends to emerge. That is to say, the repressed submergent unconscious now tends to float—or sometimes erupt—into awareness. The individual confronts his shadow (and, on occasion, primal or archaic fantasies from the archaic unconscious). An individual can spend months or even years wrestling with his shadow, and this is where orthodox therapy can certainly complement meditation. (Incidentally, notice that what is released here is the repressed submergent unconscious, and not *necessarily* the subtle or causal emergent unconscious, unless they are part of the repressed emergent unconscious screened out by the *same* defenses wielded against the shadow. This is indeed possible and even probable to a certain degree, but on the whole the defenses against the shadow and those against the subtle-causal are of a different order.)

What has happened, up to this stage in meditation, is that the individual—through the loosening of the egoic translation and embedded unconscious—has "relived" his life up to that point. He has opened himself to all the traumas, the fixations, the complexes, the imagos, and the shadows of all of the prior levels of consciousness which have so far emerged in his life—the pleromatic, the uroboric, the typhonic, the verbal, and the mental-egoic. All of that is up for review, in a sense, and especially up for review are the "sore spots"—the fixations and repressions that occurred on the first five floors of his being. Up to this point in meditation, he has seen his past, and perhaps humanity's past. From this point on, he sees his future—and humanity's future as well.

Incidentally, Washburn has suggested that only receptive meditation leads directly and immediately to the unconscious, whereas absorptive meditation "is so immersed in its object that all else, including messages from the unconscious, is unavailable to awareness; and for this reason confrontation with the unconscious can occur only after the object has been discarded, or after the practice has been concluded."[49] Again, I think that is quite true, but again I think it applies to only some aspects of the developmental unconscious, particularly the archaic, submergent, and embedded unconscious. It does not apply to, for example, the subtle emergent unconscious, because in the state of subtle absorption in the yidam, mantra, or nada, one *is* directly in touch with that previously unconscious state. Even if one doesn't cognize it as an object, which one doesn't, one is still intuitively alive to the subtle, as the subtle. The concentrative path *disclosed* this subtle-realm aspect of the emergent unconscious in a perfectly direct and immediate way.

However, while absorbed in the subtle, it is true that no other objects tend to arise in awareness, and that would include, for example, the shadow. The subtle meditation does help to break the egoic translation, however, so that when one ceases subtle absorption, one is indeed open to shadow influx, just as Washburn describes. With receptive meditation, of course, one is open to whatever arises whenever it arises, and so one "sees" the shadow on the spot as it derepresses. Thus, Washburn's points, in my opinion, apply very significantly to the shadow, but not to the emergent unconscious at all.

As the subtle emerges from the ground unconscious into awareness, various high-archetypal visions, sounds, and illuminations occur. I described the subtle realm earlier and so needn't repeat it here. The point is that subtler and subtler translations emerge and are eventually undermined, and transformation to new and subtler translations occurs. This is nothing more than *development* in the subtle realm. One version of this runs as follows:

> It is the strongest impulses that are affected first, and as they dim, the meditator begins to discern more subtle ones—just as the setting of the sun brings the stars into view. But these more subtle impulses themselves wane, which allows even more subtle ones to be discriminated. Interestingly, this is not an absolutely continuous process, for during sitting meditation there occur interludes of virtual silence during which, it seems, one passes through some kind of psychic "membrane" that divides the present level from the next, subtler level. Once this divide has been passed, psychomental activity resumes . . .; but its character is now much finer and more rarefied.[50]

The "membranes" are simply the translation processes of each level, which screen out the other levels and divide the present level from the rest; the "passing of this divide" is simply transformation to a higher, subtler, and "more rarefied" translation. "The new threshold [the new translation] that is established in this way can itself be reduced [transformed] by continued meditation, and this one too, and so on. In each case a new spectrum of lower-intensity, subtler objects becomes accessible to the meditator's inner sight."[51]

Although these subtle sounds and illuminations are the goal of the Sambhogakayas, they are all viewed as makyo (or inferior productions) by the Dharmakayas. Thus, if meditation continues into the causal realm, all prior objects, subtle or gross, are reduced to gestures of consciousness-as-such until even the transcendent witness or I-ness of the causal realm is broken in the great death of emptiness, and the unparalleled but only obvious state of sahaj is resurrected. This is called *anuttara samyak sambodhi*. It is without recourse. At this final transformation, there are no longer any exclusive translations occurring anywhere; the mirror and the reflections are one and the same.

So proceeds meditation, which is simply higher development, which is simply higher evolution, a transformation from unity to unity until there is simple Unity, whereupon Brahman, in an unnoticed shock of recognition and final remembrance, grins silently to himself, closes his eyes, breathes deeply, and throws himself outward for the millionth time, losing himself in his manifestations for the sport and play of it all. Evolution then proceeds again, transformation by transformation, remembering more and more, until each and every soul remembers Buddha, as Buddha, in Buddha—whereupon there is then no Buddha, and no soul. That is the final transformation. When Zen Master Fa-ch'ang was dying, a squirrel screeched on the roof. "It's just this," he said, "and nothing more."

REFERENCES

1. Smuts, J. *Holism and Evolution*. New York: Macmillan, 1926.
2. Welwood, J. Meditation and the unconscious. *Journal of Transpersonal Psychology*, 1977, 9(1), 1–26.
3. Werner, H. The concept of development from a comparative and organismic point of view. In *The Concept of Development* (Harris, Ed.). Minneapolis: University of Minnesota Press, 1957.
4. Jackobson, R. *Child language aphasia and phonological universals*. Quoted in Gardner, H. *The Quest for Mind*. New York: Vintage, 1974.
5. Bateson, G. *Steps to an Ecology of Mind*. New York: Ballantine, 1972.
6. See reference 4.
7. Loevinger, J. *Ego Development*. San Francisco: Jossey-Bass, 1976.
8. Arieti, S. *The Intra-psychic Self*. New York: Basic Books, 1967.
9. Maslow, A. *The Farther Reaches of Human Nature*. New York: Viking Compass, 1971.
10. Kohlberg, L. Development of moral character and moral ideology. In *Review of Child Development Research*, (M.L. Hoffman and L.W. Hoffman, Eds.), Vol. 1. New York: Russell Sage Foundation, 1964.
11. Wilber, K. *The Spectrum of Consciousness*. Wheaton: Quest, 1977.
12. Wilber, K. *No-boundary*. Colorado: Shambhala, 1980.

13. Wilber, K. *The Atman Project.* Wheaton: Quest, 1979.
14. Wilber, K. *Up from Eden.NY: Doubleday-Anchor, 1981.*
15. Gruber, H. and Vonèche, J. *The Essential Piaget.* New York: Basic Books, 1977.
16. See reference 8.
17. See reference 7.
18. Freud S. *The ego and the id. Standard Edition,* Vol. 19, London: Hogarth,
19. See reference 15.
20. Fenichel, O. *The Psychoanalytic Theory of Neurosis.* New York: Norton, 1945.
21. Sullivan, C., Grant, M.Q. and Grant, J.D. The development of interpersonal maturity: applications to delinquency. *Psychiatry,* 1957, *20,* 373–385.
22. See reference 7.
23. Fromm, E. *Escape from Freedom.* New York: Farrar, Straus and Giroux, 1941.
24. Riesman, D. *The Lonely Crowd.* New York: Doubleday, 1954.
25. See reference 7.
26. Dean, S. (Ed.). *Psychiatry and Mysticism.* Chicago: Nelson-Hall, 1975.
27. Blofeld, J. *The Tantric Mysticism of Tibet.* New York: Dutton, 1970.
28. Ibid.
29. Hixon, L. *Going Home.* New York: Anchor, 1978.
30. Bubba Free John, *Paradox of Instruction.* San Francisco: Dawn Horse, 1977.
31. Wilber, K. The ultimate state of consciousness. *JASC,* 1975-6, *2*(3).
32. Frey-Rohn, L. *From Freud to Jung.* New York: Dell, 1974.
33. See reference 18.
34. Freud, S. *A General Introduction to Psychoanalysis.* New York: Pocket Books, 1971.
35. Freud, S. From the history of an infantile neurosis. *Standard Edition,* Vol. 17. London: Hogarth,
36. See reference 32.
37. Hall, C. *A Primer of Jungian Psychology.* New York: Mentor, 1973.
38. Freud, S. Outline of psychoanalysis. *Standard Edition,* Vol. 23. London: Hogarth.
39. Ibid.
40. Ibid.
41. Jung, C. The psychological foundations of belief in spirits. *Collected Works,* Vol. 8.
42. Freud, S. Beyond the pleasure principle. *Standard Edition.,* Vol. 18. London: Hogarth,
43. Ibid.
44. Freud, S. New introductory lectures. *Standard Edition,* Vol. 22. London: Hogarth,
45. See reference 30.
46. Washburn, M. Observations relevant to a unified theory of meditation. *Journal of Transpersonal Psychology,* 1978, *10*(1).
47. Ibid.
48. Ibid.
49. Ibid.
50. Ibid.
51. Ibid.

No drives, no complusions, no needs, no attractions: Then your affairs are under control. You are a free person.

Chuang Tzu

Self-mastery, self-discipline, personal power, controlled folly, fear of loss of control, voluntary surrender, are all terms that are used in this book. The closer we look at these terms, the more subtle and elusive they may seem to become. The terms themselves raise some of the great unanswered philosophical questions, such as free will and determinism, the role of the self, the goal of optimum well-being.

Yet, although the questions themselves are extremely difficult, the frequency of the use of these related terms in traditions ranging from the health and healing sciences to philosophy and religious studies, may require at least initial efforts to try to bring increased clarity and precision to the construct of self-control. In this chapter, Deane Shapiro, using the metaphor of balance, tries to tie together different themes of self-control and optimum well-being. He suggests that (at least) two types of self-control—active control and letting-go control—may be being utilized by various authors and traditions: and that these two types of self-control may appear somewhat different, depending on the perspective (from the body to the spiritual, and including affective, cognitive, and perceptual dimensions) from which it is being viewed and for which it is being utilized.

16
Self-Control and Positive Health: Multiple Perspectives of Balance

Deane H. Shapiro, Jr., Ph. D.

Seek simplicity and distrust it.

Alfred North Whitehead

Who sees inaction in action
  and action in inaction
He is enlightened among men
  He does all actions, disciplined.[1]

Bhagavad Gita

The theme of acting with self-discipline and self-control is one which occurs in widely varying cultures and religious traditions. Examples reflecting this concept include the Hellenistic Greek's autonomous individual living in harmony with the community;[2] Muslim's ethical self-restraint;[3] Confucianism's self-sufficiency and internal self-regulation;[4] and Christianity's control and elimination of carnal desires.[5] In this book, the concept of self-control is also frequently referred to, including such terms as controlled folly, personal power, acting impeccably,[6] self-mastery,[7] voluntary surrender[8] and—with negative connotations—fear of loss of control, the anxiety of helplessness, and inappropriately wanting to be in control.[9,10]

Contemporary psychology also provides us with a variety of concepts which may be related to self-control, such as the social learning theorist's self-efficacy,[11] the existentialist's will,[12] the neoanalytic concept of competence,[13] and Seligman's learned helplessness.[14] Further, there are efforts to bring control theory[15] from mathematics, and systems[16] and cybernetic theory[17] to discussions of self-regulation. In addition to concepts of control, there are also a variety of self-regulation and self-control tecniques, which include, but are not limited to, biofeedback,[18] meditation,[19] behavioral self-management,[20] self-hypnosis,[21] cognitive self-instructions,[22] guided daydreams, and imagery.[23]

Scientific research on these self-control strategies has, for the most part, been limited to their use in specific clinical problems ranging from stress and tension management[24] to weight control,[25] hypertension,[26] pain management,[27] etc. Less attention has been directed toward the question, Self-control for what, or toward what? in terms of refining and creating a vision within which self-control strategies may be utilized to enhance optimum well-being.[28]

Depending upon the tradition, the cultural context, and the specific situation in which self-control strategies are used, their purposes may be quite different, from resolution of a specific clinical problem to quite extraordinary control of attention, body, etc. For example, if we look again at the ancient Hindu text the *Bhagavad Gita,* it is stated that for persons of wisdom there is not a hair's breadth between will (what they want to do) and action (what they do). Yet, although this provides us with an elegant vision, it also leaves unanswered a myriad of questions—some philosophical, some theoretical, some practical, and some value laden. For example, what are the areas in which individuals can gain control? Is there an optimum level of control? Can we ever have too much self-control? Are there different types of self-control; i.e., is a different type of discipline necessary to see action in inaction than to see inaction in action? Who is the "self" in self-control—is self an object of control, or the controller, or both? How does self-control relate to philosophical assumptions of free will and determinism, or nature and nurture? How do people develop discipline? Do they learn it, or are they born with it? What is the role of conscious choice, effort, and individual responsibility in self-control? Is self-control a relevant concept for everyone? Is it a useful one? Do all people need to feel in control, or do some try to escape from control and freedom?[29] Should they? Are there right or wrong answers?

A brief chapter such as this cannot hope to answer all of the above questions. However, it is intended to raise some of the critical questions, to set the soil for deeper discussion and investigation, and to seek to bring a beginning clarity and order to the field. Further, in keeping with the task of this book which is the creation of models and visions of extreme psychological health, the primary thrust of this chapter is to examine how self-control may be related to optimum well-being.

BALANCE AS A METAPHOR

In this chapter, we posit optimum well-being as the ability not to be caught exclusively by any one particular perspective, but rather to maintain a flexibility, and to have the internal control and discipline to act appropriately and skillfully, while remaining relaxed and composed, based on the demands of a given situation.[30]

Balance, which may be defined as follows: (a) harmony and pleasing integration, (b) counterbalance, (c) stability (generally between opposites), (d) equanamity or equilibrium (both physically and emotionally), is chosen as a metaphor because it implies a flexibility, a realization that there is not one right course of action. Rather, while acknowledging the metagoal of internal harmony and integration, there is a realization that this goal is sometimes achieved by a counterforce or counterbalance; sometimes by a stability between opposites; and sometimes by an equanamity. As Smith notes, regarding the wise person,

> Not invariance, but appropriateness is his hallmark, an appropriateness that has the whole repertoire of emotions at its command. . . . He can be forceful when need be, . . . he has reserves to draw on. . . . We sense him as relaxed and composed rather than charged. . . . If leadership is called for, the adept steps forward; otherwise, he is just as happy to follow. . . . Focus or periphery, limelight or shadow—it doesn't really matter. . . . Both have their opportunities; both, their limitations.[31]

Smith's statement echoes the opening line of our chapter from the *Bhagavad Gita* on action and inaction. The wise individual is able to see the action, fullness, and beauty of inaction (e.g., meditating peacefully—action in inaction) and is also able to maintain a sense of peace while performing actions in the world (inaction in action). In this way, a person may have a sense of a wide range of behavioral options available and, at the same time, a sense of peace, stillness, and fullness of activity in each. It is the Taoist yin/yang, in which yin represents the yielding, quiet, light side; and yang, the more active, dark, motion-filled side. Yet, in the diagram, yin always has a bit of yang, and vice versa, and the two are in a balanced harmony.

This balance is also reflected in the discussion of the seven factors of

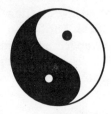

enlightenment, in which there are the arousing factors of wisdom, energy, and rapture which make the mind wakeful and alert, and the tranquilizing factors of calm, concentration, and equanimity which make the mind peaceful and still. Goldstein notes that these have to be in harmony. "The factor of mindfulness is so powerful because it not only serves to awaken and strengthen all of the other factors, but it also keeps them in their proper balance."[32]

At the risk of oversimplification, and as a means of providing additional clarity, it might be helpful to consider yang and yin, or arousing and calming factors, as reflecting two different aspects of self-control. One aspect or factor might be *active control,* reflecting the leadership components discussed by Smith, the yang, the energetic arousing factors, the action side of the *Bhagavad Gita* quote. A second construct might be called *letting-go control.* This would reflect the inaction side of the *Bhagavad Gita* quote, the calming factors, the yin, the ability to be a follower which Smith discussed, a voluntary surrender, a noninterfering mind, a certain soft quality.

Extrapolating from these two constructs, and keeping the assumption which many of the above authors make that the two constructs need to be in balance for optimum well-being to occur, we might suggest that when one of the constructs is too weak, the individual rather than being *in control,* would be out of control. For example, if there were too little arousing, active control, then an individual, rather than being in a letting-go control mode, might be in a mode more reflective of passivity, diffuseness, torpor, and sloth. Conversely, if there were too little letting-go control, and as a result too much arousal, this might lead to overactivity and restlessness. Utilizing the reversed U-shaped curve of stress research, which suggests that optimum functioning occurs when the person neither is overstressed (Figure 16–1) nor has too little arousal, we would have the following four-grid model (Figure 16–2).

Being out of balance, or out of control, in this model, would occur when there is not an appropriate balance between the two constructs (Scales 1 and 2) of self-control. For example, if we just look at the two left-hand boxes (Scales 1 and 3) we see that they represent the active side of the model. Scale 1 would be appropriate *in control* activity; Scale 3, out of control ac-

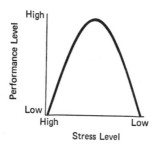

Figure 16-1.

tivity—too much pushing toward a goal, restlessness, too active effort to try to "control" the world. There is a sense in Scale 3 that balance has been lost. The stillness and lightness of Scale 2 would not seem to be present. The following lines from the Globuses in discussing don Juan, and from Rajneesh, reiterate the importance of this balance. The Globuses note that the warrior needs to be able to be in full control of himself *and* at the same time light and fluid. They discuss both control and abandon—a person being in total command of himself and at the same time able to let go without attachment to outcome.[33] Rajneesh discusses this when saying he became

strong, but strong with the strength of a rose flower—so fragile in its strength. So sensitive, so delicate. . . . Or the strength of a dewdrop on a leaf of grass, just shining in the morning sun: so beautiful, so precious, and yet it can slip any moment. So incomparable in its grace, that a small breeze can come and the dewdrop can slip and become lost forever. The power is not of that which kills; the power is that which creates.[34]

Assertive	Yielding
Active control	Letting-go control
Scale 1	Scale 2
Out of control— overactivity, restlessness	Out of control (too little control)— complacency sloth, torpor
Scale 3	Scale 4

Figure 16-2.

Without wanting to do a disservice to the Globuses or to Rajneesh by unduly oversimplifying their views to fit them into the model discussed here, it
may be possible to see a balance between an active and a letting-go control in
evidence. The yang, active side would include Rajneesh's discussion of
strong power and don Juan's total (active) command of himself; the yin side,
the letting-go control, could be seen as evidenced by Rajneesh's discussion of
fragile, sensitive, delicate and by don Juan's abandon, nonattachment to
outcome. By achieving this balance, there is a soft strength, and therefore a
Scale 3 out of control activity is not in evidence—i.e., there is not a power
which kills (Rajneesh) or as the Globuses say, "You don't use and squeeze
people until they have shrivelled to nothing." [35]

SELF-CONTROL AND BALANCE REFLECTED IN PHYSICAL AND MENTAL WELL-BEING

In this section we address the question of how the issue of balance previously
discussed is evidenced in physical and mental well-being.

Self-control and Physical Well-being

The idea of exercise, physical fitness, increasing longevity, patient self-care,
and "super (physical) health" are all gaining prominence in our medical
health care literature. Control is clearly an important and relevant concept
here. First, and now quite obvious, there is recognition that dietary habits,
alcohol consumption, smoking, drugs, and physical exercise—all variables
which can be within a person's control—are extremely critical for physical
health.[36]

Further, research is revealing that individuals have considerably more
ability to control their bodies than heretofore believed. For example,
classical neurology stated that individuals had no voluntary control over the
autonomic nervous system (heart rate, blood pressure), a fact recently
refuted.[37] Basmajian[38] has shown that individuals can learn to control the
firing of a single motor unit. Similarly, the work of adepts shows that we
have potentially quite extraordinary control over blood flow and bodily
pain.[39]

In terms of "type" of control at the body level, the person may want to
have the flexibility and ability to activate, energize, and arouse the body at
certain times, and at different times to relax and calm the body—all the while
keeping a sensitivity to when the body is becomong too activated or too
relaxed.

There are some that might disagree with this vision of balance on a
physical level. For example, a recent essay in the *New England Journal of*

Medicine[40] said that there may be dysfunctional aspects to health education, and that if we taught Type A people to be mellower, to learn an alternative life-style, these people would then have to deal with issues of job satisfaction and insecurity, as well as what to do with themselves. It seems to me that this posits a false either/or dichotomy, that either one is a Type A hard-driving executive, with the positive aspects of this such as high achievement on the job, and the negative aspects such as an unhealthy, overactive life-style; *or* one is mellow, calm, and relaxed, but also bored, passive, and insecure. In addition to positing an either/or dichotomy, this essay also mixes professional and career dimensions with physical health. By using the vision of balance that we are offering, it may be possible for individuals to "have it both ways"—a both/and—a flexibility to be active when that is skillful and appropriate, the ability to be calm and relaxed when that is appropriate, and the ability to combine the two: action in inaction, and inaction in action.

Self-control and Mental Well-being

Almost all traditions agree that the mind, no matter how defined, is largely out of control for most individuals. This mind is filled with uncontrolled internal dialogues, unwholesome factors,[41] constructed reality,[42] fantasies that occur largely without choice and often without conscious awareness. In these traditions, generally this term "mind" encompasses affective, perceptual, and cognitive areas. When the mind is out of control on an affective level, unwholesome factors such as lust, aversion, and grasping are in evidence, and according to Buddhist texts, "These powerful emotions and states such as greed, anger, or dislike . . . grip the mind and render it hard to control."[43]

The vision of "controlling the mind" involves several abilities. One is a *cognitive* self-control—the ability to choose to think or not to think, not be bound and limited by thought processes and discrimination. This cognitive self-control also includes the following: freedom to accept or reject any paradigm; to choose one's belief system;[7] to believe that we are free;[44] to believe that we have the ability to accomplish great things;[39] to watch the mind without being attached to any thoughts; to analyze a situation, evaluate it, and set a goal without being exclusively bound by the mode of analysis, or trapped and controlled by the goal which is set.[45]

On an *emotional* level, Jahoda,[46] from her review of the mental health literature, suggested that the mature person is self-reliant and has control over his or her emotions. This emotional control of carnal desires is reflected in many traditions. In the Vipassana tradition, as well as in Zen and many other Eastern disciplines,[47] the person is trained to develop an immovable wisdom, such that one can reduce (extinguish) strong affective responses. In terms of the seventh parami, Walsh notes, "Elaboration of strong affective responses is reduced, and the mind gradually becomes less reactive and more calm. As such, it becomes easy to control and remains unperturbed in the face of an increasingly broad range of experience."[48]

On the *attentional* and *perceptual realm,* the vision involves recognizing the distortions of constructed reality: "greater sensitivity to and control of this stream of dialogue and fantasy (with resultant greater range, fluidity, and voluntary control of perceptual perspectives)."[49] As Goleman notes in discussing jhana, and reflecting on the importance of the voluntary control of attention, it "may be mastered so that the meditator can enter it at will for as long as he desires."[41]

Thus, control and balance of the mind can be evidenced both in the power to use words, to discriminate between cause and effect; and in the ability not to think, to stop the internal dialogue. In Rajneesh's terms, it is the ability to become Ouspensky the intellect plus Gurdjeiff the intuitive mystic. It is also the ability to know when it is functional to let go of goals and to just experience—be in the here and now—and when it is functional to analyze the situation, evaluate it, and set a goal. In so doing, the individual learns a control of the mind and, as Goleman notes, "The practicing Buddhist embarks on a coordinated program of environmental, behavioral, and attentional control to attain his final goal, a plateau of purely healthy mental states."[41]

PHILOSOPHICAL ISSUES

Although we can discuss a model of balance, and how different constructs of control may be evidenced in both physical and mental well-being, if we are to take the term self-control to a deeper level of analysis, we need to recognize that there are many philosophical assumptions that are actually embedded in the word itself. In this section, these assumptions will be addressed and clarified.

Free Will versus Determinism

Self-control as a construct implies a process movement away from reflexive action to conscious choice and awareness. The belief system (postulate, assumption) upon which the construct is based, is that individuals are not absolutely determined, can gain more autonomy and free choice, and do have the ability to effect change in their life on some level. Even those schools that argue that free will or free choice is a misnomer, if they wish to utilize the concept of self-control, have to then argue that an illusion of freedom is important to individuals. Thus, the concept of self-control is not possible without recourse to a view of individual choice and freedom, even if only an "as if" view.[44] Further, this assumption of free choice, which is an existential given, may be increased as the individual learns additional skills of awareness, decision making, etc. These philosophical assumptions of freedom can be seen reflected in the following two examples.

In psychoanalytic theory, Freud's relatively passive ego on the id horse of passions became refined in a way to give more "control" to the individual. For example, Hartmann talks about the autonomous ego developing in a deterministic fashion, but then becoming relatively independent of, and able to regulate, the instincts from which it has arisen.[51]

Another example comes from an Eastern perspective, as evidenced in the Chinese language. The Chinese have two characters which make up their word "fate" (i.e., how one is controlled). One of these characters is heredity and the other is environment. The Chinese believe that individuals were determined (controlled) by their fate. However, the word "to learn" in the Chinese language consists of two characters, one the nose (meaning self in the East) and one wings above the nose. To learn was to have the self soar. Thus, rather than control being forever externally imposed by the environment and heredity, the individual can learn to exercise a "self" control. The Chinese language exemplifies a belief in the individual's *learning* to "rise above" or "transcend" fate by developing certain self-control skills.[45]

Responsibility

Responsibility is also a critical underpinning of self-control, a movement away from blaming others and the environment, away from an external locus of control, to an internal locus of control and assuming self-responsibility.[52-55]

Both Freud and Jung believed that, in the last analysis, it was up to the patient to change. Although the therapist could be facilitative, could lead the horse to water—in fact, the Freudian analyst trying to overcome resistance can even push the horse's mouth down toward the water—it is the horse's choice whether to drink. In a sense the issue becomes one of self-control: the choice is the individual's. As Jung noted:

> Any of my pupils could give you so much insight and understanding that you could treat yourself if you don't succumb to the prejudice that you receive healing through others. In the last resort every individual alone has to win his battle, nobody else can do it for him.[56]

Who's Doing the Controlling: The Role (or Non-Role) of Self

This may be one of the most difficult and confusing philosophical issues regarding self-control. Specifically, it is the question of who or what controls the mind, and who or what is being controlled. Are there various layers of "self"? Is it the ego that controls the mind? Or is some *part* of the mind in control, as in the "executive" control of a computer? Does self-control imply control of the self (self as object) or is it a self exercising control? What is the relationship between this self, if such an entity is posited to exist, and the mind? Does the self control the mind, or the mind control the self? Are we talking about a level of self with a small s, or a grand Self with a capital S?

There are many different and competing views with regard to this self, and at this point all they can provide are metaphors, analogies, or viewpoints, for there is not yet any definitive evidence suggesting any one right answer. Therefore, it is critical that we be quite precise in stating the viewpoint from which we are discussing the concept of self.

Some views suggest that the concept of self is not needed in understanding human behavior;[57] others, that self needs to be seen as an interaction between the person and environment, whether field theory,[58] social interaction theory,[59] reciprocal determinism,[60] or systems model.[61] Some suggest that the vision of personal autonomy and self-control is located in this "self," whether it's called the centered self as in the existentialist[62] view or the individuated self in Jungian terminology.[63]

Some traditions talk about the importance of controlling the "self," developing and enhancing this self so that there is an ability to overcome identity diffusion and low self-esteem.[64] Several traditions discuss the importance of increasing the sense of congruence between self-concept[65] and actual behavior, and increasing a positive sense of oneself (i.e., high self-esteem).[66]

Still other approaches talk about the need to lose self-importance[67] to transcend self-other dichotomies[68] and to keep the self from becoming exclusively identified (i.e., being able to disidentify).[69]

In terms of our model of balance, the task may be two fold a) to have a strong sense of self and positive self-esteem, (scale one) without becoming too egocentric and too exclusively identified with oneself. (scale three) and, when appropriate b) being able to be relatively egoless to transcend the ego from a place of conscious choice, (scale two), a state of mind quite separate and distinct from identity diffusion. (scale four)

MULTIPLE PERSPECTIVES: THE LENSES THROUGH WHICH WE PERCEIVE SELF-CONTROL

Related to the question of mind and self is the complex issue of who is doing the perceiving. Without getting caught in the philosophical difficulties of this issue, it is important, in rounding out our discussion of self-control, to be attentive to the filter or lens through which we observe.* In other words,

---

* Another related issue which is not going to be discussed here deals with the creation of a developmental model—both within the four constructs and quadrants of control that we have proposed, as well as between different perspectives for which self-control may be utilized.

when we utilize self-control, or a self-control strategy, what is the end state—goal—that we are utilizing it for? If we are trying to improve our physical health, then control strategies are used for that purpose. The mind becomes a component, or vehicle, in service of the body (e.g., mental strategies to calm the body such as autogenic training).

The body, the mind, and the self (depending upon the particular tradition's viewpoint) may be goals for which, and perspectives from which, self-control is utilized, *or* components utilized in the service of other end states and goals—whether they be professional and career, intimacy (including intimacy of adults, family),[70] and/or spiritual. The way self-control is perceived and the types of self-control utilized to attain an end state will, in large part, depend upon the particular perspective goal and lens through which we are looking.

In terms of a model of balance, other questions which need to be addressed are how the different lenses and perspectives through which life is viewed interact and interrelate with each other, and how, if, and to what extent a balance might be created between the dimensions of professional, intimate, and spiritual goals.

FINAL COMMENTS ON BALANCE AND CONTROL

On the one hand this paper has sought to "seek simplicity." In the most simple terms, I find myself arguing for the ability to choose the kind of life we would like to live and for the ability to accept when we can't make it happen—a view quite similar to the Alcoholics Anonymous prayer:

> Grant me the ability to change what I can change, the ability to accept what I can't, and the wisdom to know the difference.

We have attempted, in this chapter, to develop a vision of extreme psychological health based on the construct of control, and to posit a four-quadrant model, in which the goal or vision of extreme psychological health was to increase the amount of control whether of a Scale 1 or Scale 2 nature, and to keep these two in balance. Further, the vision involved decreasing the amount of Scale 3 restlessness (too high activity) and decreasing the amount of Scale 4 torpor, sloth, and helplessness. A (paradoxical) subcorollary of this was that at the same time we are trying to actively change (i.e., Scale 1) from Scale 3 and 4 to Scale 1 and 2, we also are accepting (Scale 2) those aspects of ourselves which are Scale 3 and 4.

An effort was also made to suggest how control may be evidenced across many different perspectives and to suggest that no one type of control provides an exclusive answer on any given level. Rather, the individual may need flexibility and appropriateness in choosing different types of control, based on a particular perspective and goal.

Taking such a complex, multifaceted issue as self-control and trying to reduce it to two positive constructs of being in control necessarily cause us to lose a great deal of information. The hope in such a task, however, is that the problems inherent in loss of information will be outweighed by the clarity we might gain in bringing a certain amount of order to a quite complex topic. The simplicity is of no use unless resultant clarity helps us to see common themes, provides a foundation for unifying or integrating models, and/or provides a construct which can support research hypotheses, leading to both construct and predictive validity.

At the same time that we have sought simplicity, there has been an effort to raise important philosophical issues which encourage us to "distrust the simplicity." Free will versus determinism, the role of responsibility, issues of self and mind, and multiple perspectives may help us see that we need great precision and sophistication on when and how to balance different self-control modes, and on matching a self-control technique to a particular person, with a particular perspective and goal.

The Tibetan Wheel of Life has a framework around it which is the ultimate state—heaven, nirvana. This state of consciousness, which is outside the circle of conditioned existence containing the six ordinary realms, is called the Buddha realm. The ultimate state in the model of control and balance suggested here is one which utilizes as a value framework words like functional, skillful, appropriate. This extreme of psychological well-being is one in which individuals have increased degrees of freedom, know how to utilize self-control techniques *appropriate* for different ends, and have the motivation, resolve, and determination to carry through on their intent and goals.[71] Appropriate means that which minimizes unnecessary suffering to oneself and others, and maximizes a sense of joyfulness and compassion—a stable, harmonious, integrated balance.

Acknowledgement. My thanks to Ben Friedman, Ken Wilber, and my coeditor for their comments and suggestions on previous drafts of this manuscript.

REFERENCES

1. *Bhagavad Gita* (F. Edgerton, translator). Cambridge, Mass.: Harvard University Press, 1964, Ch. 4, Verse 18, p. 25.
2. Shades, M. Self-control: the Greek paradigm. In *The Quest for Self-control* (S.Z. Klausner, Ed.). New York: Free Press, 1965.
3. Lapidus, I.M. Adulthood in Islam: religious maturity in the Islamic tradition. In Adulthood, *Daedalus,* 1976, 93–108.

4. Tseng, W.S. The concept of personality in Confucian thought. *Psychiatry,* 1973, *36,* 191–202.
5. Vouwsma, W.J. Christian adulthood. In Adulthood, *Daedalus,* 1976, 77–92.
6. Globus, M. and Globus, G. The man of knowledge. This book.
7. Erhard, W., Gioscia, V. and Anbender, K. Being well. This book.
8. See, for example, Rajneesh, B.S. You are it; and Kornfield, J. Higher consciousness. This book.
9. Deikman, A. Sufism and the mental health sciences. This book.
10. Walsh, R. and Vaughan, F. Toward an integration of psychological well-being. This book.
11. Bandura, A. Self-efficacy: toward a unifying theory of behavioral change. *Psychological Review,* 1977, *84,* 191–215.
12. May, R. *Existential Psychology.* New York: Random House, 1969.
13. White, R. Motivation reconsidered: a concept of competence. *Psychological Review,* 1959, *66,* 297–333.
14. Seligman, M.E. *Helplessness.* San Francisco: Freeman, 1975.
15. Carver, C.S. and Scheier, M.F. *Attention and Self-regulation: A Control Theory Approach to Human Behavior.* New York: Springer-Verlag, 1981.
16. Wiener, N. Cybernetics: *Control and Communication in the Animal and Machine.* Cambridge, Mass.: MIT Press, 1948.
17. Von Bertalanffy, L. *General Systems Theory.* New York: Braziller, 1968.
18. Shapiro, D. *Biofeedback and Behavioral Medicine.* New York: Aldine, 1981.
19. Shapiro, D. *Meditation: Self-regulation Strategy and Altered States of Consciousness.* New York: Aldine, 1980.
20. Mahoney, M.J. and Arnkoff, D. Self-management. In *Behavioral Medicine: Theory and Practice* (O.F. Pomerleau and J.P. Brady, Eds.). Baltimore: Williams and Wilkins, 1979, pp. 75–98.
21. Fromm, E. Self-hypnosis. *Psychotherapy: Theory, Research and Practice,* 1975, *12,* 295–301.
22. Meichenbaum, D. *Cognitive Behavior Modification: An Integrative Approach.* New York: Plenum, 1977.
23. Singer, J.L. Navigating the stream of consciousness: research in daydreaming and related inner experience. *American Psychologist,* 1975, *30,* 727–38.
24. Stoyva, J.M. Musculoskeletal and stress related disorders. In *Behavioral Medicine: Theory and Practice* (O.F. Pomerleau and J.P. Brady, Eds.). Baltimore: Williams and Wilkins, 1979.
25. Stunkard, A. From explanation to action: a case of obesity. *Psychosomatic Medicine,* 1975, *37,* 195–236.
26. Agras, S. and Jacob, R. Hypertension. In *Behavioral Medicine: Theory and Practice* (O.F. Pomerleau and J.P. Brady, Eds.). Baltimore: Williams and Wilkins, 1979.
27. Fordyce, W.E. and Steger, J. Chronic pain. In *Behavioral Medicine: Theory and Practice* O.F. Pomerleau and J.P. Brady, Eds.). Baltimore: Williams and Wilkins, 1979.
28. Nolan, J.D. Freedom and dignity: a functional analysis. *American Psychologist,* 1974, *29,* 157–60.
29. Fromm, E. *Escape from Freedom.* New York: Reinholt, 1941.
30. See, for example, Ram Dass. *Journey of Awakening: A Meditator's Guidebook.* New York: Doubleday, 1978; and Bohm, D. *Causality and Chance in Modern Physics.* Philadelphia: University of Pennsylvania Press, 1957.
30a. Webster's *Third International Dictionary.*
31. Smith, H. *The sacred unconscious.* This book.
32. Goldstein, J. *Experience of Insight.* Santa Cruz Calif.: Unity Press, 1976.

33. Globus, M. and Globus, G. The man of knowledge. This book.
34. Rajneesh, B.S. Then you are it. Way of the White Cloud. Poona, India: 1975.
35. Castaneda, C. *Journey to Ixtlan*. New York: Simon and Schuster, 1973, p. 69.
36. Farquhar, J. The American Way of Life Not Being Hazardous to Your Health. Stanford: Stanford University Press, 1978.
37. See, for example, the edited *Biofeedback and Self-control Annuals* (N. Miller, L. Dicara, J. Camilla, D. Shapiro et al., 1971, 1972, 1973, 1976, 1978, 1980.)
38. Basmajian, J.V. and Newton, W.J. Feedback training of parts of buccinator muscle in man. *Psychophysiology*, 1974, *11*, 92.
39. Pelletier, K. and Peper, E. The chutzpah factor in altered states of consciousness. *Journal of Humanistic Psychology*, 1977, *17*, 63–73.
40. Cohen, C.I. and Cohen, E.J. Health education: panacea or pointless. *New England Journal of Medicine*, 1978, *299*, 718–720.
41. Goleman, D. and Epstein, N. Meditation and well-being: an Eastern model of psychological health. This book.
42. See Tart, C. *States of Consciousness*. New York: Dutton, 1975. See also Ornstein, R. *The Psychology of Consciousness* (2nd ed.). New York: Harcourt, Brace, Jovanovich, Ch. 11. 1976.
43. Cited in Smith, H. This book, Ch. 11. For a further discussion of "as if" see Vaihinger H. *The Philosophy of As If*. London: Routeledge and Kegan Paul, 1924. See also William James discussion of will in which James chooses to believe in free will, "My first act of free will shall be to believe in free will. For the remainder of the year, I will . . . voluntarily cultivate the feeling of moral freedom. . . ." William James, cited in Perry, R.B. *The Thought and Character of William James*, Vol. 1. Boston: Little Brown, 1935, p. 147.
45. Shapiro, D. *Precision Nirvana*. Englewood Cliffs, N.J.: 1976.
46. Jahoda, M. *Current Concepts of Positive Mental Health*. New York: Basic Books, 1958.
47. For statements about detached self-observation, see, for example, the *Maitraya-Brahmana Upanishad* (F. Max Muller, F. translator). New York: Dover, 1962, p. 295; Herrigal, E. *Zen and the Art of Archery*. New York: Pantheon, 1953, pp. 57–58.
48. Walsh, R. The ten perfections: qualities of the fully enlightened individual as described in Buddhist psychology. This book.
49. Walsh, R.N. and Vaughan, F. Toward an integrative model of psychological well-being. This book.
50. Lefcourt, H.M. The function of the illusion of control and freedom. *American Psychologist*, 1973, *28*, 417–25.
51. Klausner, S.Z., *The Quest for Self-control*. New York: Free Press, 1965.
52. Globus, G. On I: the conceptual foundations of responsibility. *American Journal of Psychiatry*, 1980, *137*, 417–422.
53. Knowles, J.H. Responsibility in the individual. *Daedalus*, 1977, *106*, 57–80.
54. Rotter, J.B. Generalized expectancies for internal versus external control of reinforcement. *Psychological Monographs*, 1966, *80*, 609.
55. Shapiro, J. and Shapiro, D. The psychology of responsibility. *New England Journal of Medicine*, 1979, *301*, 211–212.
56. Jung, C. In *Letters* (G. Adler, Ed.). Princeton, N.J.: Princeton University Press, 1973, p. 126.
57. Skinner, B.F. *Science and Human Behavior*. New York: Macmillan, 1953.
58. Gordon, C. and Gergen, K. *Self and Social Interaction*. New York: John Wylie, 1968.
59. Mead, G.H. Genesis of the self and social control. *International Journal of Ethics*, 1925, *35*, reprinted in reference 58.

60. Bandura, A. The self system in reciprocal determinism. *American Psychologist,* 1978, *33,* 344–358.
61. Minuchin, S., Rossman, B.L. and Barker, L. *Psychosomatic Families: Anorexia Nervosa in Context.* Cambridge, Mass.: Harvard University Press, 1978.
62. May, R. *Existential Psychology.* New York: Random House, 1969.
63. Jung, C. The structure and dynamics of the psyche. In *Collected Works,* Vol. 8. Princeton: Princeton University Press, 1960.
64. Erikson, E. *Childhood and Society.* New York: Norton, 1950.
65. See, for example, Rogers, C. *Client Centered Therapy,* Boston: Houghton Mifflin, 1951; and Lecky, P. *Self-consistency.* New York: Island Press, 1945.
66. See, for example, Hannum, J.W., Thoreson, C.E. and Hubbard, D.R. The behavioral study of self-esteem with elementary teachers. In *Self-control: Power to the Person* (M. Mahoney and C. Thoreson, (Eds.). Monterey, Calif.: Brooks Cole, 1974.
67. Globus, M. and Globus, G. The man of knowledge. This book.
68. See, for example, chapters by Goleman, Walsh, and Rajneesh in this book.
69. Assagioli, R. (*Psychosynthesis: A Manual of Principles and Techniques.* New York: Hohles and Dorman) notes, "We are dominated by everything with which ourself becomes identified. We can dominate and control everything from which we disidentify."
70. Shapiro, J. and Shapiro, D. Self-control and the path of relationship: toward an intimate vision of extreme psychological well-being. This book.
71. The issue of determination and effort is cited by many authors. An example is this quote from Chapter 11, by Huston Smith, "Along with being a gift to be received, life is a task to be performed. The adept performs it: whatever his hand finds to do, he does with all his might. . . . What matters focally, as the Zen master Dogen never tired of noting, is resolve."

Every transformation of man ... has rested on a new picture of the cosmos and the nature of man.

Lewis Mumford

Western schools of psychology have been splitting and proliferating with remarkable rapidity, and there has been debate over whether or not it might be possible to construct one or more broad synthetic theories which would integrate diverse viewpoints. In Towards an Integrative Psychology of Well-being *Roger Walsh and Frances Vaughan suggest ways in which an initial integration can be begun.*

They examine the dimensions of consciousness, perception, identity, motivation, and defenses, and point to various syntheses both within and between Western and Eastern psychologies on each of these dimensions. They then use this integration to suggest how certain qualities of well-being described in Eastern traditions can be understood from the perspective of this integration.

Frances Vaughan is a clinical psychologist in private practice in Mill Valley, California, a Professor of Psychology at the California Institute of Transpersonal Psychology, and a former president of the Association for Transpersonal Psychology. She is author of Awakening Intuition *(Doubleday/Anchor, 1979) and coeditor with Roger Walsh of* Beyond Ego: Transpersonal Dimensions in Psychology *(J. Tarcher, 1980). She has both personal and theoretical knowledge of an exceptionally broad range of psychological disciplines and is thus well equipped to suggest cross-disciplinary integrations. Her current interests include both theoretical implications and practical applications of transpersonal values.*

17

Towards an Integrative
Psychology of Well-Being

*Roger Walsh
and
Frances Vaughan*

A great thorough-going man does not confine himself to one school, but
combines many schools, as well as reads and listens to the arguments of
many predecessors.

Kuo Hsi

Each year the number of psychological theories continues to expand. Even
within the major schools, different subgroups and factions multiply. As if
there were not sufficient choice within Western psychology, we have recently
seen a growing interest in Non-Western concepts and models. Such an abundance of riches has led to considerable confusion, competition, and occasional out-right internecine warfare between diffcrent schools.

Not surprisingly, along with this growing embarrassment of riches has
come a growing interest in the possibility of obtaining some broad synthesis
and overview which could make sense out of this morass of competing
claims. Unfortunately more energy has been expended by people trying to
prove that theirs is the only true way than in integrating various ways. Even
where integrative models have been attempted, they have usually been confined to syntheses among related schools, for example, among various

psychoanalytic perspectives. Indeed, some psychologists have wondered whether broad theories are premature or even appropriate to psychology. Carl Jung[1] was pessimistic about the possibilities in his time and wrote

> We know so very little about the psyche that it is positively grotesque to think we are far enough advanced to frame general theories. We have not even established the empirical extent of the psyche's phenomenology. How then can we dream of general theories?

Indeed it has been argued that the belief that we may be able to extract a single overarching integrative psychology is nothing more than naive monism. Theoretical pluralism may reflect both the vastness and the very nature of knowledge. According to Joseph Royce,[2]

> It would indeed be a miracle if the range, complexity, and richness of psychological phenomena were to be accommodated by one world view, one conceptual framework, one paradigm or one theory.

On the other hand, most scientists usually assume that large numbers of fragmented and conflicting models represent an early phase of investigation in a field and that further development and data will result in an ongoing sifting and integration of theories. Raymond Corsini[3] notes,

> Psychologists generally assume the viewpoint that personality theory is science rather than philosophy. If it is a science, there can be an eventual convergence of all theories into one final theory of human nature. The present situation is similar to that of the blind man describing the elephant: each theorist sees the truth, but not the whole truth.

Whether or not knowledge in a field as vast as psychology may be ultimately reducible to one or even a very few general theories is thus a moot point. However, it is our impression that one of the major factors presently limiting resolution of the plethora of theories and conflicts is not their inherent irreducibility, but rather psychologists' limited familiarity and depth of understanding of the different schools. With sufficient breadth and depth of understanding it may be possible to penetrate differences in language, data base, perspectives, and presuppositions to detect ways in which different theories may display underlying commonalities and complementarities.

This idea is supported by the fact that in recent years a few models of truly broad integrative scope have appeared. The works of Ken Wilber have provided far-reaching syntheses among the major psychologies of the world. In addition to attempting to map different psychologies and therapies along a spectrum of states of consciousness, he has formulated a developmental psychology encompassing the major Western and non-Western systems. His chapters in this volume and his books[4-6] are all rich sources of integrative information and synthesis.

In this chapter we are attempting a preliminary synthesis of major psychological models. We will attempt to show that many of the major psychologies may present partially overlapping and partially complementary pictures of human nature. Since Eastern psychologies have focused on well-being, the major emphasis will be on integrating Eastern and Western systems—although we will point to syntheses within these systems where possible. As much as possible we will strive for simplicity rather than detailed comprehensiveness, and we acknowledge that the suggested synthesis is tentative, preliminary, and partial. However, at the present stage even preliminary and partial attempts at integration may be useful in suggesting directions for future exploration.

The Nature of Models

In the introduction to this book it was pointed out that there has recently been an emerging appreciation of the formerly unrecognized power and influence that models of reality exert on us. Models not only uncover facts but actively create them out of the interaction among beliefs, perception, analysis, and interpretation of data by the observer.[2]

Models are necessarily relatively simple and limited by comparison with the phenomena they describe. Indeed that is the very function of models: to simplify phenomena so as to render them comprehensible to us. Models therefore collapse and order multidimensional, multilevel properties along a small number of salient dimensions. Psychologies are clearly attempts to do just this. From the awesome complexity that is a human being, a few conceptual dimensions are abstracted in an attempt to parsimoniously account for a maximal range of behavior.

This approach is central to most of Western science. However, difficulties arise when we do not recognize the ways in which models can influence our perspective once they are accepted as true. For example, they tend to reify and isolate the dimensions, leading us to see them as independent entities awaiting discovery, rather than as parts of an interconnected whole. In contrast, the emerging world view in certain areas of science, particularly physics, points to the interconnected, interdependent, holistic nature of reality whereby all components are fully dependent on all others and are tied together in an unbroken net of interdependencies and interdeterminations. Any attempt to dissect out individual components, aspects, or dimensions is therefore necessarily somewhat simplistic and artificial. In adopting any particular perspective or model, we are therefore necessarily adopting an arbitrary viewing framework which will appear to create specific "facts." In doing so, we may collapse many dimensions into a few, reduce process to stasis, view the interdependent as relatively independent, and create out of an omnideterminism in which all things determine all others, an apparent one way cause-effect relationship.

The physicist David Bohm[7] refers to the indivisible whole which he says underlies the physical world as the *holomovement* and suggests:

> In certain cases we can abstract particular aspects of the holomovement (e.g. light, electrons, sound, etc.). But more generally, all forms of the holomovement merge and are inseparable. Thus, in its totality, the holomovement is not limited in any specifiable way at all. It is not required to conform to any particular order, or to be bounded by any particular measure. Thus the holomovement is undefinable and immeasurable. To give primary significance to the undefinable and immeasurable holomovement implies that it has no meaning to talk of the *fundamental* theory on which *all* of physics could find a permanent basis, or to which *all* of the phenomena of physics could ultimately be reduced. Rather, each theory will abstract a certain aspect that is relevant only in some limited context, which is indicated by some appropriate measure.

This suggests one reason why there have been so many psychological models. Each perspective and model will abstract out certain dimensions, facts, and implications, each of which may be relatively real, partially overlapping, and partially complementary to other models. This is another reason why it may be unrealistic to expect that psychology can elucidate any single fundamental theory, dimension, or model.[8,9]

However, many psychologists have tended to assume that truth is to be found in a single, or at best a very small number, of models and have adopted an either/or attitude, assuming that if one model is correct another must be wrong. This attitude has been reinforced by a common conceptual shortcoming: namely, the failure to recognize the vastly overdetermined nature of human behavior. Since multiple factors enter into the determination of any psychological outcome, one is likely to find any particular determining factor one looks for. Thus, for example, the Freudian analyst examining patients for libido motivators, the behaviorist looking for external reinforcers, the cognitive behavior modifier searching for contributing thought patterns, the Adlerian seeking superiority strivings, and the humanist anticipating self-actualizing tendencies have all been successful in their quest. Error arises, however, when it is assumed that such findings provide exclusvie evidence for one particular theory. This is not to say that all theories are equally accurate or that testing theories is impossible. However, a fundamental tenet of the philosophy of science is that theories cannot be *proved* correct, they can only be disproved. This sometimes seems to have been forgotten by personality theorists. It must be recognized that in a complex, interdependent, overdetermined system, any and all motivational factors may be found and do not necessarily supply exclusive evidence in favor of one model over another.

Thus, in summary, we need to move towards a recognition that models and "facts" are part of a dialectical process. Facts suggest models, and models suggest validating facts. Multiple models are possible and will produce their corresponding body of supportive facts, and each will be relatively real. While broad integrative models are desirable, it may be that large-scale models are less precise in describing small subareas. We may need a dynamic epistemology in which we move between models of varying scale according to the scale of the phenomena under investigation. Synthesis is necessary whenever possible, but may not remove the need for the smaller models which it integrates.

The Process of Integration

The integration of psychological models entails several processes. The first of these may be a willingness to question existing beliefs and assumptions. Most of us tend to identify with a particular model and argue its merits over all others. However, integration demands letting go of an either/or approach in favor of openness to the possibility of a both/and perspective. One must be willing to learn not just one, but multiple, psychologies in sufficient detail to be able to translate terms, identify commonalities, and recognize relationships between the models. In the resulting synthesis, each primary model now becomes a part of the integrative one, the set becomes a subset, context becomes content, and what was the whole system becomes a subsystem.[10,11] The result tends to be the inclusion of a greater number of variables, levels, and interactions. Hopefully, this greater complexity is rendered more coherent by the recognition of common dimensions which underlie what were formerly seen as unrelated phenomena.

Criteria for an Integrative Model

Theories are easy to propose—witness the large number of them around—but good theories, and good integrative theories, are another story. What are the qualities of a good integrative theory?

Obviously it should be truly synthetic, capable of including a wide range of concepts and data from its component models without ignoring major portions of them. Broad inclusiveness is desirable; hence the integrative model may include more dimensions than any of its components. At the same time, the principle of parsimony suggests that it be able to collapse aspects of the individual models along certain dimensions, for example, by showing how different models may reflect different levels or aspects of the same dimension.

The perspective or viewing frame of the integrative model should effectively be a metaperspective. That is, it should provide a new viewpoint from which the perspectives or viewing points of the component models can be identified. Since any viewpoint stems from assumptions and beliefs, those of the component theories should be identified to see how they may account for resultant interpretations and findings.

In view of this role of beliefs and assumptions in determining perspectives, it is important that the integrative model should be as explicit as possible in identifying and describing its own assumptions. In the case of the model described here, the assumptions can be found woven into the previous discussion on the nature of models. These include, for example, the statements that all models are limited and relative (probably partially true, probably partially complementary), that "facts" are partly created by a viewing framework, that integration consists of moving to a metaperspective, etc. Identifying these statements as assumptions does not mean that they are necessarily right or wrong. To us they seem reasonable, but of course that is the nature of theoretical assumptions: they always seem reasonable to those of us who propose them.

Thus we make no claims for objectivity in proposing this integrative model. Indeed, true objectivity is probably impossible for it seems that psychologies reflect personalities, representing the projections of their founders' belief systems upon the Rorschach test we call the world. Their value systems attest to the attractions and aversions, their profundity mirrors the depth of insight, and their scope reflects the range of experience of their proponents. What lies beyond this depth and scope remains unrecognized, unattended, or pathologized. Their description of human nature is but their founders self-image "writ large" upon humankind.

> Every theory is a personal confession. It reflects a subjective bias, even in the very questions it selects to ask and how it sets out to answer them. If acknowledged openly and taken seriously into account, this personal bias may prove to be a scientific asset rather than a liability.[12]

We hope to mitigate these factors somewhat by trying to acknowledge our own assumptions and beliefs. For example, we acknowledge that models proposed here are hypotheses, that the present model is only one of many possible integrations, and that our personal experience, however preliminary, of a wide range of both Western and non-Western psychologies, therapies, meditations, and yogas, has led us to believe that much of what have been called the "mystical psychologies" are "mystical" only because of our lack of acquaintance and research of them. We therefore feel that, given sufficient study, a partial though broad integration, both within and between Western and non-Western systems, is possible. The present chapter is our attempt to suggest preliminary components of such an integration.

The major dimensions that will be covered in this model include consciousness, perception, identity, motivation, defenses, and health. Since the only branch of Western psychology to attempt an integration of Western and non-Western perspectives has been transpersonal, the model presented here shares certain transpersonal orientations.

Consciousness

Any attempt to integrate Western and non-Western psychologies must view consciousness as a central dimension since it has been the primary concern of Eastern traditions. This contrasts with the history of Western psychology and psychiatry in which consciousness has usually been either excluded from consideration (e.g., radical behaviorism) or examined indirectly through focusing on its contents (e.g., thoughts, emotions, sensations, and behavioral manifestations).

An integrative perspective must acknowledge a broad spectrum of states of consciousness. Both Eastern and Western models recognize our usual waking consciousness, sleep and dream states, as well as various pathological and dysfunctional states such as intoxication, delirium, and various psychoses. However to these the Eastern models add a variety of other states, some of which are said to be "functionally specific" and a few to be true "higher" states. The term "functionally specific" is used to indicate states in which certain capacities are enhanced above and beyond the usual waking condition whereas others are reduced. The term "higher" indicates states possessing all the capacities of the usual waking condition plus additional ones.[13]

Some Asian psychologies contain detailed cartographies and descriptions of these states. For example, Buddhist psychology contains detailed descriptions of the processes involved in attaining, and the phenomenology of, various functionally specific states of extreme concentration and mental imperturbability called *jhanas* as well as true higher states.[14] Because of differences in culture, language, philosophy, and practice, it has traditionally been very difficult to determine the precise relationship between the states described by one tradition and those described by others. However, it now seems possible to make meaningful comparisons and to abstract some of the underlying commonalities (see Chapter 16).[15] At the farther end of this spectrum lies a family of states variously described as enlightenment, liberation, etc. Actually the farthest reaches or "ultimate state of consciousness" is probably not a state per se but rather the ground of all states.[9,11] Thus an integrative model acknowledges the possibility of the existence of a broad range of states of consciousness from the most severely pathological and dysfunctional, through the usual waking condition, to a range of functionally specific states, intermediate higher states, to enlightenment. Some of these states will be discussed further in the section on identity.

An integrative model must also recognize state dependency which suggests that some functions may be limited by the state in which they occur. This is a concept enunciated thousands of years ago in various non-Western psychologies[16] and recently explored experimentally in the West in both animal[17] and human[13] subjects. The concept is important to any model which encompasses a broad range of states and seeks to indicate relationships among them. For example, in state dependent learning, what is learned in one state may not necessarily be remembered or comprehended in another. Similarly, in state dependent communication, the insights of an individual in a particular state may not be comprehensible to another in a different state. On the other hand, cross state retention suggests that an individual may attain information or insights in one state and retain at least part of them in other states in which they would not normally be accessible.

State dependency is particularly important in any integration of Western and non-Western psychologies since several non-Western disciplines involve specific training in altered states.[15] The limits of cross state communication may therefore apply, and failure to recognize this appears to have led a number of Western investigators to misinterpret and dismiss Eastern claims.[18]

One of the most radical implications of higher states and an integrative model is that, contrary to traditional Western assumptions, our usual waking state may be suboptimal. The perennial psychologies such as Buddhist, Hindu, and Sufi psychologies, are unanimous in agreeing that our usual state is filled to a remarkable and unrecognized extent with a continuous flow of largely uncontrollable thoughts and fantasies which exert an extremely powerful but usually unappreciated influence on perception, cognition, and behavior. Trained self-observation such as that employed in a variety of meditative practices reveals that our usual experience is perceptually distorted by the continuous, automatic, and unconscious blending of input from reality and fantasy in accordance with our needs and defenses. These distortions are discussed in more detail in the section on perception.

We are all prisoners of our minds. This realization is the first step on the journey to freedom.[19]

Viewing our usual state from this expanded context of a spectrum of states of consciousness results in some unexpected implications. The traditional Western model defines psychosis as a distorted perception of reality which does not recognize the distortion. From the perspective of this multiple states model, our usual model fits this definition, being suboptimal, providing a distorted perception of reality, and failing to recognize that distortion. Indeed, any one state of consciousness is necessarily limited and only relatively real. Hence from the broader perspective, psychosis might be defined as entrapment in any single state of consciousness and the failure to recognize its relative and distorted picture of reality.

Since perceptual distortions, insensitivity, and defenses are self-masking, they obscure their own nature and effects. Thus, unless an individual examines his or her own consciousness with meticulous rigor, the true nature of this condition can go unrecognized throughout a lifetime. This claim, though radical from the perspective of traditional Western psychology, has actually been made repeatedly across cultures and centuries by a variety of disciplines whose central claim is that our usual state is suboptimal and distorted yet these distortions can be removed by mental training. These disciplines and their theories have been described as the perennial philosopy,[20] the perennial religion,[21] and the perennial psychology.[4]

In summary, the perennial psychologies suggest that in addition to the states of consciousness which Western psychology usually recognizes there exists a spectrum of other states which are attainable through specific mental training. Certain of these are said to be "functionally specific" or "higher," and it is said that understanding of them by those without direct experience is necessarily limited. Recent Western research and concepts such as state dependency are beginning to make these claims more understandable.

PERCEPTION

Projection makes perception. The world you see is what you gave it, nothing more than that. . . . It is the witness to your state of mind, the outside picture of an inward condition. As a man thinketh, so does he perceive. Therefore, seek not to change the world, but choose to change your mind about the world.

Anonymous[22]

To understand the claim that perception is distorted to an unrecognized degree, it is necessary to draw a distinction between awareness and what we will call here, mind. In this context, *mind* refers to the contents and processes involved in the production of thoughts, emotions, images, memories, and fantasies. In order to provide an integration of Western and Eastern perspectives on perception, it will be necessary to introduce a number of claims about the mind which are widespread in various Eastern psychologies and meditative practices. Many of the claims do not actually run counter to traditional Western assumptions but rather extend them to more pervasive and subtle levels.

Both Western and non-Western psychologies would agree that the mind is continuously active, producing an ongoing stream of mental content. Eastern psychologies have claimed that this continuous creativity is more prolific than Western models recognize and that much of the flux of thoughts, emotions, images, etc., goes unrecognized. Furthermore, the untrained person is said to spend a large percentage of time lost in unrecognized fantasy.[4,6,23] While in the fantasy, the person does not realize that he or she is in it; at the moment one is in it, it appears real. Recognition, if it occurs at all, happens only retrospectively.

A further claim is that the mind is largely outside voluntary control. The continuous stream of mental contents is said to be produced by conditioned automaticity and to trap awareness to an unrecognized degree. Like smokers who feel in control of their habit until they try to stop it, we as individuals without specific mental training are said to be unaware of the extent to which we are controlled by, and unable to control, our own minds. Part of this fragmentation and lack of control of awareness has also been noted by some Western psychologists. Carl Jung[24] remarked that

> ... the so called unity of consciousness is an illusion. It is really a wish-dream. We like to think that we are one; but we are not, most decidedly not. We are not really masters in our house. We like to believe in our energy and in what we can do; but when it comes to a real showdown we find that we can do it only to a certain extent. ...

Several Western behavioral scientists have reported their amazement, on beginning meditation practice, at discovering the extent of this lack of control.[11,25-30] Thus in the words of Duane Elgin,[30] a social scientist with considerable experience of meditative practices,

> We tend not to notice or appreciate the degree to which we run on automatic—largely because we live in an almost constant state of mental distraction. Our minds are constantly moving about at a lightening fast-pace—thinking about the future, replaying conversations from the past, engaging in inner role playing, and so on. Without sustained attention, it

is difficult to appreciate the extent to which we live in an automated, reflexive, and dreamlike reality that is a subtle and continuously changing blend of fantasy, inner dialogue, memory, planning, and so on. The fact that we spend years acquiring vast amounts of *mental content* does not mean that we are thereby either substantially aware of, or in control of, our mental process.

In our usual state of consciousness, this everflowing stream of mindstuff distorts and reduces the sensitivity of perception. When a stimulus enters awareness, it elicits a chain of conditioned associations, emotions, fantasies, etc.,[31,32] and it is these which are experienced rather than the stimulus per se which elicited them. Our inability to differentiate between raw percepts and the mental elaborations which they elicit means that we unknowingly perceive an illusory, fantasy-distorted image of the world.

This illusory distortion has been described for centuries by all the major consciousness disciplines and has been called by many names including "maya" or "samsara." The description of perception as illusory has often been misunderstood as implying that the world does not really exist. Rather, what is implied is that perception is distorted to such an extent that we do not perceive things as they really are, but instead see them colored by our own mental filters and projections. Thus our experience of the world and of ourselves is not a clear perception but rather an actively constructed interpretation or illusion—passive, but actively created and constructed.

Since perception is a function of the attendant state of consciousness, one's view of the world and one's sense of self may shift radically in different states. Thus what was taken to be fixed and absolute in one state may be perceived as relative in another. Experiences of altered states reveal that perception and the sense of self are far more fluid than usually recognized.

This suggests the potential for attaining perception which is clearer and more veridical than that of our usual state, and indeed this is one of the major aims of the consciousness disciplines. As Duane Elgin[30] comments,

The crucial importance of penetrating behind our continuous stream of thought (as largely unconscious and lightening fast flows of inner fantasy-dialogue) is stressed by every major consciousness tradition in the world: Buddhist, Taoist, Hindu, Sufi, Zen, etc. Yet, western cultures have fostered the inclusive understanding that a state of continual mental distraction is in the natural order of things. Consequently, by virtue of a largely unconscious social agreement as to the nature of our inner thought processes we live, individually and collectively, almost totally imbedded within our mental constructive reality.

As Fritz Perls[33] remarked, "I would say the majority of modern man lives in a verbal trance."

Training perception so as to free awareness from entrapment in the distorting influence of mind is a central method employed in many consciousness disciplines. For example, in Buddhist insight meditation, the practitioner is trained to focus bare attention on each stimulus.[14,23,31,32] Meditators state that with practice, they can observe the bare stimulus prior to the elaboration of mental associations to it. With further practice, the number and extent of these elaborations tend to be reduced so that the mind begins to become less reactive and agitated, thus allowing a clearer, less cluttered, and less distorted perception of one's moment-by-moment experience. This perceptual training, when carried to deeper and deeper levels, results in a progressive freeing of perception, thought, and behavior from the uncontrollable, unrecognized, conditioned automaticity which formerly affected one's every waking moment.

When the inner fantasy-dialogue ceases, then awareness is no longer captured, filled, distorted, and reduced by it. There is remarkable unanimity among the consciousness disciplines that at this point whole new realms of experience, perception, concentration, states of consciousness, and sense of self may emerge. Now there is the possibility of entering the "subtle realms" described by Hindu psychology—states in which one becomes aware of ranges of experience whose subtlety or faintness are such that they cannot be sensed above the noise of the usual, by comparison very loud, gross, or intense, inner fantasy-dialogue. Here also is the possibility of states such as the jhanas and samadhi of concentration meditations, the stages of insight of Vipassana meditation, and beyond these the still more refined "causal realms" described by Ken Wilber in his chapter on the evolution of consciousness.[15] This process appears to be an example of "perceptual release," the phenomenon in which the removal of intense stimulation allows the recognition of more subtle phenomena.

Consider the remarkable unanimity of the following quotations (more can be found in Chapter 15) taken from a range of disciplines and cultures.

The fundamental task which gives the key to many realizations is the silence of the mind. . . . All kinds of discoveries are made, in truth, when the mental machinery stops, and the first is that if the power to think is a remarkable gift, the power not to think is even more so.

Satprem[35]

Of all the hard facts of science, I know of none more solid and fundamental than the fact that if you inhibit thought and persevere, you come at length to a region of consciousness below or behind thought, and different from ordinary thought in its nature and character. A consciousness of quasi-universal quality, and a realization of an altogether vaster self than that to which we are accustomed. And since the ordinary consciousness with which we are concerned in ordinary life is before all things founded on the local little self, it follows that to pass out of that is to die to the ordinary self and the ordinary world. It is to die in the ordinary state, but in another sense, it is to wake up and find that the I, one's real, most intimate self, pervades the universe and all other beings. That the mountains, and the sea, and the stars are a part of one's body, and that one's soul is in touch with the souls of all creatures. It is to be assured of an indestructible and immortal life and of a joy immense and inexpressible.

Edward Carpenter[36]

Whenever the dialogue stops, the world collapses and extraordinary facets of ourselves surface, as though they have been kept heavily guarded by our words.

Castaneda[37]

Thus, in summary, Western[38] and perennial psychologies are in agreement that perception is an active constructive process which yields a less than totally accurate picture of the world. The perennial psychologies extend this to say that the inaccuracies are more subtle, pervasive, and illusion producing than is appreciated without specific mental training.[39] Moreover, they suggest that it is possible to train attention and perceptual processes through specific practices such as meditation so as to greatly reduce or even eradicate these distortions, finally resulting in what Huston Smith[40] calls "the fully realized human being . . . whose doors of perception have been cleansed."

IDENTITY

Perhaps the most fundamental question we can ask is, "What are we?" Deeper even than the question Who are we? (which essentially asks what type of people we are), What are we? takes us below implicit assumptions into the deepest realms of being. We might say that this question addresses the issue of what exactly it is which assumes itself to be a (particular type of) person.

The answer we give to this question seems awesome in its power to determine our view of both our self and our world. Everything we do, think, or feel, is touched by it, for all behavior seems at least partly based on our beliefs about what we are.

With few exceptions, Western psychology has tended to address the "who" level of this question and has answered in terms of such things as personality, intellectual capacity, etc. This too may be the first response of most people when asked, "What are you?" Yet this particular range of answers appears to reflect the nature and limitations of our perceptual sensitivity and cultural beliefs, rather than the most fundamental levels of self-knowing.

Like perception in general, it appears that the self-sense is constructed. Furthermore, there appears to be not merely one possible self-sense which can be constructed, or even a narrow range, but rather an awesome breadth of possible identities. For what the perennial psychologies are unanimous in claiming is that as the perceptual processes involved in the formation of our constructed self-sense are recognized, halted, or seen through, which occurs in meditation,[15,41] then a deepening recognition of more and more fundamental levels of self occurs.

It appears, then, that we may have considerably underestimated the possible range of responses to the questions of who and what we are. Indeed, the self-sense apears to be vastly more fluid than previously recognized, perhaps infinitely so. It may be that this self-sense can attach to, or identify with, anything. In the material world, it can become identified with specific objects, the body, the environment, or even the entire universe,[42] and in the mental realm, with any mental content such as thoughts or emotions, or with consciousness itself.[15] Identification is defined here as the process by which consciousness assumes a thing to be self. That is, identification occurs when awareness, the faculty of knowing, does not differentiate itself from the object it knows.[23,43] (When awareness identifies with an object exclusively and differentially, then the me/not-me dichotomy occurs and the isolated, separate self-sense of the existentialist is created.)

One of the major demarcating points between traditional Western assumptions on the one hand, and transpersonal and Eastern perspectives on the other, is a recognition of the process of the identification of awareness with intrapsychic contents and processes. Traditionally, identification has been considered in terms of externals as when a person feels the same as, or like, someone or something else.[44] However, the non-Western perspective, while it recognizes this, also recognizes that awareness can identify with mental contents such as thoughts and emotions.

Furthermore, this type of identification goes unrecognized by most of us including psychologists, therapists, and behavioral scientists, because we are all so involved in it. That is, while one may ask "Who am I?" consensually validated identifications tend to go unrecognized because they are not called into question. Indeed any attempt to question them may meet with considerable resistance from others.

Attempts to awake before our time are often punished, especially by those who love us most. Because they, bless them, are asleep. They think anyone who wakes up, or . . . realizes that what is taken to be real, is a dream, is going crazy.[45]

The process of identification has far-reaching implications. The identification of awareness with mental content renders the individual unconscious of the broader context of consciousness which holds this content. When awareness identifies with mental content, this content becomes the context from which all other mental content and experience are viewed. That is, what was the object of awareness now becomes the subject, the seen becomes an attribute of the seer, and what was being perceived becomes the perspective, framework, and filter from which perception occurs. Thus the content-become-context may now interpret other content, and determine meaning, perception, belief, motivation, and behavior—all in a manner which is consistent with, and reinforces, this context. Furthermore, the context sets in motion psychological processes which also reinforce it.[27]

For example, if the thought "I'm scared" arises, and this thought is observed and seen to be what it is (i.e., just another thought), then it exerts little influence. However, if it is identified with, then the reality at that moment is that the individual is scared and is likely to generate and identify with a whole series of fearful thoughts and emotions, to interpret nondescript feelings as fear, to perceive the world as frightening, and to act in a fearful manner.[46] Thus identification sets in train a self-fulfilling, self-prophetic process in which experience and psychological processes validate the reality of that with which it was identified. For the person identified with the thought "I'm scared" everything seems to prove the reality and validity of his or her fear. Remember that with identification, the person is unaware of the fact that his perception stems from the thought "I'm scared." This thought is now not something which can be seen, rather it is that from which everything else is seen and interpreted. Awareness, which would be transcendent and positionless, has now been constricted to viewing the world from a single self-validating perspective. This is similar to the process which occurs with unrecognized models as described earlier.

> We are dominated by everything with which our self becomes identified. We can dominate and control everything from which we disidentify.[47]

As long as we are identified with an object, that is bondage.[48]

It may be that thoughts and beliefs constitute the operators or algorithms which construct, mediate, guide, and maintain the identificatory constriction of consciousness and act as limiting models of who we believe ourselves to be. As such, they must be opened to review in order to allow growth. It may be that beliefs are adopted as strategic, defensive decisions about who and what we must be in order to survive and function optimally.

When it is remembered that the mind is usually filled with thoughts with which we are unwittingly identified, it becomes apparent that our usual state of consciousness is one in which we are, quite literally, hypnotized. As in any hypnotic state, there need not be any recognition of the trance and its attendant constriction of awareness, or any memory of the sense of identity prior to hypnosis. While in the trance, we think we are the thoughts with which we are identified. Put another way, those thoughts from which we have not yet disidentified create our state of consciousness, identity, and reality. As Globus and Globus said in Chapter 14, this internal dialogue "serves to maintain an order we know as the world.)"[49]

The most commonly assumed identity of most adults is the ego. Presumably this has not always been so, and in *Up from Eden,* Ken Wilber has recently put forward a broad-ranging view of the historical and ongoing evolution of humanity through a sequence of progressive refinements of identity.[50] Ego appears to come into existence when awareness identifies with thought, and this process is described with great clarity by Wilber in "The Evolution of Consciousness" (Chapter 16).[51] Thus the nature of ego is essentially conceptual. Ego might therefore be defined as the self-sense which arises from the identification of awareness with a constellation of thoughts. Ken Wilber[6] describes it as follows:

> The ego is a self-concept, a constellation of self-concepts, along with the images, fantasies, identifications, memories, sub-personalities, motivations, ideas and information related or bound to the separate self-concept.

Existential and psychoanalytic schools have pointed out that the ego perceives itself as an isolated entity, unalterably separate from the remainder of the universe, and locked in a perpetual and insurmountable struggle with both psychodynamic forces and existential limits. While it may adjust to, and cope with, these conflicts and limits and their attendant suffering, it can never ultimately escape them at this level of consciousness. Many psychologies recognize this problem but not the possibility of states in which it is not operative, e.g., Freudian psychoanalysis, existentialism, and behaviorism. From this perspective the human condition is seen as a no-exit situation to be met with courage, authenticity, problem solving, and acceptance. These psychologies are in agreement with Buddhism's first noble truth which notes the pervasiveness of suffering, but not with the subsequent truths which describe a way out.

Suffering may attend any state of consciousness where exclusive identification results in a self/not-self dichotomy. As soon as there is a distinction between subject and object, between me and not-me, fear and suffering are inevitable say the consciousness disciplines. In the words of the millenia old Upanishads, "Wherever there is other there is fear." The key to escape is said to lie in the transcendence of this dichotomy.

If transcendence of the self/not-self dichotomy and freedom from suffering are actually possible, then how are they attained? All the major consciousness disciplines offer answers to this question. In fact, teaching the means for escape from suffering constitutes the reason for their existence. The key feature of all of them is mental training in which formerly uncontrolled processes are brought under increasing voluntary control.

All scriptures without any exception proclaim that for attaining Salvation mind should be subdued.[51]

Ramana Maharshi

The mind of a yogi is under his control; he is not under the control of his mind.[52]

Shree Ramakrishna

As this occurs, it induces a sequence of states of consciousness in which awareness disidentifies from more and more subtle mental phenomena. A detailed account of the process is provided by Ken Wilber in Chapter 16.

Finally, states of consciousness may emerge in which identification of awareness with some objects to the exclusion of others is permanently dismantled. When it endures, such a state of consciousness is known by a variety of names such as enlightenment, liberation, etc. Freed of any exclusivity, the me/not-me dichotomy collapses or is transcended. Awareness now experiences itself as both nothing (no thing, i.e., pure awareness) and everything (the entire universe). Detached from any identification with material or mental objects, it now experiences itself as being nonspatial, nowhere and everywhere, and outside time, eternal, always in the unchanging now. That is, shorn of dualism and exclusivity, awareness now experiences itself as transcendent to both time and space, as pure consciousness and yet one with the universe, transcendent to the limitations and suffering which seemed so real, absolute, and inescapable from its former perspective.

In the utmost depths of the human psyche, when all dualism and exclusivity have been dropped, awareness finds no limits to identity and directly experiences itself as beyond both time and space: that which humanity has traditionally called God.

To me God is a word used to point to our ineffable subjectivity, to the unimaginable potential which lies within each of us.[53]

Now we can begin to understand from a psychological perspective some of the statements of the world's great mystics and religious figures, all of whom have been unanimous in claiming that the source of true religious experience is internal. Note the convergence or "transcendent unity"[54] of religions evidenced in the following statements.

The kingdom of heaven is within you.

Christianity

Look within, thou art the Buddha.

Buddhism

Atman (individual consciousness) and Brahman (universal consciousness) are one.

Hinduism

By understanding the Self all this universe is known.

Brihad-aranyaka Upanishad, 4, 5

God dwells within you as you.

Siddha Yoga

I am God. This is a statement of total humility.

Sufism

He who knows himself, knows his Lord.

Islam (Muhammad)

He who knows himself knows God.

Christianity (St. Clement)

Recalling that our usual self-sense is egoic and hence primarily conceptual or thought based,[15] we can now understand the startling claim which mystics have made for millennia that "who you think you are is a thought in the mind of God." This is reminiscent of William James:[55]

> Out of my experience . . . one fixed conclusion dogmatically emerges . . . . there is a continuum of cosmic consciousness, against which our individuality builds but accidental forces, and into which our several minds plunge as into a mother-sea.

MOTIVATION

The integrative perspective proposed here recognizes a broad hierarchical organization of motivation which encompasses most motives recognized in

Western psychology. This model does not necessarily deny the validity of other psychological models. Rather, it attempts to set them in a broader context which recognizes that behavior is overdetermined (many motives enter into any behavioral outcome), that motivational systems may be organized hierarchically in that motives tend to emerge sequentially, and that this hierarchy includes motives towards "higher" goals such as aesthetics, self-actualization, and self-transcendence.

The Hierarchy of Needs

This model owes a great deal to Abraham Maslow who was the first Western psychologist to explicitly formulate a hierarchical model encompassing "higher" motives. However, analogous ideas can be found in other schools, both East and West. For example, Gestalt psychology acknowledges that increasingly subtle incomplete gestalts arise and predominate in awareness whenever a preceeding gestalt is completed.

One of Maslow's major contributions was his recognition of the hierarchical organization of needs according to their potency and primacy. He identified a broad range of needs which he felt were present in everyone, and he therefore called them basic or instinctual. The most powerful and prepotent were fundamental survival needs with a clear physiological basis, such as hunger or thirst. When these needs were fulfilled, other less powerful ones such as needs for shelter, sex, affection, and self-esteem could become effective motivators in their turn. Only after these prepotent deficiency or D-needs were filled could more subtle, growth-oriented Being needs, or metaneeds, play a primary motivational role.

To this second group Maslow assigned such uniquely human desires as impulses to freedom, beauty, goodness, unity, justice, and self-actualization. These higher needs are initially weak, subtle, and easily disrupted by adverse environments, attitudes, and habits. For most people, they require considerable nurturing if they are to flourish, but flourish they must if the individual is to find full expression for his or her basic humanity and avoid what Maslow termed the "metapathologies" such as boredom, cynicism, and lack of inspiration.[56]

In ascending this hierarchy the needs appear to shift from clearly physiological to apparently more psychological in nature, from strong to subtle, from prepotent to less potent and more easily disrupted, from spontaneous to requiring cultivation, from deficiency to sufficiency, from egocentric to selfless, from avoidance to approach, from external to internal reinforcement, from field dependence to field independence, and from frequent to rare in occurrence in the population.

"Higher" Needs

In his later years Maslow added a still higher need beyond self-actualization: namely, the need for self-transcendence.[56,57] In this Maslow saw a drive towards a mode of experiencing and being which transcended the usual egoic states of consciousness and limits of experience and identity, i.e., the drive towards the transpersonal realms. Similar hierarchical models incorporating transcendent components are to be found in a number of non-Western psychologies such as Sufism and Hinduism.

Thus in recent decades there has been an interesting trend in Western psychology towards the recognition of increasingly "higher" motives. Early psychoanalytic formulations emphasized libido. Self-actualization was initially placed at the peak of Maslow's hierarchy, but subsequently gave way to self-transcendence. Thus self-transcendence has been suggested as the summa of human motivation.

However, in examining various non-Western psychologies and consciousness disciplines, another possibility appears. All of these disciplines are in agreement about the motivation of the fully enlightened master, the person firmly ensconced in the highest realms of transcendent states of consciousness, the arahat of Hinayana Buddhism and the bodhisattva of Mahayana Buddhism, the master of Zen, the jivanmukti of Hinduism, the sage of Taoism, the tzaddik of Hassidic Judaism, the prototypic saint of all traditions. This person, they agree, is totally unmoved by egocentric desires. "There is no motivation without ignorance."[58] Rather, such a person is held to act "in accord with the Tao," that is, to respond effortlessly, appropriately, compassionately, and selflessly to the needs of the situation, in such a way as to most effectively contribute to the well-being of others. In the words of the third Zen patriarch, "Sengtsan" writing in the sixth century, "For the unified mind in accord with the Way all self centered striving ceases."[59] In these rare individuals, it is said that

> whatever is, or is thought to be, necessary for sentient beings happens all the time of its own accord.
>
> Gampopa[58](p. 271)

In these people it seems that selfless service may be the prepotent guiding principle.

> Fools think only of their own interest,
> While the Sage is concerned with the benefit of others.
> What a world of difference between them.
>
> Mahayana[58] (p. 195)

In addition to emerging spontaneously in the fully realized master, selfless service may also be consciously cultivated by any individual. As such it can be used as a means of reducing egocentric motivation ("purification") and as a pathway to the transpersonal; it is then called karma yoga, the yoga of service.

Even the motivation towards self-transcendence can apparently be sublimated in favor of selfless service. For example, a major division in Buddhism is between the Hinayana and the Mahayana schools. In the Mahayana tradition, the ideal prototype is the bodhisattva, the individual who renounces the pursuit of his or her personal enlightenment in favor of first facilitating the liberation of others. In the Hinayana tradition on the other hand, the individual is encouraged to strive first for personal liberation, thus eradicating egocentric hindrances in order to become a more effective teacher and instrument of service.

> One should not be over-anxious and hasty in setting out to serve others before one hath oneself realized Truth in its fullness; to do so, would be like the blind leading the blind. As long as the sky endureth, so long will there be no end of sentient beings for one to serve; and to every one cometh the opportunity for such service. Till the opportunity come, I exhort each of you to have but one resolve, namely, to attain Buddhahood for the good of all living things.
>
> Milarepa[60]

> Thus it is that the highest aim of every sincere yogi, be he Hindu, Buddhist, Jain, Taoist, Sufi, or Gnostic Christian, is first to fit himself to become a World-Teacher and then to return to human society.
>
> Evans-Wentz[60]

Thus, whether it emerges spontaneously in the enlightened individual or whether it is consciously cultivated either as a means to, or even in favor of, personal enlightenment, it seems possible that selfless service may warrant a position above self-transcendence as the highest of the hierarchy of motives.

The cultivation or free expression of selfless service suggests a general principle: namely, that the hierarchy may actually reverse such that the highest experienced motive tends to become predominant. Individuals who have either tasted the fruit of higher motives or sufficiently satisfied the lower ones may begin to experience such a shift, finding satisfaction of the lower needs now less fulfilling than the higher. Even an intellectual discovery of the existence, nature, and attainability of higher motives may be sufficient to initiate such a shift, and suggests the importance of disseminating information about their existence. In other cases individuals may engage in a discipline of one type or another (e.g., meditation, yoga, service, or study) with the specific intention of cultivating higher motives and making them predominant. For example, a strong creative drive may supersede a need for acquiring wealth. Likewise, a desire for transcendence may predominate over a desire for esteem and recognition.

Such a model makes comprehensible some of the concepts which are central to a variety of consciousness disciplines and the esoteric core of the great religions. Among these are statements about "attachment," "purification," "giving up the world," and the ultimately unsatisfying nature of lower needs.

Most such disciplines state that the lower needs can provide no ultimate or permanent satisfaction. Rather, such lower needs as desire for prestige and material possessions are said to result in only transient satisfaction (rapid habituation) with each new acquisition, and to be addicting in that their transiency demands a continual supply of novel possessions and stimuli. The individual is thus dependent for his or her sense of well-being on access to a regular supply of external objects which, in order to counteract the tendency to habituation, should preferably be of increasing intensity or value. Such a situation is obviously self-limiting and ultimately frustrating. Yet the failure to recognize this fact can lead to the familiar syndrome of compulsively increasing consumption and decreasing satisfaction so characteristic of affluent cultures.

This discussion leads automatically to another central concept of many disciplines—namely, "attachment"—for which the closest Western term is addiction. Attachment signifies a condition in which the failure to fulfill a desire results in suffering. For example, if one wants or desires an ice cream but is not attached to having it, then one can be happy and enjoy the ice cream if it arrives but also be quite content if it doesn't. On the other hand, if one is *attached* to having the ice cream, then again one can be happy and enjoy it if it is available, but if it isn't the result will be frustration and pain.

Attachment is held by many disciplines to be a central cause of human suffering. For example, Buddhist psychology states quite explicitly, in the Buddha's second noble truth, that "the cause of suffering is craving." The path to liberation from suffering is said to lie in the third noble truth: reducing craving. The means for this is described in detail in the fourth noble truth as "the eightfold path," a prescription for ethical living and mental training. While stating it less explicitly, a variety of both Western and non-Western psychologies would agree with these principles.

Whenever there is attachment
Association with it
Brings endless misery

Gampopa[58]

Whenever we are still attached, we are still possessed; And when one is possessed, it means the existence of something stronger than oneself.

Jung[61]

The power to reduce our wants is all we have to oppose the forces of our lives . . . without it we are dust in the winds.

Castaneda[62]

However, in most cultures, including our Western ones, the lower-order motives predominate and there is little recognition of the existence and attainability of higher ones. Certain lower-order motives such as the acquisition of wealth and many material possessions are culturally valued and reinforced, and attachment to them is regarded as normal and even necessary for psychological well-being.[63] Whether the satisfaction of these desires is viewed in terms of tension release, positive reinforcement, gestalt completion, or other alternate models, Western psychologies have generally confused desire and attachment, and a certain degree of attachment is regarded as normal and necessary for motivation.

From this it can be seen that traditional Western psychologies and cultural beliefs differ significantly and centrally from non-Western psychologies and the consciousness disciplines. The latter differentiate between desires and the attachment to fulfillment of desires, stating that attachments represent the source of suffering. The indiscriminate satisfaction of lower-order needs is held to reinforce attachments, producing temporary satisfaction but a residual tendency towards stronger attachments and resultant suffering. Psychological well-being is thus seen as involving the relinquishment of attachments.

If you drop motivation there is no frustration in life. Then nothing can make you unhappy. . . . A Buddha becomes a Buddha only when all desires have disappeared. If you ask what motivates a Buddha you are asking him an absurd question. Nothing can motivate him. That's why he is a Buddha.

Rajneesh[64]

Higher-order motives however are held to be ultimately less entrapping, although it is said to be quite possible to become attached to desires such as self-transcendence and to suffer accordingly. In the words of the sixth century Zen monk Sengtsan,[59] "Even to be attached to the idea of enlightenment is to go astray." However what is different is that behavior motivated by such higher-order desires tends to ultimately reduce the number and strength of attachments rather than reinforce them. For example, it is reported by many individuals and disciplines that for persons attempting to train the mind and develop transcendent states of consciousness, the pull of such attachments as wealth, power, and fame is now experienced as agitating, disruptive, and hence aversive. Thus they are likely to be voluntarily and happily relinquished without any sense of sacrifice.

This allows an understanding of the concepts of "purification" and "letting go the world." From this integrative hierarchical model of motivation, "purification" can be seen as a conscious attempt to cultivate higher desires, especially those aimed at self-transcendence, and to extinguish lower ones. This is usually done by the simultaneous and long-term frustration and nonreinforcement of lower-order attachments (extinction), emulating advanced practitioners (modeling), and the practice of behaviors and attitudes which are increasingly consistent with the desired motives (successive approximation).

Since lower- and higher-order desires are externally and internally oriented, respectively, purification involves relinquishment of seeking external objects, situations, and reinforcement as the primary sources of satisfaction (letting go the world), in favor of internal reinforcers. From other perspective and models, this transition may be seen as involving shifts from gross to subtle realms (Hinduism), from field dependence to field independence (perception theory), from predominantly egocentric to predominantly selfless motivation, from attachment to nonattachment, and from environmental to self-control.

The hierarchy of motives and the concept of purification also relate to the Buddhist model of mental health. The central constitutents of this model are the so-called mental factors. These are said to be psychological factors which determine the relationship between consciousness and its stimuli. For example, the mental factor of greed is said to result in a state of consciousness in which the individual tends to grasp and cling to the stimulus. The factor of aversion results in a state in which consciousness seeks to avoid awareness of the stimulus. Most systems list some 50-odd mental factors of which some are said to be associated with psychological health and others, such as greed and aversion, are said to be unhealthy (see Chapter 9).[14]

Healthy and unhealthy factors are said to counteract one another by a type of reciprocal inhibition. Healthy factors include some motives which clearly belong at the upper end of the hierarchy, e.g., compassion, loving kindness, and altruistic joy, the joy which occurs with awareness of another's pleasure. Certain unhealthy factors clearly correspond to lower-order motives, e.g., avarice.

Purification and growth in the Buddhist tradition is said to involve "skillful means," the adoption of those behaviors, attitudes, motives, and meditative practices prescribed by the eightfold path. This path is designed to cultivate healthy mental factors and inhibit unhealthy ones, a goal that could also be described as cultivating the higher-order needs and inhibiting the lower.

The Major Human Motive

The nature of motivation has been a central concern for most psychologies, which have frequently centered on the question, What is the central human motive? Many have assumed that there is one fundamental motive and, having settled on what they believe this to be, have interpreted other motives as expressions, distortions, or denials of this fundamental drive. In doing so, different schools of psychology have thus focused on different levels of the hierarchy of needs. For example, Freud assumed sexual libido was the prime motivator of human behavior; Adler felt it was superiority-esteem striving; Becker thought it was heroics, the desire for central importance and "cosmic significance." While not denying the role of other motives, humanistic psychologists have emphasized that even the most neurotic defensiveness represents unskillful thwarted attempts towards self-actualization. For Carl Rogers,[65] "the basic actualizing tendency is the only motive which is postulated in this system." Transpersonalists have recognized the pull towards self-transcendence, while behaviorists have tended to focus on reinforcers more than on the nature of the desires with which they interact.

In general, there has been a tendency for each school to recognize and acknowledge as valid and independently real, motives lying below theirs on the hierarchy. On the other hand, they have tended to deny the independent validity of, and to explain and diagnose away, motives above their own. For example, in psychoanalysis the drive towards self-actualization might be perceived as a sublimation or defense against repressed sexuality, while some humanistic psychologists might deny the independent validity of the pulls towards self-transcendence and selfless service.

On the other hand, some Western (e.g., Jungian) and non-Western psychologies view the fundamental human motivator as essentially open, formless, transcendent, not attached to any particular object, a kind of free-floating available energy. In the perennial psychology, specific needs are said to represent constrictive expressions of the objectless transcendent energy, which is focused, constricted, shaped, and funneled towards specific objects. These then function as inherently less satisfying, substitute gratifications for the transcendent.

We thus have two divergent sets of views. In the traditional Western set, a specific motive is often seen as primary and others as secondary expressions of it, yet schools differ in what they see as the primary need. In the Eastern set, the primary component is seen as essentially formless and transcendent yet capable of expression as any specific motive. How are we to integrate these divergent perspectives?

Western psychologies clearly agree that there are many things that most of us desire but there is little agreement on what we desire most. Here we must ask a radical question. Is it really a thing or object that we desire? Is it really sex, power, prestige, cosmocentricity, self-actualization that we want, per se, or is it the state of consciousness and affect that they produce in us? Have we confused the object and the state of mind which the object elicits? For example, would one want sex if it elicited a state of deep depression? At the opposite extreme, would one want sex if one were already blissfully happy? This latter question suggests one reason why the Eastern traditions say that desires such as sex and power tend to extinguish as one begins to experience the extreme pleasure of transcendent states. That is, there is little desire for objects, activities, and experiences which elicit states of mind that one is already experiencing.

The next question is, What is the state of consciousness and accompanying affect that is most strongly desired? Simple logic would suggest a state of total positivity, of total bliss. Here we are in agreement with the perennial psychology which says that is exactly what is desired. That state and its attributes are described in many ways, but one of the most familiar is *sat-chit-ananda,* translated as total unbounded unlimited awareness, being, and bliss.[4,66] This is the condition occurring in the states of nirvana, formless jhana, samadhi, fana, etc. We are now in a position to suggest an integrating answer to the question which has divided so many schools of Western psychology: What is the fundamental human motive, what is it that men and women most deeply want? The answer is simple: a totally positive state of consciousness.

Eastern psychologies are unanimous in agreeing that this state of sat-chit-ananda can only be attained through mental training. It cannot be elicited or obtained by means of any object or thing. If this is so, why do most of us spend so much of our lives struggling to acquire objects, persons, or experiences which are so much less fulfilling? Why do we spend our lives desperately attached to what are, by comparison, relatively trivial concerns? Several answers suggest themselves.

Failing to appreciate that we really want the states of mind and not the objects which elicit them, we look outside rather than within for our sources of satisfaction. Unable to control our own minds to any significant degree, we have no experience, and in Western cultures usually no knowledge, of any transcendent states except orgasm and occasional brief peak experiences.

We seek then those stimuli which elicit the most positive experiences we know and think we can attain. However, as Norman O. Brown points out, "Mankind is unconscious of its real desires, and therefore unable to obtain satisfaction.''[67] The paradox, according to Sri Nisargadatta Majaraj,[68] is that "you do not ask for too much but for too little." Our pleasures are partial and substitute gratifications, and leave us with a sense, no matter how subtle, of unsatisfactoriness. This corresponds to the Buddha's first noble truth which stated that life is inherently unsatisfying for the untrained mind.

As soon as one desire is satisfied, another arises to take its place. The perennial psychologies are unanimous in agreeing that desires can be insatiable. Desires are likened metaphorically to an all-consuming fire, or a treadmill in which the pursuit itself maintains the illusion that one could be happy "if only one had. . . ." It seems one can never get enough of what one doesn't really want and that no *thing* can ever be fully satisfying. Satisfaction is said to come only to the person who recognizes the futility of looking outside him or herself for the source of satisfaction, who frees the mind from attachments to substitute gratifications and brings it under voluntary control, free from the distorting effects of uncontrolled fantasy-dialogue. The natural experience of such a mind, it is said, is that which is most desired, namely *sat-chit-ananda*.

Is the Hierarchy of Motives a Hierarchy of Desires, Needs, or Attachments?

Having differentiated desires from attachments to fulfilling desires, we can examine more closely the nature of the motives discussed in the hierarchy of motives. To what extent do these motives represent true needs whose lack of satisfaction will be pathogenic, to what extent do so-called needs derive from attachment, and to what extent to they represent only desire or wanting independent of need or attachment?

Maslow called his model a hierarchy of needs, arguing that the fulfillment of both lower needs and metaneeds was necessary for the avoidance of pathology and the development of the fullest human potentials. The failure to satisfy lower needs led to obvious physical and psychological pathology. For the metaneeds he suggested the existence of metapathologies such as loss of meaning and direction, cynicism, and anomie.

The question then arises as to whether the failure to fulfill the self-transcendent and selfless service motives also results in metapathologies. Here we are outside the realm of traditional Western psychological theorizing and research. We can, however, examine some of the non-Western psychologies in which there has been extensive discussion of this question, especially with regard to self-transcendence.

What we find in these psychologies is a broad consensus of far-reaching implications. The fulfillment of the drive towards self-transcendence is equivalent to the attainment of those states of consciousness described earlier as enlightenment.

From the perspective of those states, the absence of self-transcendence results in identification with the ego and its sense of isolation, aloneness, and angst. In this view, *all* states short of transcendence are viewed as relatively pathological, and the motivation towards transcendence would be labeled as a true need whose nonfulfillment results in the pathology and suffering of maya or samsara.

When we ask to what extent the strength of individual motives, and hence their position in the hierarchy, springs from desire and to what extent from attachment, we are on difficult grounds. The concept of attachment is so new to Western psychology that we can find no information here. Nor to our knowledge are the relative strengths of the two in determining overall motivation explicitly differentiated in non-Western systems. Presumably the two factors interact, but how is less certain.

One source of possible preliminary information is the phenomenological reports of advanced meditators and of individuals who are supposedly free of attachments. They suggest that desires without attachment function more as signs or indicators of need, rather than having any inherent compelling power. The sense of compulsion or being driven is said to be a function of attachment.

DEFENSES

Our prevailing cultural beliefs about defenses are largely psychoanalytic in nature. In general, defenses are held to be universal, essential, and part of a necessary, continuous, vigilant, self-monitoring to guard against an essentially untrustworthy self-nature. Some models hold that all motivation is basically defensive, and that conflict and defenses are essential to motivation and creativity. However, other perspectives are possible. In order to examine them fully it is necessary to first examine the fundamental nature, cause, and aim of defenses.

Let us begin with a definition as follows: defenses are processes in which we attempt to protect what we think we are by reducing or distorting awareness. Like all behavior, defenses originate from our beliefs about who and what we are. We defend whatever we think we are, our self-image or identity, against whatever we think we are not, including objectified, alienated parts of our psyche. We especially defend any perceived deficits or vulnerabilities in what we assume ourselves to be. Since most of us assume ourselves to be an ego, that is what we defend, and we defend it against anything and everything nonegoic, both intra- and extrapsychic.

Categorization of Defenses

Let us now consider how we can categorize defenses. Here there are four main dimensions to be considered.

1. What is defended (this is always an aspect of the self-image or identity, i.e., that which one thinks one is)
2. What is being defended against
3. The mode of distortion of awareness
4. Intensity of defense

Reducing and Distorting Awareness

One of the characteristics of defenses used in the definition was that they employ reductions or distortions in awareness. This differentiates them from more adaptive coping strategies which attain their ends without compromising awareness.

While it is probably true that all defenses exert both reducing and distorting effects, they differ in the relative amounts of these effects. Thus, for example, repression and denial clearly operate predominantly by reducing awareness. On the other hand, displacement and projection show marked distorting effects.

It is possible to rank defenses in a hierarchical order depending on the degree to which they compromise awareness. For example, rationalization involves explaining behavior in socially acceptable terms and tends to result in relatively little distortion. However, at the other end of the scale, denial involves a blotting out of reality, a traumatic reduction in awareness. A number of studies[69-72] have reported that healthier individuals tend to employ defenses which result in milder compromises of awareness, whereas more severe pathology is associated with more frequent use of grosser defenses.

> The most important criterion which determines whether a defense is relatively sophisticated or primitive is the amount of reality testing the defense retains.
>
> Giobacchini[73] (p. 29)

From this discussion, it is possible to point to some bridges between non-Western and our traditional Western conceptualizations of defenses. In the consciousness disciplines, the major problem confronting humanity is said to be distorted and reduced awareness resulting in suboptimal states of consciousness. The task of these disciplines is, very simply, to enhance awareness to optimal levels. What reduces awareness and what must be counteracted by these disciplines are defenses which have been mapped and categorized in considerably more detail by our traditional Western psychologies than by the non-Western traditions.

Again, according to the Buddhist model of mental factors,

> Of the fourteen basic unhealthy factors the major perceptual factor is delusion, a perceptual cloudiness causing misperception of the object of awareness. Delusion is seen as the fundamental source of unhealthy mental states.[74]

Delusion then, in this model, corresponds to a basic tendency towards misperception which underlies distortions of awareness produced by defenses.

In this system, delusion is counteracted by the major healthy factor of insight or understanding, which is "clear perception of the object as it really is." Delusion and insight cannot coexist in a single mental state. Thus, meditative training in the Buddhist system places great emphasis on the practice and cultivation of insight.

Creator/Victim of Defenses

A close examination of the dynamics of defenses suggests that they are actively, intentionally, and specifically created. Yet we perceive ourselves as their passive experiencers and helpless victims rather than as their creators.

Two possible explanations for this lack of awareness suggest themselves. The first is that defenses may originate in deep levels of the unconscious and hence remain inaccessible to us. Another possibility is that the awareness-compromising nature of defenses involves an active repression of awareness of their creation. There is some evidence from the consciousness disciplines that the latter perspective is correct. In deep meditation it is possible to observe an extraordinarily rapid process by which stimuli are recognized and evaluated for their threat potential, and defenses are chosen and constructed.[26,27] Similarly, some of the consciousness disciplines state that defenses are created intentionally but that the awareness of this process is repressed. For example, the following quotation is taken from an anonymous mystical Christian text:

> Defenses are not unintentional, nor are they made without awareness. They are secret, magic wands you wave when truth appears to threaten what you would believe. They seem to be unconscious but because of that rapidity with which you choose to use them. In that second, even less, in

which the choice is made, you recognize exactly what you would attempt to do, and then proceed to think that it is done.

Who but yourself evaluates a threat, decides escape is necessary, and sets up a series of defenses to reduce the threat that has been judged as real? All this cannot be done unconsciously. But afterwards, your plan requires that you must forget you made it, so it seems to be external to your own intent; a happening beyond your state of mind, an outcome with a real effect on you, instead of one effected by yourself.

It is this quick forgetting of the part you play in making your "reality" that makes defense seem to be beyond your own control. But what you have forgot can be remembered, given willingness to reconsider the decision which is doubly shielded by oblivion. Your not remembering is but the sign that this decision still remains in force, as far as your desires are concerned. Mistake not this for fact. Defenses must make facts unrecognizable. They aim at doing this, and it is this they do.

Anonymous[75] (pp. 250–251)

What Are We Defending?

We defend what we believe ourselves to be. Since most of us assume ourselves to be our ego, or more precisely our persona or acceptable self-image, that is what we defend.

Let us now recall the earlier discussion of the fundamental nature of the ego as a self-concept. That is, the ego is a conceptual self-image, a constellation of thoughts about the attributes we assume ourselves to be. At the most fundamental level then, *what we defend are our thoughts about who and what we are.*

As discussed earlier, the sense of self as ego appears to be created when consciousness identifies exclusively with thought. Moreover, precise trained observation such as in advanced meditation reveals that there is no abiding ego but rather a continuous shifting flux or succession of thoughts. The sense of a solid, permanent, and relatively unchanging ego or self is experienced as a result of imprecise perception and hence is fundamentally illusory. This is a key concept of most consciousness disciplines.[14,23]

This sense of self as ego therefore reflects a compromised awareness, and we then compromise awareness further in order to defend this illusory ego. This then may be the fundamental nature of defenses: *that they are distortions of awareness designed to protect distortions of awareness—illusions defending illusion!*

If the ego is a product of, and is maintained by, distortions of awareness, and if such distortions are the modus operandi of defenses, then is the ego itself a defense or defense system? Most Western developmental psychologies agree that the ego is constructed as a coping strategy. Could we argue then that the ego is that constructed self-sense which we believe we need to be in order to cope optimally?

If this is so why would we not construct a self-sense which was perfect, self-assured, and conflict free? The answer may lie in the belief systems that we adopt. The vast majority of us introject numerous limiting beliefs about who and what we are, can be, and what we need to do and be in order to survive and cope. Once these limiting beliefs are accepted, then the ego constructed in response to them may represent a perfectly logical response, an apparently appropriate self-construction for dealing with reality as it is believed to be. Within the context and matrix of the psychological reality created by our overall belief system, we may construct a subset of concepts and beliefs about who and what we are and what we need to believe in order to cope most effectively. Furthermore, once this ego self-sense is constructed, then the specific pattern of defenses which the individual creates to protect it may also follow quite logically and consistently. The total patterning of distortions of awareness, of both the ego self-sense and the defenses designed to protect it, may therefore represent perfectly logical responses to reality as it is believed to exist. From within the thought system each step may seem not only logical and appropriate but optimal.

> You cannot evaluate an insane belief system from within it. Its range precludes this. You can only go beyond it, look back from a point where sanity exists and *see the contrast*. Only by this contrast can insanity be judged as insane.
>
> Anonymous[75] (p. 164)

What Do We Defend Against?

We defend ourselves against anything which we perceive as threatening the survival or integrity of our self-image. Potentially this includes anything conceived to be "not-self," including alienated components of our psyche.

Deeper analysis into the fundamental nature of the mental processes involved in defense leads to some radical conclusions. The first question we must ask is, "What is it we defend against?" The answer is one which will be surprising, even unbelievable, to some and perhaps perfectly obvious to others, particularly those who have explored any of the non-Western psychologies or personally examined their own mental processes under the microscope of meditation. For what these divergent sources of information point to is that we do not defend ourselves against what actually exists at any given moment. That is, we do not defend ourselves against reality but rather against our interpretations and expectations of it, against our thoughts, fantasies, interpretations, and projections about the past and the future.

Let us take fear as a cogent example since fear is perhaps the primary emotional motivator for defense. At first glance it seems obvious that what we fear are aspects of reality, but a few moments' thought, and particularly a period of trained intensive introspection, reveals that we do not fear reality but rather our thoughts and fantasies about the possible future effects of that reality on us. What we fear are our own mental products, our own thoughts! Thus we are drawn to the far-reaching conclusion that both what we defend and what we defend against are none other than the creations of our own mind. We defend those thoughts we assume to be self against those we assume to be not-self.

The Cost of Defenses

Much has been written about the cost of defenses. Anxiety, fear, perceptual insensitivity, and symptoms of every kind are but some of the obvious effects. Here we will not go further into those costs which have been so fully described elsewhere. Rather, we will examine certain aspects which have not been clearly recognized in traditional models.

Defenses function by escape-avoidance learning. That is, we learn to reduce our experience of aversive stimuli by avoiding or escaping from them. One of the characteristics of escape-avoidance learning is that by virtue of its effectiveness it is very long lasting.[76] We can be so successful in avoiding experiences which we once found threatening that we may not give ourselves a chance to reexperience them and find out whether they remain threatening. Defenses therefore perpetuate the belief in the existence of vulnerability, illusory deficits, the aversiveness of the stimuli against which we defend, and the belief that defenses are necessary. Defenses may therefore maintain the very deficits they are meant to protect.

The State Specific Nature of Defenses

In our traditional Western psychological models, we have usually assumed defenses to be an inescapable part of human existence. However, in the non-Western psychologies we find frequent suggestions that defenses may be state specific. In those states where awareness no longer identifies exclusively with some aspects of self or reality to the exclusion of others, defenses are said to no longer operate.

In advanced stages of the consciousness disciplines, defenses and their attendant distortions of awareness are gradually pared away, the ego is recognized as a limited and illusory self-sense, and awareness starts to detach from this exclusive identity with ego to a new, more encompassing self-sense. This process is detailed in Chapter 16.

In the most extreme cases of detachment, such as various states of satori or nirvana, awareness no longer exclusively identifies with anything. With no exclusive identification, there is no dichotomy between self and not-self. There is only pure awareness which identifies itself with no thing, and because there is now no dichotomy, also with everything. Being no thing there is nothing to defend, being everything there is nothing to defend against. "Who is NOTHING will be afraid of no thing." [77] Indeed, with the realization of this state, there is the recognition that there never was anything that needed defense, the former self-sense and its perceived limitations and vulnerabilities are now recognized as illusory. Defenses are now seen as not only superfluous but as impediments to clear awareness and well-being.

Insights of this nature may underlie some of the long-lasting beneficial effects reported to follow even very brief transcendental states such as satori or peak experiences. [56,78] For example, even an instant of direct experience of the state of nirvana is said to permanently eradicate the belief in the existence of a solid, permanent ego and to result in corresponding personality changes (see Chapter 9).

Thus, defenses may not be the universal, essential, and creative coping devices they are sometimes thought to be. Rather, they may represent coping strategies designed to maintain a self-sense constructed in response to limiting and distorting beliefs about who and what we are and need to be. In states of consciousness and well-being in which these beliefs are recognized as incorrect, or when the me/not-me dichotomy is transcended, defenses may be recognized as superfluous and counterproductive maintainers of an unnecessarily constricted self-sense.

PSYCHOLOGICAL HEALTH AND WELL-BEING

Having presented a preliminary integrative model of the person, how can we use this to gain some insight into the nature of psychological well-being? At first glance it seems relatively simple. Theoretically, we simply examine the model and describe the positive ends of the dimensions which the model suggests. Experimentally, we examine groups of people, identify the characteristics of the most healthy, and see how they fit with the theoretical predictions. However, in both cases it is obvious that assumptions have already been made as to what health is. How else could we identify the healthy subpopulation? So it seems that we bring unexamined assumptions to our attempts to describe models of health, a point detailed in Chapters 5 and 6.

We therefore begin our examination of psychological well-being by probing one of the most fundamental assumptions of all and asking the question, What is it that is healthy? We have seen that our usual concepts of what we are dissolve upon deeper examination, and we therefore approach a model of health in terms of the deeper structures which such examination reveals. For example, to define health in terms of personality types as most Western psychologies have done is clearly insufficient. Remember that who we experience ourselves to be in the ultimate depths of our being, when all constricting limitations and exclusive identifications have been dropped, is both no thing or pure awareness, and everything, or the entire universe, transcendent to space, form, and time. From this realm of identity we can acknowledge a corresponding realm of very different possibilities for defining health. From this perspective, ego and personality are viewed as either subcomponents of self or illusory identifications. They do not define health at this transpersonal level.

Thus what we experience ourselves to be in the depths of the psyche is clearly transcendent to any dimension or concept of health. Like so many, perhaps all, subjective dichotomies, that of health and illness collapses in the deepest levels of being. In other words, who we experience ourselves to be behind our selective and partial identifications is beyond both health and illness, indeed beyond all definition. We are what we are, and any attempted definition, as the sages of the consciousness disciplines have told us for centuries, is meaningless.

Such paradoxes are familiar to those who explore the consciousness disciplines since paradox commonly results from comparing observations from different perspectives and levels. It is sometimes said that the twin lions which guard many Eastern temples represent confusion and paradox, and that the person who would have true wisdom must be willing to pass through both. Let us see how we can clarify this paradox of the nature of psychological well-being by integrating perspectives and levels.

If, as the perennial psychology claims, our true nature is pure awareness, transcendent to all definitions and dichotomies including that of health/illness, then what are we to make of the vast and incomprehensible amount of suffering which human beings endure and of our usual concepts of psychopathology and well-being? How are we to integrate these apparently radically oppositional viewpoints of Eastern and Western psychologies? An answer seems possible by contrasting the nature of the self which these psychologies assume to be real.

For the perennial psychology only the state of pure transcendent awareness is consistent with any true definition of mental health; all else is pathological. That is, all states of consciousness in which awareness undergoes selective, constricted identification are regarded as pathological. The result is seen as a case of mistaken identity (i.e., the ego). Awareness can experience itself as transcendent, unconditioned, unattached, and enjoying unlimited being, awareness, and bliss (sat-chit-ananda). However, awareness can also mistakenly and illusorily experience itself at the mercy of the distorting and suffering mind-body system and as a victim of emotion, thought, and sensation. This is the defining characteristic of psychopathology according to the perennial psychology.

Our traditional Western perspective, on the other hand, usually takes the ego to be the true self. Health is therefore logically defined in terms of the ego's adjustment and coping with its perceived nature and limitations. Western and non-Western discussions of health are therefore operating from different identity baselines, and many apparent contradictions and paradoxes can be attributed to this fact. In both systems, major pathology is seen as a function of disturbances in what is taken to be our true self. In both systems, a constriction of the self-sense through exclusive identification is viewed as pathological. For example, in the model of Carl Jung, when unfavorable aspects of the ego are denied and alienated as the shadow, what is left is a shrunken self-sense: the persona. It is thus possible to recognize a spectrum of states of identity and consciousness, at each level of which constriction of the self-sense represents pathology.[4]

From this it follows that movement towards health will be viewed differently by Eastern and Western systems. In the West, changes in psychological well-being are almost invariably measured in terms of ego or personality change. From the Eastern perspective, on the other hand, health is seen most fundamentally as a shift in identity away from ego. Here, ego and personality change may be regarded as useful or necessary preliminaries and facilitators but are seen as of secondary importance to this shift. From this perspective, our usual egoic state of consciousness is seen as a dream (maya, samsara), and the various psychopathologies with which we are familiar in the West are regarded as nightmares. The well-adjusted ego and the functional personality may indeed by less painful and more functional but at bottom remain a happy dream. Since one can awaken from any type of dream, it is not always necessary to change it. As the perennial philosophy would have it, "There is nothing to do, nothing to change, nothing to be." On the other hand, certain dreams are usually easier to awaken from than others. The aim of the consciousness disciplines could be described as developing lucid dreaming in which one knows that one dreams and is able to create that dream from which awakening is most easy.

Let us now turn to the integrative model of the person as outlined earlier and attempt to define the characteristics of those dimensions associated with well-being.

The first two dimensions of the model were consciousness and perception. Enhanced voluntary control of mental processes, which includes simple noninterfering awareness or mindfulness (Krishnamurti's choiceless awareness), would probably be a hallmark of well-being. This control might extend to a range of psychophysiological processes as in some of the reports of voluntary control of cardiovascular and other systems.[81] A less extreme example of this is the simple relaxation response.

One of the skills of an advanced practitioner of a consciousness discipline such as meditation is the ability to enter and hold specific states at will. For example, the expert meditator who is proficient in directing attention may be able to elicit a range of states of extreme concentration, known as jhanas in Buddhist psychology or samadhi in Hindu traditions, and to move between various states within this general family of concentrative conditions.

In addition to being able to enter a wider range of states, the very healthy individual may be able to elicit a wider range of functionally specific and true higher states and to use them to further enhance well-being. For example, Buddhist psychology provides detailed instructions for inducing states characterized by the predominance of mental factors such as compassion, loving kindness, or joy, and using them to counteract personality traits such as greed or anger.[81] Thus the attainment of such experiences can be used as a tool for further purification.

In the area of perception, attributes of health might include sensitivity, clarity, and relative freedom from distortion. "The fully realized human is one whose doors of perception have been cleansed."[40] Since these distortions appear to arise from the largely uncontrolled and unrecognized internal dialogue and fantasy, it might be expected that psychological well-being and its concomitant perceptual enhancement would be accompanied by a greater sensitivity to, and control of, this stream of dialogue and fantasy. This is indeed a common aim of most consciousness disciplines and is equivalent to stopping the internal dialogue which Maria and Gordon Globus[49] describe as a central component of the training of a man of knowledge.

Most psychologies of both East and West are unanimous in agreeing that perception is not a passive registration of reality but rather an active constructive process.[38] Since different states of consciousness may reveal different pictures of reality, it follows that we learn to construct *a* reality, not *the* reality. However, most of us learn to construct only one "reality," see it as "the truth," become attached to it, defend it, and panic if we experience perceptual shifts.[26,52] Nevertheless, it is clearly possible to cultivate other perceptual perspectives. For example, certain consciousness disciplines train their practitioners to view the world in selective ways, such as seeing all people as fundamentally loving. Such perceptual shifts also occur as concomitants of the states of consciousness which these disciplines elicit.

In summary then, we might expect extreme psychological well-being to be associated with certain perceptual characteristics. We might predict enhanced clarity, domination by positive mental factors, reduced attachment to any one viewpoint, and a greater range, fluidity, and voluntary control of perceptual perspectives (multiperspectivism).

In the earlier discussion on consciousness, it was pointed out that from the perspective of a multiple states model our usual state of consciousness fits the definition of psychosis, being suboptimal, providing a distorted perception of reality, and failing to recognize that distortion. Since any one perceptual perspective and its attendant state of consciousness are necessarily limited and only relatively real, from the broader perspective psychosis might be defined as attachment to, or being trapped in, any single state of consciousness or perception.[25,52] Thus the ability to perceive clearly, without attachment to any one perspective, represents awakening from psychosis.

> We grow up with one plane of existence we call real. We identify totally with that reality as absolute, and we discount experiences that are inconsistent with it. . . . What Einstein demonstrated in physics is equally true of all other aspects of the cosmos: all reality is relative. Each reality is true only within given limits. It is only one possible version of the way things are. There are always multiple versions of reality. To awaken from any single reality is to recognize its relative reality.
>
> Ram Dass[52] (p. 21)

Identity

For identity, perhaps the most relevant dimension for health would be the degree of conscious and choiceful relinquishment of self-other dualism. In most cases this would involve a choiceful inclusivity of identification in which what was formerly seen as other is now identified as self. That is, the more inclusive one's identity, the greater is the degree of health that would be expected. It should be noted that this inclusiveness involves both intra- and extrapsychic components. Intrapsychically we would expect that the individual who has recognized, owned, and integrated the shadow would be healthier than the person who has denied it. Similarly the individual who has recognized, owned, and integrated multiple personas (the social masks which we display to the world) and subpersonalities would be healthier than someone locked into a single one.

The perennial psychology extends this expansion of identity to the entire universe. The more highly developed individual is seen as one who identifies with others, with humanity at large, and with the cosmos rather than with self as an isolated entity. Ultimately the self-sense is said to transcend all dualisms and result in an all-encompassing sense of *tat tvam asi* (I am that also). At this level there comes the final recognition that, in the words of Norman O. Brown,[82]

The rents, the tears, splits and divisions, are mind made: They are not based on the truth but on what the Buddhists call illusion.

The concept of the healing of self-other splits as central to growth is found in a diverse range of psychological systems. This is the movement "from separation to oneness," one of the "classical metaphors of transformation."[83] The process is one of integrating and blending dichotomies, the classical *coincidentia oppositorum,* the alchemical *coniuncitio,* and the perennial psychologies' transcendence of dualism. As Wilber pointed out in "Where It Was, There I Shall Become," the process is also consistent with a range of Western therapies, e.g., Freudian, Jungian, and Gestalt. Freud stated[88] that he "decided to assume the existence of only two basic instincts, *Eros* and the destructive instinct. . . . The aim of these basic instincts is to establish ever greater unities." For Plato,[88] "this becoming one instead of two is the very expression of mankind's need. . . . and the desire and pursuit of the whole is called love."

This unification usually occurs by stages. For example, the first alchemical level is that of the *unio mentalis* (mental union),[84] corresponding to Wilber's[42] integration of persona and shadow; secondly, the *unio in corpore* and Wilber's mind-body or centaur level; and finally, the union of the individual with the *unus mundus* or Wilber's level of merger with the environment or cosmos.

Speaking of the difficulty that many Westerners experience in accepting the validity of this last level, Carl Jung[85] wrote:

I have studied these psychic processes under all possible conditions and have assured myself that the alchemists as well as the great philosophies of the East are referring to just such experiences, and that it is chiefly our ignorance of the psyche if these experiences appear "mystic."

Paradoxically this same realization may be attained by a process of progressive disidentification. For example in one technique of jana yoga, the practice which employs a refinement of discriminating intellect, one may minutely observe one's experience, noting that no component of experience contains a "self." This is the path of "neti, neti" (I am not this, not this), in which one progressively detaches the self-sense from the elements of experience with which it had formerly identified. By this process, said to be one of the most rapid but also one of the most demanding paths, one may eventually disrupt all self-other dualisms and arrive at the same nondualistic state of consciousness as revealed by the opposite path. This is an example of the adage that all paths converge at the top of the mountain.

Motivation

We would expect healthier individuals to be motivated more by higher-order needs and less by basic survival and security ones. Pulls towards self-actualization, self-transcendence, and selfless service might predominate along with concomitant behaviors and experiences such as ethicality, compassion, and commitment to humanitarian concerns. Maslow[56] pointed out that the lower-order needs were basically deficiency motivated, while the higher order needs or metaneeds were what he termed "being" needs or values. He suggested that when deficiency motivation predominates, an individual tends to react defensively and cling to current or former modes of coping, whereas when being needs predominate, the individual is open to novelty and growth. He, therefore, pointed to the possibility that the ratio of being needs to deficiency needs might provide an index of actualization. Since lower-order needs are basically aversive or avoidance motivators and metamotives are primarily approach motivators, the approach:avoidance ratio may be a similar measure.[86] Finally, a ratio of service-oriented to egocentric behavior might be a further indicator of psychological development.

Healthy individuals would probably be expected to display fewer and weaker attachments. One might predict from this that such individuals would be happier, experience less suffering, and be less caught up in the so-called material triumvirate—the desire for wealth, power, and prestige. With less desire for material acquisitions, one might anticipate greater voluntary simplicity. This is the term given to a life-style in which people consciously choose to simplify their lives, relinquishing those activities and possessions experienced as superficial and less satisfying so as to deepen and intensify those aspects of life felt to be most central and significant.[30]

> To have but few desires and satisfaction with simple things is the sign of a superior man.
>
> Precepts of the Gurus[87]

It is interesting to note that a similar shift has been observed at a cultural level by the noted historian Arnold Toynbee.[30] He found that the flowering and height of a civilization could not be measured solely by material parameters such as the degree of mastery over the physical world. Rather, an essential corollary and index of cultural development manifests as what he called "the law of progressive simplification," a trend towards reduced concern with grosser physical stimulation accompanied by a refinement of attention and interest in more subtle realms of experience. This may reflect movement up the hierarchy of needs at a cultural level.

As a concomitant of a clearer perception, expanded self-sense, and reduced attachment, one might also expect fewer and weaker defenses. In accordance with the finding that some defenses are more likely to be associated with relatively less perceptual distortion and with healthier modes of adjustment (e.g., intellectualization) and others with more distortion and pathological modes (e.g., denial and projection), then it would be expected that healthier individuals would display a corresponding pattern of defenses. This has in fact been found.[69-73] At the upper extreme, all defenses might be relinquished as unnecessary and burdening anachronisms.

Closely related to both perception and motivation are the Buddhist mental factors which were discussed earlier. Buddhist psychology provides an explicit and articulate description of factors said to be conducive to psychological well-being (e.g., concentration, calm, and equanimity) and their unhealthy opposites (agitation, anger, and greed). Mental health is said to be determined by the prevailing balance between healthy and unhealthy factors.

Summary

These then are some of the attributes which this preliminary integrative model suggests might characterize extreme psychological well-being. Although these attributes appear consistent with the suggestions of the major non-Western and some Western psychologies, they are largely lacking in empirical data. At the present time therefore, they must be considered preliminary hypotheses for future thinking and research rather than established principles.

This has been a partial and preliminary description which necessarily cannot do justice to the full range of the human potential. Perhaps no description can. On the other hand, however preliminary it may be, it does point to the possibility of future broad-ranging integrations between Western and non-Western psychologies. Each can contribute something to the other, and together they may be able to span the range of human development. We have only just begun.

> What lies behind us and what lies before us are tiny matters compared to what lies within us.
>
> Ralph Waldo Emerson

REFERENCES

1. Jung, C. *Collected Works,* Vol. 17. Princeton: Princeton University Press, 1970, p. 7.
2. Royce, J. Psychology is mutli-: methodological, variate, epistemic, world view, systemic, paradigmatic, theoretic, and disciplinary. In *Nebraska Symposium on Motivation 1975: Conceptual Foundations of Psychology.* Lincoln, Nebr: University of Nebraska Press, 1976, p. 38.
3. Corsini, R. *Current Personality Theories.* Itasca, Ill.: Peacock, 1977, p. 8.
4. Wilber, K. *The Spectrum of Consciousness.* Wheaton, Ill.: Quest, 1977.
5. Wilber, K. *No Boundary.* Los Angeles: Center Press, 1979.
6. Wilber, K. *The Atman Project.* Wheaton, Ill.: Quest, 1980.
7. Bohm, D. Quantum theory as an indication of a new order in physics: B. Implicate and explicate order in pysical law. *Foundations Physics,* 1973, *3,* 139–168.
8. Royce, J. How can we best advance the construction of theory in psychology? *Canadian Psychological Review,* 1978, *19,* 259–276.
9. Welwood, J. Self knowledge as the basis for an integrative psychology. *Journal of Transpersonal Psychology,* 1979, *11,* 23–40.
10. Erhard, W., Gioscia, V. and Anbender, K. Being well. This book.
11. Wilber, K. Odyssey. *Journal of Humanistic Psychology,* 1982, *22,* 57–90.
12. Maduro, F. and Wheelwright, R. Carl Jung. In *Current Personality Theories* (R. Corsini, Ed.). Itasca, Ill.: Peacock, 1977, p. 84.
13. Tart, C. *States of Consciousness.* New York: Dutton, 1975.
14. Goleman, D. and Epstein, M. Meditation and well-being: an Eastern model of psychological health. This book.
15. Wilber, K. The evolution of consciousness. This book.
16. Buddhagosa. *The Path of Purity* (P.M. Tin, translator). Sri Lanka: Pali Text Society, 1923.
17. Overton, D.A. Discriminative control of behavior by drug states. In *Stimulus Properties of Drugs* T. Thompson and R. Pickens, Eds.). New York: Appleton-Century-Crofts, 1971.
18. Walsh, R. The psychologies of East and West. This book.
19. Ram Dass. *Association of Transpersonal Psychology Newsletter,* 1975 (winter), p. 9.
20. Huxley, A. *The Perennial Philosophy.* New York: Harper & Row, 1944.
21. Smith, H. *Forgotten Truth.* New York: Harper & Row, 1976.
22. Anonymous. *A Course in Miracles, I: Text.* Tiburon, Calif.: Foundation for Inner Peace, 1975.
23. Goldstein, J. *The Experience of Insight.* Santa Cruz, Calif.: Unity Press, 1976.
24. Jung, C. *Analytic Psychology: Its Theory and Practice.* New York: Pantheon, 1968.
25. Ram Dass. *Grist for the Mill.* Santa Cruz, Calif.: Unity Press, 1977.
26. Walsh, R. Initial meditative experiences: I. *Journal of Transpersonal Psychology,* 1977, *9,* 151–192.
27. Walsh, R. Initial meditative experiences: II. *Journal of Transpersonal Psychology,* 1978, *10,* 1–28.
28. Kornfield, J. Meditation: theory and practice. In *Beyond Ego: Transpersonal Dimensions in Psychology* (R. Walsh and F. Vaughan, Eds.) Los Angeles: J. Tarcner, 1980.
29. Hendlin, S. Initial Zen intensive (sesshin): a subjective account. *J. Pastoral Counsel* (in press).
30. Elgin, D. *Voluntary Simplicity.* New York: Morrow, 1981.
31. Mahasi Sayadaw. *Practical Insight Meditation.* Kandy, Sri Lanka: Buddhist Publication Society, 1976.
32. Mahasi Sayadaw. *The Progress of Insight.* Kandy, Sri Lanka: Buddhist Publication Society, 1978.

33. Perls, F. *Gestalt Therapy Verbatim.* Lafayette, Calif.: Real People Press, 1969, p. 124.
34. Kornfield, J. Higher consciousness: an inside view. This book.
35. Satprem. *Sri Aurobindo, or the Adventure of Consciousness.* New York: Harper & Row, 1968.
36. Harmon, W. An evolving society to fit an evolving consciousness. *Integral View,* 1979, *1,* 14.
37. Castaneda, C. *Tales of Power.* New York: Simon Schuster, 1974, p. 33.
38. Royce, J., Coward, C., Egan, E., Kessel, F. and Mos, L. Psychological epistemology: a critical review of the empirical literature and the theoretical issues. *Genetic Psychological Monographs,* 1978, *97,* 265-353.
39. Tart, C. (Ed.). *Transpersonal Psychologies.* New York: Harper & Row, 1975.
40. Smith, H. The sacred unconscious. This book.
41. Brown, D. A model for the levels of concentrative meditation. *International Journal of Clinical and Experimental Hypnosis,* 1977, *25,* 236-273.
42. Wilber, K. Where it was, there I shall become. This book.
43. Walsh, R. and Vaughan, F. Beyond the ego: toward transpersonal models of the person and psychotherapy. *Journal of Humanistic Psychology,* 1980, *20,* 5-31.
44. Brenner, C. *An Elementary Textbook of Psychoanalysis.* New York: Anchor, 1974.
45. Laing, R.D. *The Politics of the Family.* New York: Pantheon, 1971.
46. Keisler, S. Emotions in groups. *Journal of Humanistic Psychology,* 1973, *13,* 19-31.
47. Assagioli, R. *Psychosynthesis: A manual of Principles and Techniques.* New York: Hohles and Dorman, 1965.
48. Wei Wu Wei. *All Else Is Bondage.* Hong Kong: Hong Kong University Press, 1970.
49. Globus, M. and Globus, G. The man of knowledge. This book.
50. Wilber, K. *Up From Eden.* New York: Doubleday, 1981.
51. Ramana Maharshi. In *Who Am I?* (T. Venkataraman, Ed.; 8th ed.). India, 1955.
52. Ram Dass. *Journey of Awakening: A Meditator's Guidebook.* New York: Doubleday, 1978.
53. Bugental, J. *Psychotherapy and Process.* New York: Addison Wesley, 1978, p. 139.
54. Schuon, F. *The Transcendent Unity of Religions.* New York: Harper & Row, 1975.
55. Murphy, G. and Ballou, R. (Eds.). *William James on Psychical Research.* New York: Viking, 1960, p. 324.
56. Maslow, A.H. *The Farther Reaches of Human Nature.* New York: Viking Press, 1971.
57. Roberts, T. Beyond Self actualization. *ReVision,* 1978, *1,* 42-46.
58. Gampopa. *The Jewel Ornament of Liberation* (H. Guenther, translator). Boulder, Colo.: Shambhala, 1971.
59. Sengtsan. *Verses on the Faith Mind* (R.B. Clarke, translator). Sharon Springs, N.Y.: Zen Center, 1975.
60. Evans-Wentz, W. (translator) *Tibetan Yogas and Secret Doctrines.* London: Oxford University Press, 1951.
61. Jung, C. *Collected Works,* Vol. Princeton: Princeton University Press, 1962.
62. Castaneda, C. *A Separate Reality: Further Conversations with Don Juan.* New York: Simon and Schuster, 1971.
63. Maslow, A.H. *Toward a Psychology of Being* (2nd ed.). Princeton: Van Nostrand, 1968.
64. Rajneesh, B.S. *The Alpha and the Omega* (tape recording). Poona, India: Shree Rajneesh Ashram, 1977.
65. Rogers, C. A theory of therapy, personality, and interpersonal relationships as developed in the client—centered framework. In *Psychology: The Study of a Science* (S. Koch, Ed.), Vol. 3: Formulations of the Person and the Social Context. New York: McGraw-Hill, 1959, pp. 184-256.

66. Smith, H. *The Religions of Man*. New York: Harper & Row, 1958.
67. Brown, N.O. *Life against Death: The Psychoanalytic Meaning of History*. Middletown, Conn.: Wesleyan University Press, 1959.
68. Sri Nisargadatta Maharaj. *I Am That*. Bombay, India: Chetana Publishers, 1973.
69. Vaillant, G.E. Theoretical hierarchy of adaptive age mechanisms. *Archives of General Psychiatry*, 1971, *24*, 107–118.
70. Vaillant, G.E. Natural history of male psychological health, II: Some antecedents of healthy adult adjustment. *Archives of General Psychiatry*, 1974, *31*, 15–22.
71. Vaillant, G.E. Natural history of male psychological health, III: Empirical dimensions of mental health. *Archives of General Psychiatry*, 1975, *32*, 420–426.
72. Vaillant, G.E. Natural history of male psychological health, V: The relation of choice of ego mechanisms of defense to adult adjustment. *Archives of General Psychiatry*, 1976, *33*, 535–545.
73. Giovacchini, P. Psychoanalysis. In *Current Personality Theories* (R. Corsini, Ed.). Itasca, Ill.: Peacock, 1977, pp. 15–44.
74. Goleman, D. A guide to inner space. In *Beyond Ego: Transpersonal Dimensions in Psychology* R. Walsh and F. Vaughan, Eds.). Los Angeles: J. Tarcher, 1980, p. 131.
75. Anonymous. *A Course in Miracles, II: Workbook*. Tiburon, Calif.: Foundation for Inner Peace, 1975.
76. Bandura, A. *Principles of Behavior Modification*. New York: Holt, Rinehart, and Winston, 1969.
77. Pant, A. Foreword. In Maharaj, N. *I Am That*, Vol. 2. Bombay India: Chetana Publishers, 1973, pp. ix-x.
78. Livingston, D. Transcendental states of consciousness and the healthy personality: an overview. Ph.D. thesis, University of Arizona, 1975.
79. Heath, D. The maturing person. This book.
80. Shapiro, D. *Meditation: Self Regulation Strategy and Altered States of Consciousness*. New York: Aldine, 1980.
81. Walsh, R. The ten perfections. This book.
82. Brown, N.O. *Love's Body*. New York: Random House, 1966.
83. Metzner, R. Ten classical metaphors of self-transformation. *Journal of Transpersonal Psychology*, 1980, *12*, 47–62.
84. Dorn, G. *Physica Trismegisti, Theatrum Chemicum, IV*. Ursel, 1920.
85. Jung, C. *Mysterium Coniunctionis, Collected Works*, Vol. 14. Princeton, N.J.: Princeton University Press, 1955, p. 535.
86. Walsh, R. and Davidson, P. Towards a behavioral estimate of mental health. *Proc. Cong. Roy. Aust. New Zealand College Psychiat.*, 1977.
87. Evans-Wentz, W.Y. (Ed.). *Tibetan Yoga and Secret Doctrines* (Lama Kazi Dawa-Samdup, translator). New York: Oxford University Press, 1935, p. 80.
88. Wilber, K. The pre-trans fallacy. *Re Vision*, 1980, *3*, No. 2.

Psychotherapeutic and healing approaches abound, and additional ones seem to be springing up with regularity. Further, as those in the health sciences look to religious and spiritual dsciplines for their healing potential, we are confronted with a maze of different practices, languages, and often cultural contexts which makes it difficult to know how to evaluate the claims and counterclaims of the different traditions.

In this chapter, Deane Shapiro attempts to systematically compare and contrast each of the traditions within this book with three Western traditions not included in this book—id psychology, ego psychology, and behavior therapy. By trying to order and evaluate these traditions along certain common dimensions—view of the person, goal of therapy, view of disease etiology, motivation, awareness, use of techniques, and qualities of the teacher and therapist—this chapter helps facilitate an understanding of where there are real differences between traditions and where differences are merely semantic distinctions. In so doing, it makes an effort to remove the "mysticism" from various approaches and to provide a foundation for subsequent integrative efforts.

18

A Content Analysis of Eastern and Western, Traditional and New-Age, Approaches to Therapy, Health, And Healing

Deane H. Shapiro, Jr., Ph.D

A Zen master asks his student, "Which would you rather be, a lowly stonecutter chipping away at the base of a mountain, or the mountain itself?" As he asks the question, he taps his foot on the stone floor, representing the clanging sound of the stonecutter chipping away at the mountain.

"I would rather be the stonecutter for he is stronger and chips away at the mountain."

"Very good. And now there is a nobleman for whom the stonecutter works. Which would you rather be, the stonecutter or the nobleman?"

"I would rather be the nobleman for he is the boss and master of the stonecutter."

"Very good," the master replied. "Now the nobleman has many fields which are being scorched by the hot blazing sun. Which would you rather be, the sun, or the nobleman?"

"I would rather be the sun which is more powerful than the nobleman."

"Again, very good. And now a cloud comes and blocks the rays of the sun. Which would you rather be, the cloud, or the sun?"

"I would rather be the cloud, for it is stronger than the rays of the sun."

"Now the cloud moves across the sky and runs into a large mountain which divides the cloud and makes it scatter into many pieces. Now which would you rather be, the cloud, or the mountain?"

"The mountain, of course, because it is stronger than the cloud."

And with that, the master smiles, again taps his foot on the stone floor, and bows.

A Japanese Folktale

The battle between competing viewpoints which attempt to gain supremacy in the marketplace is not limited to the political realm. The history of religion, psychology, and other disciplines is replete with battles, symbolic, mental, and/or actual, between different schools of thought. In terms of Eastern and Western traditions, traditional and new-age psychotherapies, there seems to be an endless number of alternatives, each making claims, at least along certain dimensions, for a certain supremacy. How is it possible to make sense out of what appears to be a myriad of approaches—each with its own assumptions, and often different language, cultural contrasts, and practices?

Given our current state of knowledge, there does not yet appear to be any particular orientation or school which has a complete hold on "truth." Almost every school has internal weaknesses and inconsistencies which need to be honestly faced. Unfortunately, if you ask adherents of any particular approach about this, all too often it seems that their school is defended, and "naive preconceptions" of the other schools are cited and then attacked. One can't help feeling, however, that "straw persons" are being generated without real understanding. Therefore, a prime task with which we are faced is to try to begin to look critically yet fairly at different psychotherapies and religious traditions, to compare one against the other, and to begin to see the strengths and weaknesses of each.

The consideration of such an undertaking raises several important concerns. First, it may be that some of the traditions are so different that to try to find a common interface may be impossible.[1] Second, there is often no common language, and therefore a selection of dimensions upon which to make comparisons feels, at least at this stage in our knowledge, somewhat arbitrary, artificial, and inadequate. Third, for some, an analytical, intellectual approach, comparing different traditions, may seem distasteful. There may be a feeling that an exciting, beautiful, and mysterious quest for new visions is being reduced to precise little boxes of analysis.

While not denying the above concerns, there may be several benefits in utilizing a systematic methodology to review each chapter. First, we can begin to see differences and similarities in the traditions. For example, we can see that all traditions have theories of human nature and that these theories may be quite different. We can see that although all approaches involve the role of awareness, the type of awareness utilized and the focus of that awareness may be radically different.

Second, if the dimensions we have posited are accurate across different therapeutic approaches, this systematic presentation may help us to specifically note weaknesses along certain dimensions of a therapeutic approach. For example, as we shall see, some approaches lump certain dimensions together, equating a vision of health with the person in his or her natural state. Other traditions have less to say about the nature of disease etiology, or in religious terms, the concept of evil.

Third, hopefully we can begin to see the strengths and weaknesses of each tradition more clearly. Fourth, we as consumers may begin to see which approaches from a philosophical "gut" level are more attractive to us and perhaps investigate some of our personal biases that cause us to be more attracted by certain traditions. Fifth, we may begin to look toward an integration, drawing from the strengths of each of the different traditions. Sixth, this content analysis may help us see where there are real differences between schools, and whether differences are actually semantic distinctions. Finally, this chapter may help us to remove some of the preconceptions that major schools have, one about the other. Some preconceptions are accurate; there may be real differences between the schools, and some of those differences may be disadvantages. However, some of the preconceptions are not accurate and seem to serve no useful purpose other than group affiliation.

Yet, even if we agreed to the worth of the project, and even if knowledge permitted, it would be nearly impossible to compare all traditions in detail along all the multiple dimensions which have been considered in both psychological and religious traditions. Therefore, certain choices must be made, and the biases inherent in these choices need to be made explicit.

In terms of selection of therapy approaches, I believe that all of the approaches discussed in this paper, Eastern and Western, traditional and new-age, may be viewed as schools of psychotherapy or change. To some it may seem confusing that religious or philosophical teachings (e.g., Zen and Sufism) are being considered as therapeutic approaches. I am looking at religions (Eastern or Western) as types of psychotherapy insofar as they represent attempts at healing. Regardless of whether religious systems are willing to evaluate their efficacy scientifically, the fact that they may enable a healing to occur and the fact that they may posit elegant visions toward which we might aim in our efforts at healing, I believe justify their inclusion here.

"New-age therapies" is a summary term which I am using to include the new awakening of Western interest in Eastern religious, transpersonal psychotherapy, and esoteric and mystical healing practices. Traditional refers to those "established" Western psychotherapies: classical id psychology, ego psychology, and behavior therapy.*

In this chapter, I will compare the different traditions discussed in this book, with these three "traditional" schools. I selected these three schools (a biased selection which may be considered arbitrary by some) because they provided different viewpoints about the nature of the person and, therefore, offer interesting contrasts with each other, as well as with the traditions in this book.

The next issue which needed to be tackled was which dimensions to utilize for comparison. The dimensions which I selected were those which seemed important because they appeared salient across many of the different approaches. Further refinement, however, may suggest that they could be clustered into fewer dimensions, or perhaps the grouping is too small and limiting and more may be necessary. As Walsh and Vaughan note,[2] the function of models is to "simplify phenomena so as to render them comprehensible to us. Models therefore collapse and order multidimensional, multilevel properties along a small number of salient dimensions." In so doing, this chapter will provide a method by which comparisons can be made in order to extract commonalities and differences between traditions along these certain dimensions.

Table 18-1. Dimensions for Comparison: An Overview.

Section I: Structure of the Theory
    1.1 View of the "person": human nature "as it is"
    1.2 Definition of enlightenment: view of psychological health
    1.3 Etiology of disease: barriers, obstacles, defenses, resistances

Section II: The Process of Change—Dynamics of the Theory
    2.1 Motivation
    2.2 Awareness/consciousness
    2.3 Qualities of the therapist or teacher
    2.4 Role of techniques

*The reader is asked to bear with and/or excuse this admittedly Western viewpoint; i.e., the Freudian id analysis is traditional and classic, although only 90 years old, and Zen and Eastern strategies are *new-age* although several thousand years old!

SECTION I: STRUCTURE OF THE APPROACHES

In this section, we will look at the view of the individual, the goal of therapy, and the etiology of disease. This section is divided into five parts. The first part explains these three dimensions. The second part describes more specifically the "traditional" Western approaches which are being utilized: id and ego psychology and behavior therapy. This detail is provided because those traditions are not included in this book and may not all be equally familiar to the reader. The final three parts look exclusively at each of our three dimensions as evidenced in the various chapters in this book. In those parts, an effort is made to be quite precise, in order to see how consistent a given theory is and to point out where theory and belief may be inappropriately stated as fact.

PART ONE: OVERVIEW OF THE THREE DIMENSIONS

View of the Individual

Each tradition's view of the individual is a *belief system* (implicit or explicit) describing how it views human nature "as is," i.e., at birth. All of us have, implicitly or explicitly, a theory of human nature. Yet up to this point in our knowledge, we do not yet know as fact what this human nature is. Rather, we all have beliefs about it. In this section, I would like to list different possible beliefs about human nature, and then suggest how the different authors/schools in this book portray their beliefs.* Basically, there are four broadly conceived beliefs about human nature as it is, summarized in Table 18.2.

Table 18-2.

THEORY	VIEW OF HUMAN NATURE
1	Innately evil/amoral
2	Innately good, self-actualizing nature
3	Tabulae rasae: existence precedes essence
4	Innately good and an essence in harmony with the divine

* I will also attempt to examine whether what is actually a belief is ever stated as proven fact (see Chapter 2 on demand characteristics).

Theory 1 states that the person is evil or basically amoral. Christians talk about this in terms of original sin; Freud talks about it in terms of the basic angry, aggressive, warring, amoral id. Theory 2 says that people are good. This view posits as innate nature a self-actualizing inner self which is good and positive. Theory 3 includes the blank slate or tabulae rasae view. In its most extreme form, argued by radical behaviorists, or the philosopher John Locke, it suggests that people are neither good nor bad. In an existential sense, it is existence preceding essence. There is no essence to the person. Essence is created by how people act. Theory 4 states that people have self-actualizing innate natures which not only are personal (as in Theory 2), but in fact reflect a spark of the divine or cosmic or transpersonal that is intrinsic to everyone. Finally, as we shall note, there are also combination theories.

The Goal of Teaching (Therapy, Discipline, etc.)

The goal of the teaching refers to the vision of psychological health and reflects the model of human nature from which it springs (see Table 18–3). Let us look at each of these in turn:

Table 18-3.

THEORY	VIEW OF HUMAN NATURE	VISION OF HEALTH
1	Innately evil/amoral ⟶	Lessen the evil and/or seek salvation
2	Innately good, self- ⟶ actualizing nature	Uncover the self
3	Tabulae rasae: existence ⟶ precedes essence	Create self
4	Innately good and in ⟶ essence in harmony with the divine	Uncover the essence of Self

1. *The Amoral Theory of Human Nature.* Since the person is basically evil, sinful, and amoral, the vision can only be to make them "less so." In Freudian terms, the goal is to give the individual more control over the id impulses; in traditional Christianity, the goal is to have the person seek salvation and God, realizing their basically evil nature.
2. *The Good Theory.* This theory suggests that a concept of health is having the individual uncover his or her own self-actualizing nature. "To move away from the facades, oughts, pleasing others, and to move toward self direction—being more autonomous, increasingly trusting and valuing the process which is himself."[78]

3. *The Blank Slate Existence Precedes Essence Theory.* The vision of this theory, in a relativistic world, is to choose one's self, to stand forth (existential), and to learn skills necessary for optimal cultural functioning (behavioral).
4. *Transpersonal Approach.* The vision is an awakening, nirvana, kensho to one's true self, which is "no-self" but rather part of the larger Self.

Thus, the first theory seeks to lessen the evil, the second and fourth theories seek to uncover the small self (Theory 2) and large Self (Theory 4), and the third theory seeks to create one's self.

Etiology of Disease

Why do mental health problems occur? Why are people evil? What prevents people from reaching the vision of health as posited by the respective approaches?

Our first theory of human nature, the evil theory, has the simplest explanation. Basically, individuals are starting from such a difficult place, are unwilling to acknowledge themselves and how bad they are, and don't have the potential (at best) to overcome that. The "good" theories (Theories 2 and 4) have a more difficult time explaining the issue of evil and obstacles, but they too have explanations as we shall see, including trying to meet external standards, oughts, and shoulds (Theory 2) and the mode of consciousness, impurity, ignorance, and desire (Theory 4). Theory 3 viewpoints such as the existential (existence precedes essence) or behavioral (blank slate) suggest that disease or mental health problems occur because of improper

Table 18-4.

THEORY	VIEW OF HUMAN NATURE	VISION OF HEALTH	DISEASE ETIOLOGY: BARRIERS, OBSTACLES
1	Innately evil/amoral	Lessen the evil and/or seek salvation →	One's basic nature
2	Innately good, self-actualizing nature	Uncover the self →	Shoulds, oughts, externals
3	Tabulae rasae: existence precedes essence	Create self →	Ignorance, poor choices, bad learning
4	Innately good and in essence in harmony with the divine	Uncover the essence of Self →	Attachments, greed, desire

learning or lack of learning, ignorance, and bad habits (behavioral approach), or from the recognition of our existential angst, bad choices, meaninglessness, and lack of purpose in the world (existential approach).

PART TWO: ADDITIONAL COMMENTS ON THE THREE WESTERN APPROACHES

There are two cautions which need to be stated as part of an introduction to these three approaches—id psychology, ego psychology, and behavior therapy. The first is an elegant statement made by Walsh and Vaughan about comparing approaches.[3] They note, "All therapies share considerable areas of commonality and any comparison risks magnifying and solidifying differences without acknowledging the overlap. Then too, there are often major discrepancies between therapy as it is idealistically described and as it is practiced. Furthermore, therapists of different theoretical persuasions will exhibit selective and differing perception when viewing the same therapeutic interaction. Finally, biases are hard to eradicate, no matter how objective authors attempt to be."

A second problem is that any lumping of traditions, although it creates simplicity in labeling and is useful to illustrate points, also obscures differences. Thus, attempts to make general statements about a tradition in the space of this chapter must be taken with a certain degree of caution. However, I am taking that risk because I believe that any effort to destroy naive conceptions on one side or the other provides a sufficient service which will outweigh the disservice that may similarly be performed by the lumping of traditions.

With that in mind, I would like to comment briefly on the three Western approaches which are being utilized here and to view them along the three dimensions discussed in Part One. As will be seen, Freudian (id) psychology is a close approximation of Theory 1; ego psychology is an example of Theory 2; and behavior therapy is an example of Theory 3.

Freudian (Id) Psychology

Because of the influence of Freud's writings on the history of Western therapy, this approach is discussed first. Here, id psychology and (historical) Freudian theory are used synonymously for this approach.*

*For purposes of a sharp comparison between different approaches, historical Freud's (pre-1920) libido-instinctual drive theory is used in this paper as synonymous with id theory. Freud himself, as well as later neo-analysts expanded beyond this id psychology approach, (cf. Freud, *Beyond the Pleasure Principle*) or Rosenblatt, A. and Thickstun, J. Modern Psychoanalytic concepts in General Psychology. *Psychological Issues,* 1977, *42/43,* 42-77.

View of Human Nature.   As an example of Theory 1, classical id psychology, represented by historical Freud, is a basically bleak picture of human nature. At a fundamental level, Freud believed that the individual is ruled by an amoral, pleasure-seeking id, is innately filled with anger and aggression, and is relatively helpless to effect change. As Freud noted, man is "lived by unknown and uncontrolled forces,"[4] which originate in the id. Further, he noted that the Christian commandment "Love thy neighbor as thyself" is justified only by the fact that "nothing else runs so strongly counter to the original nature of man. The stranger is in general unworthy of my love; I must honestly confess that he has more claim to my hostility and even my hatred; men are not gentle creatures who want to be loved; they are on the contrary creatures among whose instinctual endowments is to be reckoned a powerful share of aggression. . . ."[5]

The son hates the father and wants to kill him; the father and son vie for the mother's affection; the son fears castration from the father; siblings compete with each other; and often the individual dreams the death of those of whom he is fond, the dreams representing a repressed wish.[7] Although the ego struggles to control these amoral impulses which originate in the unconscious, id psychologists believe that the ego is in fact a passive rider on the back of the horse of id passions.[4] Thus, although the ego attempts to substitute the reality principle for the pleasure principle by means of secondary process thinking which involves words, logic, and the emotions kept within bounds, the ego is in fact according to Freud merely a differentiation from the id, that part of the id which has had to face reality.[91]

Goal of Therapy.   For those that begin with the Theory 1 view of human nature, the best they can do is come to some kind of resolution, i.e., the "best possible" conditions for the ego. For psychoanalytically oriented therapists, the task of therapy is to uncover and understand initial traumatic events, "to make the unconscious conscious, to recover warded-off memories, and overcome infantile amnesia."[65] Freud noted that the primary goal of psychoanalytic therapy was "where id was, ego shall be,"[92] and as he noted in his preliminary communications to Breuer,[77] "Each individual hysterical symptom immediately and permanently disappears when we have succeeded in bringing clearly to light the memory of the event by which it was provoked, and in arousing its accompanying affect, and when the patient has described that event in the greatest possible detail and has put the affect into words." In his *Interpretation of Dreams,* Freud said that normality/abnormality was a continuum based on the repression of the unconscious. The more insight a person had about himself, the less he had to repress and therefore the more normal he was. The healthier the individual, according to Freud therefore, the less material he still had repressed in his unconscious and the more self-awareness he had about his past. Thus, for Freud, the goal of psychotherapy is to secure the best possible psychological conditions for the function of the ego: "With that, it has discharged its task".[7]

Disease Etiology. As in all Theory 1 views of human nature, mental health problems are seen as inevitable. For example, as noted, the Christian viewpoint is expressed in the doctrine of original sin, suggesting that there will always be mental health problems because of the individual's separation from God.

From a Freudian perspective, mental health problems are really innate and built into the structure of the organism. Freud believed that the ego uses various defense mechanisms such as repression, reaction formation, intellectualization, sublimation, projection, and regression, to protect itself from the instinctual demands of the id. The etiology of disease or mental health problems is thus held to lie with the instinctual impulses of the id and the ego's attempts to repress them.[8]

Ego Psychology

Ego psychology is used by different individuals, at different times, to describe a wide variety of approaches. These range along a continuum from neoanalytic viewpoints of the conflict-free sphere of the ego (e.g., Hartmann, Kris, and Lowenstein)[9] to those believing in an innate, self-actualizing, intrapsychic ego (e.g., Rogers,[10] Maslow,[11] Angyal,[12] Goldstein,[13] etc.). In between there are, of course, Jung and his concept of the individuated self,[14] and R. White[15] and the concept of competence, etc. To delineate the differences most clearly, when I use the term "ego psychology," I am referring to Carl Rogers' client-centered therapy which reflects the "humanistic psychology" viewpoint of an intrapsychic self-actualizing nature (a Theory 2 viewpoint).*

View of the Individual. Rogers believes that the individual is not a warring battleground between forces of the id, ego, and superego. Rather, he believes that the individual's basic need is to constantly strive toward positive growth and, if given a choice between progressive and regressive behavior, the person will choose the former. As Rogers noted, "The organism has one basic tendency in striving—to actualize, maintain, and enhance the experience of the organism."[17]

*It is important that the reader not confuse humanistic psychology with the American Humanist Association, which defines "humanist" as follows. "Any account of nature should pass the test of scientific evidence. . . . We find insufficient evidence for the belief in the existence of a Supernatural. As non-theist we begin with humans, not God, and nature, not deity."[16]

Goal of Therapy. Theory 2, represented by Rogers, believes there is an innate, self-actualizing quality within each individual. Therefore, the goal of therapy is merely to provide a warm, supportive, trusting environment to allow the person to see and accept that innate self. In this way, the client can perceive experiences which are inconsistent with the self-structure under conditions involving the complete absence of threat. The inconsistent experiences can be examined objectively and the structure of the self revised to assimilate and include such experiences.[18] Thus, the client can see that he/she "is a person who is competent to direct himself and who can experience all of himself without guilt."[19] The goal of therapy is therefore for the person to feel and experience who he/she already is.

Disease Etiology. Since, according to Rogers, individuals already have self-actualizing natures, they "fall" from their state of self-actualization because they try to meet external oughts and shoulds.

Since in ego psychology the organism strives to be consistent with its self-image, experiences inconsistent with the self may be perceived as threats. The more threats, the more rigid the self-structure may become in order to protect itself and maintain itself. Thus, many experiences may be denied to awareness because they may damage the self-concept.

Behavioral Approach

This approach is used as an example of a Theory 3 viewpoint. Within a behavioral approach, however, we again have many different groupings, among them the radical behaviorists, the cognitive behaviorists, and the social learning theorists, and within each of these groupings there are additional subgroupings. When referring to behavior therapy here, I refer to principles derived from the experimental analysis of behavior[20] and social learning theory[21] to modify maladaptive behavior, teach new skills, and/or inculcate more adaptive behaviors. Behavior therapy consists of activities implying a contractual agreement between therapist and patient to modify a designated problem behavior, with particular application to neurosis and affective disorders.[22,23]

View of the Individual. The "blank slate theory" of behaviorism is similar to that posited by John Locke in which the individual is primarily conditioned by the environment, and it is the environment which has therefore been behaviorism's focus. The reason for this concern with the "externally observable" is that behaviorists hypothesize that there is neither the uncontrollable passionate unconscious of the id psychologists nor the self-actualizing intrapsychic nature posited by the ego psychologists. Watson, reacting against the introspectionist school of psychology, said, "Behavior can be investigated without appeal to consciousness . . . for the behaviorist recognizes no dividing line between man and brute." [24] The individual, according to social learning theory, is not motivated by the intrapsychic forces of ego and id, but by the environmental stimuli and contingencies. Therefore, Skinner says that the concept of self is not essential in the analysis of behavior (20, p. 285) and that the self is nothing more than a "repertoire of behavior appropriate to a given set of contingencies" [25] These behaviors have been learned, performed, and transmitted because of their survival value to the species. Skinner says that to speak of drives and internal states is not to focus on the cause of behavior but only on a mental way station. "A disturbance in behavior is not explained by relating it to felt anxiety until the anxiety has in turn been explained. An action is not explained by attributing it to expectations until the expectations have in turn been accounted for." [26] Later formulations [21] as well as the work of cognitive psychologists [27-29] suggest that internal behaviors (cognitions, images, etc.) have an effect on external behaviors, and also follow the same laws as external behaviors. Further, social learning theorists suggest that both behavior and environment can influence each other. [30]

Goal of Therapy and Disease Etiology

The goal of therapy historically has been social adaptation and has involved the following: a) to teach skills that haven't been learned; b) to decrease behavioral excesses; and/or c) to increase behaviors where there is a deficit or absence.

Behaviorists suggest that to be free, people need to have knowledge of the internal and external factors which control them. This means a) having more accurate knowledge of the consequences of alternative behaviors; b) learning more skills necessary for achieving objectives; and c) diminishing anxieties which restrict participation in the alternatives chosen. Freedom also involves having precise awareness of the internal and external environments, and arranging these environments in such a way as to maximize individual choices.

Table 18-5 summarizes these three different viewpoints—id psychology, ego psychology, and behavior therapy—across the three dimensions. These viewpoints represent Theories 1, 2, and 3, respectively, as described in Part Two. In the next section, we will look at the articles of this book which, for the most part, are representative of Theory 4 viewpoints. For comparative and illustrative purposes, one of these theories, Zen Buddhism, is included in Table 18-5 as an example of a Theory 4 viewpoint and transpersonal psychology. [31]

Table 18-5. Comparison and Contrast of Four Schools of Psychotherapy.

SUBJECT	PSYCHODYNAMIC (ID PSYCHOLOGY: FREUD)	CLIENT-CENTERED THERAPY (EGO PSYCHOLOGY: ROGERS)	SOCIAL LEARNING THEORY (BEHAVIORAL PSYCHOLOGY)	ZEN BUDDHISM
View of human nature	Aggressive; hostile, life out of control; ruled by unconscious	Innately good; intrapsychic self which is self-actualizing	Person is tabulae rasae at birth; with no "essence"	Humans possess pure, innate, good, unconscious "Self" that is like Buddha nature and is within all
Goal of psychotherapy	To make the unconscious conscious; overcome childhood amnesia; recover warded-off memories	To let the person experience that self which it inwardly and knowingly is	The target behavior: if deficit, teach it; if excess, decrease it; make it appropriate	To make the unconscious conscious; to hear the bird in the breast sing
Etiology of disease	Repression of sexual and hostile childhood wishes by superego and ego	Trying to meet external shoulds and oughts; inability to assimilate experiences into one's self-concept	Environmental variables; learning deficiency	Believing there is such a thing as the "self"; greed; ego; attachments

PART THREE: THEORY OF HUMAN NATURE

With the clear exception of the Globuses' article on don Juan, most of the approaches in this book fall into some version of our Theory 4 of human nature. This theory, as we noted, suggests that there is an innate, self-actualizing intrapsychic self within each of us, and this "self" is really part of a larger, divine Self. Unfortunately, however, the language of these Theory 4 proponents often appears to be imprecise, and sometimes it appears the author is positing a Theory 4 view, but talking from Theory 1 and Theory 3 viewpoints.

Theory 4

Some examples of statements from advocates of the Theory 4 view of human nature are as follows:

There is but *one* immortal Self common in and to us all.

There is an "essence" of being, sacred, divine, a transpersonal *Self* which is immortal, timeless, nonhistorical—not the individual ego.

Wilber[32]

For now, the point is that *great potentials are not so much created as remembered.*

Wilber[33]

It is generally agreed that one does not learn to become a Buddha, one simply discovers or remembers that one is already Buddha.

Wilber[32]

The journey itself is illusory, unnecessary, and ends where it begins and the recognition that what we are looking for is that which was looking.

Walsh[34]

The truth is here right now; things are as they are and nothing need be changed.

Kornfield[36]

We are well .... a paradigm which accords us our full and entire dignity. . . . For true mastery lies not in things or in paradigms, but in our ability to cause life to be serenely, magnificently, completely, what it is.

Being well *is* the awareness of the miracle that we are and that we are aware, and that we come *to* experience, wholly, entirely, and completely able to be.

In our most fundamental being, we *are* well. Each of us comes *to* experience whole, entire, and complete, well able to cause experience.

Erhard et al.[37]

Our real nature is liberation, but we imagine that we are bound to make strenuous efforts to get free, although all the while we are free. . . . In a sense, speaking of Self-realization is a delusion. It is only because people have been under the delusion that the non-Self is the Self and the unreal the Real that they have to be weaned out of it by other delusions called self-realization; because actually the Self always is the Self and there is no such thing as realizing it. Who is to realize what, and how, when all that exists is the Self and nothing but the Self.

Ramana Maharshi (cited in Kornfield[36])

The above examples suggest, as per a Theory 4 view that individuals have within them a core which is already perfect and that enlightenment is their natural state. *These views suggest that the view of human nature and the vision of extreme psychological health are the same.* Individuals are already enlightened and nothing needs to be done. However, at least for some authors, the metaphors become less clear, and theories appear to be "nonconsciously" mixed. Before citing examples of this, let me state that I believe "combination" theories may be quite important to help us understand all the complexities of a human. My concern here, however, is only to point out where metaphors may be being mixed without awareness on the author's part.

Theory 4 + 3

Some authors state Theory 4 (we are already there), but then discuss Theory 3 (we need to create, cultivate, and learn it); i.e., there *are* tasks we need to undertake.

Smith[38] and Erhard et al.[37] mix models in this way. Erhard says that people are fundamentally well, and that this wellness or "being well" is the experience of the awareness "I am cause." It appears that Erhard is saying that we are biologically determined to be "aware" *and* that we at the same time have the existential responsibility to create ourselves and chart our evolutionary futures.

Smith talks of the sacred unconscious within us, saying there is no mountain between us and our wholeness. However, he later says, "As human beings we are made to surpass ourselves and are truly ourselves only when transcending ourselves."[38] Wilber tries to get around these issues by saying that we need to distinguish between surface structures which are learned, conditioned, historically contingent, and culturally molded (Theory 3), and deep structures, which are cross-cultural, given, and invariant (Theory 4). He also suggests that "It's a person's ultimate condition and radical potential. It's your present nature and the end result of your development. Both goal and condition, the process of its own becoming."[32] Wilber is positing a teleological model, very similar to Teilhard de Chardin,[39] that individuals must inevitably move toward an omega point of higher consciousness, both individually and as a species. Everything ultimately is for the good, being pulled forward. He says, "Consciousness was not just conditioning as orthodox psychology maintains, but creative emergence and teleological striving, neither of which can be explained by reinforcement theory."[40]

Elsewhere, Wilber posits another variation.[32] He asks the interesting question about whether this "self" is something lost and then regained. Most transpersonalists, he notes, said yes and believed that one changes from unconscious transpersonal union to conscious personal self to conscious transpersonal union. However, Wilber suggests that the self may not have been there to begin with, but is created through various developmental stages.

With some theories, there is a hedging of bets between Theories 3 and 4. For example, Walsh[4] says "In any case, whether or not we think such qualities are fully perfectable, they can act as signposts and guiding values for our own lives." This line suggests that Theory 4 may be a vision to strive for, qualities to learn and work toward perfecting (*rather than* already being innately perfect).

Deikman[42] says that our current scientific culture suggests that "man imposes meaning; he does not discover it. That this assumption may be incorrect and productive of pathology is a possibility that needs to be considered." Is Deikman saying that it's bad to existentially create meaning (Theory 3)? Would it be better to uncover it or discover it (Theory 4)? If so, why does he say that? Deikman remains unclear as to whether he is positing a Theory 3 or Theory 4 view. He says that by developing our intuition and the third eye, as per the Sufi tradition, we can "create the conditions that will permit the development of man's full capacities as yet unrealized."[42] We need to ask whether these capacities are internal and not yet realized or are simply to be developed.

The above viewpoints reflect a combination of Theories 4 and 3. We now turn to those viewpoints that combine Theories 4, 3, and 1.

Theory 4 + 3 + 1

Theory 1 (the innately evil theory) is an embarrassment to many Theory 4 views, yet it has to slip in somewhere because even if people are innately "divine," it doesn't appear that very many people evidence this very much of the time. We talk about specific issues of "evil" in Part Five. Here, we discuss briefly the "innate" view of it suggested by certain authors in this book.

Goleman and Epstein are most clear in raising these issues, saying, "One common feature of these psychologies is *that they find fault with man as he is,* positing an ideal mode of being that anyone can attain who seeks with diligence to do so. . . . The Abhidhamma assumes as a starting point a person whose mind is bound by unwholesome factors"[43] (italics mine).

This is not a pure Theory 4 view of innate goodness. Rather, it appears both good *and* evil are innate. Further, there are aspects of Theory 3, in that an individual, with practice of techniques such as meditation, "increases the amount of healthy factors in his mental state."[43] Thus, one learns to cultivate and increase healthy factors in this model, which is different from uncovering those which are already there.

Less clearly stated, but also involving an implied combination of Theories 4, 3, and 1, are the following quotes.

From this integrative, hierarchical model of motivation, "purification" can be seen as a *conscious attempt to cultivate* higher desires, especially those aimed at self-transcendence, and to extinguish lower ones. (italics mine)

Walsh and Vaughan[2]

If you want to become wise, you will have to go through transformation. You will have to pass through fire. Only then, whatsoever ugly and useless is there, will be burnt! And you will come out as pure gold."

Rajneesh[35]

In this quote, Rajneesh is talking of our becoming wise rather than stating that we are already wise. Second, there is implied a Theory 1 "evil model" (e.g., "extinguish lower ones";[2] "ugly and useless"[35]). Where does this "ugly and useless" come from? Is ugly and useless something innate or something that's tacked on later? This is never made clear. Finally, is this a theory suggesting gold inside to begin with (Theory 4), or suggesting gold through transformation (Theory 4 + 3)?

Theory 3

Chapter 14, "The Man of Knowledge," is a clear Theory 3 viewpoint. There is no a *priori* essence to an individual. Rather, through assuming responsibility, one learns to *cultivate* personal power. The Globuses talk about believing without believing, or following a path of heart. They note that there is functionality in choosing one's beliefs. They have "usefulness as a force applied to his actions. . . . Once an action is completed, the belief is no longer relevant. . . . He uses the power of believing while remaining free of any belief. . . . He follows his "path with heart" fully committed to the end, yet knowing that the path is arbitrary. . . . rather than wanting life to be easy, the warrior *chooses* to take life as a continual struggle and a challenge. He chooses to believe that the world is unpredictable and mysterious."[44] Thus, the man of knowledge is not uncovering anything innate. Rather, he creates it with his beliefs: existence precedes essence.

Some Final Issues on Theories of Human Nature

We need to be careful of stating theories as facts. Otherwise, problems of imprecision and/or evangelism can occur.

One of the confusing areas is whether a theory posits an innate positive view of human nature (Theory 4) or the ability to create that vision (Theory 3). If a person believes Theory 3, then they may want to choose a variety of "paths of heart." If a person believes Theory 4, they may feel the "path" is already chosen, is within, and/or is teleologically determined (e.g., Wilber).

For example, Wilber[32] says that consciousness differentiates itself from the ordinary mind "and thus can be called an 'over-self,' 'over-mind,' or 'supra-mind.' It embodies a transcendence of all mental forms, and discloses, at its summit, the intuition of that which is above and prior to mind, self, world, and body," and this is a feeling of oneness with God. While acknowledging that these phenomenological perceptions are "true" (for those who have them), one still needs to question whether a person is uncovering an *a priori* truth (one that is true for all people), or experiencing a phenomenological "truth" and then creating a belief system based on that experience which worked for that person. If the former, does this mean that don Juan is wrong or that don Juan's path is of lower value?

Walsh and Vaughan note, "Even an intellectual discovery of the existence, nature, and attainability of higher motives may be sufficient to initiate such a shift, and suggests the importance of disseminating information about their existence."[2] If the will to transcendence is innate, then the Eastern and transpersonalists' belief system is right, and many in the West are resisting and blocking. If it's not innate but cultivated, then it's a choice, and they're prosyletizing their own values. For example, both Walsh and Wilber talk about existential angst which the "spiritual approach" says it subsumes. This, however, may in reality be a value judgment. One could argue that from a Theory 3 viewpoint—don Juan, Camus, or Sartre—that an existential reaction to the world is a legitimate, equally "valid" reaction. Because one has a belief system of oneness, à la Teilhard Chardin, does that necessarily mean that one has a *truer* belief system? If a belief system helps one cope, does that mean it's truer? Does it mean it will be effective for *all* people to believe it? Many of the authors in this book suggest, and one of the assumptions of the book is, that we need more ennobling visions, but ennobling visions may be different from statements of human nature.

A second interesting issue is, quite apart from the "truth" of these views of human nature, why some people are attracted to some viewpoints and others to different ones. Are there advantages and disadvantages for individuals in choosing different belief systems about the view of the person?

For example, to speculate, some may be attracted to an innate, humanistic, self-actualizing nature (Theory 2), or to a transpersonal, Zen good self, in harmony with other individuals and the divine (Theory 4). The belief in our innate self (or Self) may be quite comforting, a view that we are already good and perfect as we are. This may give some people a sense of acceptance of themselves (Theory 2) and a view of being in harmony with others (Theory 4). Yet, for others, those theories, if believed too strongly, may not allow for dealing with human frailty.

Some people may be more pleased with the belief that we are basically evil. That way, when they aren't good or when they have evil thoughts, they can be more accepting because it's part of their nature. Also, when they overcome this and act in ways they feel are virtuous, they can feel they have overcome enormous obstacles. To believe themselves already there, for some, may feel too simple.

Still others may get pleasure out of existentially choosing who they might become (Theory 3) and not like a theory which suggests that they are already determined, even if that determinism is a wonderful, self-actualizing nature. They might feel that they are stronger if they can say that there is no God, there is no life after death, and existentially we need to choose who we are.

Contrariwise, some people might find the existential viewpoint too pessimistic. If the world is meaningless and there is "no exit," what escape is there? Are we condemned to nothing but day after day of meaninglessness? Deikman discusses the importance for many individuals of having the belief that there is meaning in the world. Those individuals, therefore, would find the existential viewpoint somewhat despairing and would prefer a world view which suggests that things are positive and upbeat, and that everything is moving toward Teilhard de Chardin's omega point, getting better and better. Indeed there is something to the optimistic viewpoint about life, even if it is "mushy." Where is the ritual of celebration for the existentialists? Which view is most appealing to you? Do you prefer to existentially choose (Theory 3), to overcome odds (Freud; Theory 1), or to believe yourself there already (Theory 2)? Is a spiritual dimension important to you (Theory 4)?

Again, it should be noted that we don't yet know what the truth is. One thing that further research could clarify is how the different choices affect us, or why different people are attracted to different belief systems (and then support and cling to that belief system so strongly).

A final issue which needs to be addressed with regard to a theory of human nature is a differentiation which may be made between different levels of self. Theory 4 posits a view of a spiritual Self that is perfect and whole just as it is. Theory 4 may also posit that there is an egoic or false self, with which individuals may mistakenly and illusorily identify. This doesn't eliminate the issues, however, of whether the Self already exists in whole and perfect form (Theory 4) or as a potential which needs to be cultivated and to grow (Theory 3),[45] or of how (if) Theory 4 would differentiate between the illusory self and the already whole (even though not part of the spiritual oneness) self which Theory 2 posits.

PART FOUR: VISIONS OF PSYCHOLOGICAL HEALTH AND THE GOALS OF THERAPY

Although research has not yet, and ultimately may never be able to, resolve the issue of which view of human nature is "correct," ultimately it can be framed as an empirical question. Theoretically, therefore, it should not be an issue of "values" but of science. The view of the goal of therapy, however, is more in the middle. As we noted in Chapter 2, ennobling visions may serve many functional purposes. But can this vision of health ever be totally defined? Smith notes with a wry humor that the project of finding out what is the vision of health "must fail, of course, but that doesn't keep it from being interesting."[38] Let us turn to this view of health, what Wilber describes as an effort of looking for "the highest stage of unity to which one may aspire"[32] or, as Smith[38] says, "the kind of person we would like it [genetic engineering] to produce." What is the highest good for the human being?

Relationship of the Goal of Therapy to Different Views of Human Nature

The views of health in this book are based on either a Theory 4 view (in which case the goal of health is the same as the view of human nature, i.e., who we are is who we can be); a combination of Theories 4 and 3 (i.e., we can learn and cultivate certain qualities whose *potentials* are within); or Theory 3 alone (i.e., we can create this vision of health, *if* we choose to).

Heath and the Globuses argue from a Theory 3 viewpoint. Heath says that the vision of extreme health, what he calls "maturing," is a process whose end state is determined by survival and cultural adaptability. Heath posits an empirical survival view of why people arrive at the good life as opposed to an a priori biological/teleological view as posited by several authors in this book.

As societies have evolved, their survival as well as the psychological well-being of their members has depended upon the quality of adaptations that the group and its leaders made. We have seen that the attributes of maturity are consistently related to the effectiveness with which adults adapt to diverse and varying situations and roles. Might not the different religions have identified and valued as virtues those core universal qualities found to be desirable for the psychological survival and well-being of their society's members? The values that we identify with the good life—Enlightenment, the great man, the wise person, samadhi, salvation—find their roots in the collective experience of mankind, the facts of living fully and happily. These adaptive facts are human virtues.[46]

Chapter 14, by Maria and Gordon Globus, is an example of an existential belief system suggesting that "paths lead nowhere" and that individuals, while realizing the insignificance of life, need to act with personal impeccability, not because it leads to a spiritual harmony or uncovering a oneness, but because that's what the individual chooses as his dance. The Globuses state that this person has a joyful spirit, which "results from having accepted his fate, and from having truthfully assessed what lies ahead of him."[47] This is quite different from the Eastern viewpoint of harmony and oneness, and more similar to Heidegger and Camus' description of the existentialist person seeing the vulnerability of life and choosing to confront it. As the Globuses noted, "Seeing...makes one realize the unimportance of it all'.... 'nothing is pending in the world ... nothing is finished, yet nothing is unresolved,' ... all victories and defeats are equal."[44]

Erhard and Smith, among others, are representative of a combined Theory 4 + 3 view, although they argue that we are already well (Theory 4). As Erhard notes, "The phrase 'human potential' is not wholly satisfactory since it tends to imply the fixed existence of predetermined potentialities and possibilities, which we ought thus to fulfill. It may be that we ourselves are now required to generate and manage our own evolutionary options and opportunities."

The Qualities of the Healthy Person

What are the qualities of this wise person as suggested by the authors of this book? Determination and effort are mentioned by several (Globus and Globus; Shapiro; Smith; Walsh, along with flexibility and adaptability (Heath; Shapiro; Smith); developing a sense of meaning (Deikman) and affirmation to life (Smith); dying to a finite ego (Goleman and Epstein; Kornfield, Smith; Walsh; Wilber) and losing self-importance (Globus and Globus); developing compassion and selfless service (Kornfield; Goleman and Eptstein; Smith; increased depth of intimate relationships (Heath; Shapiro and Shapiro); and developing "control" of one's mind and body (Globus and Globus; Shapiro; Walsh; Wilber).

One group of these qualities suggests religious, spiritual, or sacred values, a sense of affirmation about life. Smith suggests that the fully realized person knows the human conscious is sacred, "for true holiness has something to do with the whole" and seeing it in the ordinary. Smith describes the truly healthy person as "someone who has a honed sense of the astounding mystery of everything and lives in the numinous."[38] He suggests that the opposite of the sense of the sacred is drabness and taken-for-grantedness. Smith continues by saying that for this person there is an affirmation of life even while realizing its pain. "A realized soul is more in touch with the grief and sorrow that is part and parcel of the human condition, knowing that it too needs to be accepted and lived as all life needs to be lived." There is a sense of affirmation. "The peace that *passeth* understanding comes when the pain of life is not relieved." He notes that the Eastern masters "did not erode the yes-experience of the East's 'it is as it should be' and the West's 'Thy will be done.'"

Ethical virtues are another frequently mentioned group of qualities. Heath says, "I suggest that honesty, compassion, integrity, commitment, steadfastness, and courage are universally valued among the great religious traditions, that they are the behavior/virtues we educate for when we are furthering the maturing of youth, and that they are the values central to the 'good life.'"[46] As Wilber states, "We can see phenomenologically that these people experience a growth in love and balance of mind as a result of a radically new vision of the world."[32]

These virtures are echoed for Buddhism by Goleman and Epstein[43] who describe "the four illimitables" or measureless states—compassion, sympathetic joy, all-embracing kindness, and equanimity—some of which are among the ten paramis (the ten perfections of Buddhism) which Walsh discusses.[41]

Dramatic shifts in the experience of self also seem to be central to many discussions. Rajneesh gives a beautiful first-person account of his experience of this enlightenment, of letting go of his individual "self," and finding himself with a feeling of oneness.

> Everything was unreal, because now there was, for the first time, reality.
> For the first time, I was not alone.
> For the first time I was no more an individual, for the first time the drop had come and fallen into the ocean. Now, the whole ocean was mine, I was the ocean; there was no limitation. A tremendous power arose, as if I could do anything whatsoever. I was not there, only the power was there. I was relaxed, I was in a let-go, I was not there. It was there, call it God.[35]

Further, it is frequently suggested that the extremely healthy person is said to be less dependent on reinforcement and hence less attached to having specific outcomes occur. According to Chogyam Trungpa Rinpoche, as quoted by Kornfield:[36]

> An enlightened being has no such attitude [need for reinforcement]. Whenever someone requires his help, he just gives it; there is no self-gratification involved.

Or, as Lao-tse[48] noted:

> Truly, only he that rids himself forever of desire can see the secret essence; he that has never rid himself of desire can only see the outcome.

Final Comments on the Goal of Therapy

There are two final comments of the goal of therapy that are worth noting. The first has to do with how some theories (particularly Theories 2 and 4) may be confusing (and combining) their view of human nature as is with the goal of therapy. Let me give an illustration of a potential problem with this.

The existential vision of individuals as free to choose their own goals with personal autonomy is clearly an elegant one, and it values important qualities such as individual responsibility, autonomy, and choosing meaning in a meaningless world. Yet even though the vision is elegant, does that mean *in fact* that individuals are born a priori with that freedom or with the skills necessary to realize that vision? Perhaps as Nasrudin,[49] the wise fool of the Sufi stories suggests, individuals may initially live in a drunken awareness and, as Skinner[50] noted, be quite conditioned by their social environment, thereby living in an illusion of freedom. Perhaps through techniques of both East and West, individuals can *learn* skills for personal freedom and can attain the existential vision of freedom. If we assume that people are born with existential freedom, however, we may be doing a disservice to reality. We may be attributing skills that are not there. This is not to say that we shouldn't have a vision of people learning to become free, autonomous, and inner directed. However, we should not merely automatically assume that our vision of health is necessarily synonymous with our view of basic human nature. In fact, I would argue that the existentialists offer a weak theory of human nature and a strong vision for the goal of therapy.

A second interesting issue in terms of the goal of health is whether it in fact makes a difference if one's theory of human nature is like Theory 3 (learned and created), or like Theory 2 or 4 (one is already there). Carl Rogers, reflecting a Theory 2 view, suggests individuals have a natural inclination to learn and, when given the freedom, will do so. Homme, a student of Skinner's, reflecting a Theory 3 view, believes that there is not an a priori drive to learn; rather the student has been reinforced for exhibiting behaviors that someone has decided are representative of the desire to learn.

Yet, although reflecting different views of human nature, both discuss the same types of strategies for increasing individual freedom. Homme talks about a five-step method of transferring goal setting and reinforcement from the teacher's control to the student's control. In this way the student has to be his own manager, set his own goals, be his own evaluator. Carl Rogers points out that ways to increase freedom to learn include encouragement of self-evaluation and a concomitant removal of the threats of grade (external evaluation), as well as the use of contracts, having the pupil set goals for himself and make plans of how to reach those goals. Thus, in terms of a vision of education and giving more "control" to the student, both Homme and Rogers would agree that when a student chooses his own direction, discovers his own resources, formulates his own goals and his own problems, decides his own actions, and lives with the consequences of his choices, significant learning is maximized. Therefore, the question we must ask is whether given different views of human nature, two approaches might end up with the same goal of therapy.

For example, if we believe in a vision of graceful beauty, of divinity, of a self-actualizing nature, and *act as if* we had that within us, and if other people are also "divine beings" who should be respected, this may influence our behavior and become a self-fulfilling prophecy. Whether it is innately there or not may be only an academic question. This may be similar to the issue illustrated by Michelangelo, who believed that the sculptures he created were actually encased in the rough marble, waiting to be freed by him. Were they really? Or was it Michelangelo's *belief* that they were, his vision of what the sculptures would look like, and his training and skill which allowed him to reach the vision?

PART FIVE: DISEASE ETIOLOGY

Every theory, including Theories 2 and 4, is sufficiently reality-based to see that the world isn't the best of all possible places, that evil exists, that not all people are fully realized or at least don't act as if they are and, in most cases, don't feel as if they are. Thus, even though Smith says there is no mountain separating us from who we are and who we wish to be, nevertheless he acknowledges that this is a lesson most of us never learn. What are the mountains (or no-mountains) that keep people from reaching their full potential? There are really two issues here. The first is a question of what initially causes people to "become sick," defined here as failing to reach optimal psychological health as defined by the respective approach. As noted for Freud, this disease etiology is rooted in a view of human nature as ruled by an amoral id. Therefore, disease is built in. For Christians, the concept of original sin again makes the battle one from birth. The second issue is a question of what defenses, barriers, and resistances *subsequently* occur as the person strives to reach his full potential. It is to these issues that we now turn.

Theory 1, suggesting that "evil" is built in, and Theory 3, suggesting that poor habits are learned (behaviorism) or that choices are made in bad faith (existentialism), provide clear and understandable theories as to disease etiology or barriers to health. The other theories (2 and 4) don't really give much explanation about why, if we already have a self-actualizing nature (Theory 2) or spiritual, perfect natures within (Theory 4), so many problems subsequently occur such as identification with the egoic self, development of "the three poisons" of desire, ignorance, and aversion, etc.

Goleman, discussing the Abhidhamma, provide one of the few views to specifically account for these problems. Reflecting aspects of a Theory 1 view, he state that, one reason few people achieve ideal mental health is due to *anusayas,* latent tendencies of the mind toward unhealthy states. These unhealthy factors both cause suffering and are barriers to positive health. He notes that seven unhealthy factors are particularly strong anusayas: greed, false view, delusion, aversion, doubt, pride, and agitation, and he also discusses the unhealthy factors of agitation, worry, torpor, remorselessness, egoism, and the five hindrances, including lust, ill will, sloth and torpor, agitation and worry, and doubt.[43] These unhealthy factors cited above, are reflected by many of the traditions in this book. These obstacles to reaching the goal of therapy may be summarized as affective, perceptual, cognitive, and attentional. Before discussing the specific problems which can occur in each of these areas, it seems important to give a brief description and definition of each of these terms, particularly because they are often used without being precisely defined, and since they also overlap and influence each other.

Cognitions, as used here, refer to thoughts and images. Affect refers to emotional response, and may involve a combination of physiological cues and cognitive interpretation of those cues. Perception refers to the intake of sensory data, and may be influenced by our affective state and/or our cognitive labeling of experience. Attention refers to a conscious effort applied to perception, and involves both what we focus on (content or context) and how we focus (active or passive; concentrative or mindful; analytical or holistic). Attention may influence, or be influenced by, cognitions, affect, and perception.

Although the traditions acknowledge the interconnectedness of the above issues, there is no effort made (or any indication that there is any need) to label one of the variables as a prime cause. Smith and Deikman, like Goleman and Epstein, refer to unhealthy affective factors such as desire (including lust, greed, and grasping) and aversion (fear, hatred and anger), and how these color and influence our perceptions of the world and cause us to see it less veridically. What we take as facts, Smith notes, are largely psychological constructs as the Latin *factum* (that which is made) reminds us. In addition to affective barriers, there are also cognitive ones, such as ignorance, which Smith notes is separating ourselves from others. This ignorance causes us to divide the world into what we like and dislike, involves the use of analytical attention, and further leads us away from understanding our true selves and the world around us. For these reasons, Deikman suggests the need for nonanalytical, intuitive modes of attention, stripped of affect,[42] and Smith points out that perceptual barriers, colored by personal affect and cognition, lead us to believe that there is in fact a mountain separating us from our true selves.

For many of the authors, affective, perceptual, cognitive, and attentional issues converge and cause great difficulty around identification with the "ego" or self, and efforts to defend this self.

Many of the authors in this book suggest that the ego or self is that which keeps us from seeing our large Self, the Buddha nature within. As soon as we can let go of our sense of separate self, including labels, cognitions, analysis, and affect associated with it, we can see our "divine Selves." The egoic self, point out these authors, is really an illusion, a series of events, and the relationship between mental states and sense objects. It is this self, according to the Theory 4 viewpoint, which keeps us from seeing our true Self.

It should be noted, however, that not all of the authors and traditions in this book, have the same view of the self. For example, for don Juan, there is no such thing as the large Self, and the discussion revolves around the importance of developing personal power and, at the same time, losing self-importance.[44] Heath[46] stresses the importance of personal autonomy and developing a strong sense of self. These different views of self can partly be understood with reference to the theory of human nature from which they are evolved. A Theory 3 view of human nature, reflected by Heath and the Globuses, does not believe in the larger *Self* and therefore may come from different assumptions about what does or does not assist that human nature in developing its full potential.

A summary of the different views of human nature, the vision of health (goal of therapy), and the disease etiology is illustrated in Table 18-6.

SECTION II: THE DYNAMICS OF THE THEORY— THE PROCESS OF CHANGE

Each school in this book, as well as the Western therapeutic approaches, has a theory about the *process* by which people can change and evolve toward their respective visions of psychological health. Even "pure" Theory 2 and 4 viewpoints, which say that the individual is already innately perfect, work toward getting people to change attitudes, and thus to become more aware and accepting of that perfection.

This section will examine the process of change, by looking at four specific components which are considered important (in varying degrees) by all traditions: qualities and role of the teacher/therapist; role of techniques; awareness/consciousness; and motivation. Clearly there are other components in the process of change—responsibility, decision making, commitment, etc.—and therefore the list of components, though important, is not meant to be exclusive. Rather its inclusion is a function of personal interest and space limitations, as well as the fact that these dimensions often reflect substantial disagreement, confusion, and varying positions between traditions.

MOTIVATION

Why do people have a desire to change? How strong does that desire need to be in order for change to actually be effected? How can individuals develop the determination, energy (the first two of the ten paramis), and commitment to follow through on their desire? These questions all relate to the issue of motivation, which may be one of the central areas that needs to be addressed in all therapeutic (and religious) orientations. It is one thing to create a vision of extreme psychological health, yet quite another to understand the dynamics by which a person strives in order to achieve that vision. Why do people go to the confessional, to monasteries, into psychoanalysis? Each of the views of human nature has a theory about motivation, about what causes people to act and change. These include tension reduction model (Freud, Theory 1); environmental cues and consequences, negative and positive rein-

Table 18-6.

AUTHOR/ARTICLE	VIEW OF HUMAN NATURE	VISION OF HEALTH	DISEASE ETIOLOGY: BARRIERS/DEFENSES (INCLUDING EGO)
		PART I	
Walsh	Leaning toward 4, but no clear	Not Discussed	Not Discussed
		PART II	
Wilber	4 (remembered, not created)	Eastern "holistic," causal and subtle realms; spiritual unity	Expand the ego to include all; hierarchy of defenses
Erhard, Gioscia, and Anbender	4: being well, awareness "I am cause," plus existential choosing (3)	Existential mastery	Develop the ego and transcend it; dichotomous consciousness; content/context
Heath	Not stated	Integrity, empirical survival view, compassion, courage	The need for a strong ego is important but can be a problem
Shapiro and Shapiro	3	Relationship as a context for intimacy	"Out of control" feelings; personally and relationally
		PART III	
Walsh	4, but also mentions 1 and 3	Ten *paramis*	Greed and unhealthy factors
Goleman and Epstein	4, 1, 3	Healthy mental factors, four illimitables: compassion, kindness, sympathy, and equanimity	The anusayas: lust, torpor, sloth, doubt, ego
Shapiro	4	Buddha nature; the mirror	The belief in "I"
Smith	4 primarily: we are already at vision; no mountain exists; slips into 3s; "surpass ourselves"	Sacred unconscious: assertive and yielding; accepting, compassionate; affirming	"No mountain" exists—but; the three poisons: greed, ego, our finite self; poor perceptual awareness

Deikman	Uses Theory 4 (person discovers but doesn't impose) but also seems to imply Theory 3 model	Intuition and the third eye; sense of meaning	Let go of ego, vanity, greed, intellect, emotion over intuition
Globus and Globus	3	Existential path of heart	Fear; power; clarity; old age; feeling one's self equal to everyone; but not self-important
Kornfield	4	No "self"; but Self is God; Compassion; not needing rewards	Ego, intellect, unwillingness to surrender; need for reinforcement
PART IV			
Wilber	4 on essence of being; in-depth structure; 3 (on surface?)	A Chinese puzzle with the spiritual realm at the top	Fear of transcendence; death terror
Shapiro	3	A person who is "in control" on multilevels of reality, mind, body, self; and is able to balance these levels as well as "active" and "letting-go" control	Lack of a "crisis" to make one reflect upon one's life; lack of models to illustrate the vision of health; and lack of skills to achieve the vision
Walsh and Vaughan	4 and 3, some 1?	Reduce exclusive identification with self; cleaning perceptions; reducing defenses; increasing mindfulness and consciousness; toward an integration of different dimensions	Exclusive identification; misperception; defenses
Shapiro	Uses 3 as theory, but also tries to act " as if" 4	Doesn't posit a position, but tries to summarize other's views	Tries to summarize other's views Not Discussed

forcement (Theory 3, behavioral); attempts to create meaning and order in a meaningless universe (Theory 3, existential); and a hierarchy of motives ranging from deficit to being motivation (humanistic/spiritual, Theories 2 and 4).

As we shall see, great precision may be necessary in discussing these issues of motivation. Some theories speak in undimensional terms of motivation or of a steady progression up the ladder from the lower to higher motivations. However, it may be that different motivations are functioning at different times within the same individual, and at the same time within the same individual. Therefore we may be dealing with quite complex multilevel criteria, all under the rubric of "motivation."

Suffering or Crisis as a Motivator

Almost all traditions within this book agree that the recognition of some type of crisis or suffering is a primary issue that can catapult us into efforts to change. Each vision, however, may have different views about what causes the suffering. Freud said suffering occurs when affect attaches itself to a neutral idea, i.e., a compulsion neurosis. from an existential viewpoint, suffering occurs in recognizing the meaninglessness and emptiness of the world. In Theory 2, suffering occurs when one tries to follow shoulds and oughts that are externally imposed. The behavioral viewpoint suggests that suffering occurs when an individual receives a paucity of reinforcement, engages in maladaptive behaviors, and/or doesn't have the skills to function effectively. Theory 4 viewpoints provide a variety of causes for suffering, such as the Buddhist's discussion of the causation of pathology (samsara), the chain of dependent origination, ignorance which causes craving, etc.

These traditions seem to be suggesting, at some level, that people don't change naturally, but need a jolt, whether personal, interpersonal, professional, or spiritual, to make them question their habits and recognize the "suffering" in their lives. A metaphor which may be used is the term "crisis" borrowed from the Chinese word *wei-ji,* meaning turning point. *Wei-ji* consists of two characters, meaning danger and opportunity. Crisis, which causes suffering, can be a motivator to increase the opportunity for the person to be willing to change. Rajneesh says, for example, "Some foreign element is needed to give you a shot, to jog you out. It is just as if you are asleep and you have been asleep for many, many lives."[35] Rajneesh notes, "This spiritual anxiety is the first step toward understanding true reality, or liberation." The Globuses, echoing a similar theme, state that the warrior begins with a certainty that his spirit is off balance, and that "too much wanting and needing makes for unhappiness and loss of well-being."[44]

The Buddhist's first noble truth states that life as normally lived is suffering, and awakening to this is the first step on the path to liberation.

Elaboration of the Four Theories' Views of Motivation

Theory 1. Freudian theory posits a drive reduction model of motivation, in which certain instinctual drives originate in the id. Once these primary drives—hunger, thirst, sex, and agression—were reduced, the individual was satiated.[53] However, how is it possible to integrate this theory of motivation which suggests that energy comes from the id trying to cathect objects on the basis of the pleasure principle, with a theory of human nature suggesting that the ego is passive and has no strength of its own? Although Freud stated that psychoanalysis had a goal of "enabling the ego to achieve a progressive conquest of the id"[4] and to "transform what is unconscious into what is conscious, enlarge the ego at the cost of the unconscious,"[54] because the ego had no energy in his model of motivation, he became tied by his own Gordian knot.

Further, since Freud believed, based on the Helmholtz school of medicine, that the id and the libido were of limited and fixed size, there was therefore only a limited amount of energy available to motivate the individual. Since all motivation was drive reduction, Freud stated that in order to develop and advance civilization, it was necessary for the individual to sublimate his sexual energy.[5]

Theories 2 and 4. Freud's tension reduction model was modified by Hartmann, Kris, and Lowenstein, who suggested that the ego, rather than merely reacting to the id's impulses, may in fact be a "conflict-free sphere."[9] Still later formulations suggested not only that the ego may have an energy of its own—a drive toward competence[55,56]—but also that there was not a fixed amount of libido to motivate a person which, if given up, could not be reclaimed.[57] This provided the soil for the ego psychologist and the organismic psychologist, who reacted against the traditional psychoanalytic concepts of motivation coming entirely from the id and being of fixed size. They argued that since the ego had an energy of its own, a new conception of the person and of the human potential was possible. Maslow characterized motivations into two types: deficit and growth motivation. Deficit motivation included such things as (1) physiological and physical needs; (2) safety and security needs; (3) love and belongingness needs. These were analogous to primary drives, and their satisfaction served as a reinforcement by reducing tension. Maslow also posited, however, (4) esteem needs and (5) self-actualization needs: the needs of an organism to become what it has the potential to become.[11]

The above formulation helped break the Gordian knot that Freud had created, for now there was a healthy aspect of the person, an ego which strove toward self-actualization and, most importantly, had its own energy for so doing. The goal of therapy then became to remove the obstacles to self-knowledge and self-realization so that the innate real self could freely develop.[58] When motivations such as self-transcendence[59] and selfless service[2] are added to this hierarchy of motivations, we have a Theory 4 viewpoint.

Theory 3. Social learning views of motivation range along a continuum, with the primary emphasis being on social and environmental variables, contingencies, cultural stereotypes, models which are reinforced, and other conditioning. Motivation, according to Skinner,[20] comes primarily from the environment. Since behavior is a function of environmental variables,[60] Skinner noted that he was not concerned with concepts like drive reduction and did not want to infer learned drives or any other internal motivational force or traits. He noted, for example, that he was less interested in hunger as a drive than he was in the environment which kept food from the organism.[20] Drive was a convenient way of referring to the observable effects of such deprivation of food, but it is unnecessary, he noted, in a functional analysis of behavior. A behavioral position suggests our behavior is a function of reinforcement, either positive reinforcement or negative reinforcement (the removal of an aversive stimulus).

Some Final Comments on Motivation

Visions of extreme psychological health may serve as helpful motivators for individuals. If one extrapolates from the research on vicarious modeling, it could be suggested that individuals who espouse and live noble causes can teach us new ways of acting and, particularly if they are reinforced for their beliefs and behavior, can serve as motivators for us. We may need to distinguish, however, whether these "being" motivators are examples of drives and needs which are innate (Theories 2 and 4), or whether they are consciously cultivated choices which a person existentially chooses (Theory 3).

If we take a Theory 2 or Theory 4 viewpoint, as a belief system, we might want to be sensitive to whether our desire and effort to live by being motivations—self-actualization, self-transcendence, selfless service, approach behavior—might cause one to deny, be less sensitive to, or try to positively reformulate lower motivations. Cognitive relabeling of "negative reinforcer" or avoidance learning to growth or approach learning may be a useful technique and strategy, and may in fact serve as a beneficial motivator, but we might want to again distinguish between beliefs of these as innate motivators rather than as techniques to cultivate specific types of motivation. In this regard, we can see that a similar principle may be utilized, and called quite different things, by each of the traditions. For example, a tension reduction model (Freud) may be referred to in social learning terms as negative reinforcement (i.e., removal of an aversive stimulus). Similarly, part of the Buddha's four noble truths and eightfold path is in fact an effort to reduce tension (suffering), again what social learning theorist's would call negative reinforcement. Similarly, nonattachment, transcending ego, and losing desire may be seen as effective because they also remove the aversive stimuli (i.e., the attachments, the desires, etc.) that cause suffering.

Finally, if we were to look toward an integrated theory of motivation, we would again realize the great difficulty and complexity of the task. Others have tried to integrate specific aspects of different theories' motivational systems. For example, Dollard and Miller[53] among others[61] have tried to combine Freudian views of primary drive with behavioral views that environmental cues determine when, where, and how the person will respond. Similarly, it could be suggested that the Theory 2 viewpoint—that individuals are motivated by more than tension reduction and have an innate hierarchy of motives (needs)—could be integrated with the behavioral view which would suggest that the expression of these needs would be very much dependent upon past conditioning and present reinforcers.

To add a further level of complexity to the issue of motivation, let us look at the following two issues. First, let us assume that there are several aspects of reality: body, mind (attention, cognition), self (ego), professional, intimate, and spiritual. Let us further assume that multiple motivations (deficit and being) can occur on each of these levels: survival, belonging, sex, fame, money, power, intimacy, self-actualization. Then let us add one more assumption: the need to have a sense of control (including creation and creativity as an effort to have more order and perceived meaning).[62]

Therefore, might we not consider that there could be multiple motivations (sometimes conflicting) within each level and that these motivations might change over time. Might there also be a way to determine percentage of variance of motivation in order to determine, at a given time, the different factors that motivate an individual for a particular action? For example, on a professional level, how much of one's motivation at a given time might be to enhance one's ego, to make money, to give to others, to make an impact on humanity, etc.?

Might the percentage of a certain type of motivation on one level (e.g., ego) be different than on another (e.g., intimate or spiritual)? Perhaps we could even begin to plot and eventually predict when a certain context, or motivator, has been overused, is too high, and is ready to be habituated for one that has been too low and needs attention (e.g., when power needs might give way to intimacy needs.)[63] This is to suggest that motivation may not be a linear, unidimensional, ascending hierarchy and that so-called higher motives may not always develop last. Perhaps we can "skip" steps or levels of reality, and later have to fill them in. In terms of Maslow's need hierarchy, certain refinements might seem useful. Some deficit motivations may be seen as necessary (i.e., survival, physical needs) and others may be seen as questionable from any standpoint (i.e., desire, craving, greed, aversion, the world of samsara). So-called deficit motives may be functional at certain levels and dysfunctional at other (so-called higher) levels. A strong sense of ego may be functional at an ego or professional level, but not as functional at a spiritual or intimate level. From a teleological or religious point of view, higher motivation may be selfless service, giving to others, being relatively egoless and more in harmony with the world and oneself. However, this may need to be seen as a value, and again may be a product of multiple variables (e.g., to help reduce one's own suffering and egocentric motivation by increasing the amount of healthy factors in the mind, the active joy of giving to others, etc.) Moreover, we might need to be careful of the battles which can occur over whose motivation is higher (e.g., the arahat of Hinayana Buddhism versus the bodhisattva of Mahayana Buddhism). Otherwise there may be danger of rhetorical debates and belief systems clouding the very real complexity, intricacy, and subtlety of the dimension of motivation.

AWARENESS/CONSCIOUSNESS

Each of the traditions, therapeutic schools, and disciplines described in this book acknowledges that consciousness, or awareness, is a cornerstone of its approach. Different traditions, depending upon their view of human nature, suggest different types of awareness strategies to reach a vision of health. As we shall see, awareness is a quite complex, multifaceted issue involving the potential for multiple states of consciousness depending on questions such as a) *where* one focuses attention [e.g. on historical content, current content, specific context, metacontext, attention itself]; *how* one focuses attention— [e.g. holistic awareness, precision discrimination (of a single object; of whatever arises) with subsequent nonreactive awareness or with subsequent analytic awareness]; as well as *depth* of attentional absorption and focus. Further, different approaches argue that certain aspects of reality are more important to perceive clearly than others, and suggest what they believe to be the best type of awareness for that task. Finally, quite different words are used to describe that of which we are not aware—nonconscious,[64] selective inattention, repressed unconscious,[8] even a range of five different types of unconscious.[32]

In terms of words used to describe awareness itself, the task becomes even more difficult, since different words are used by different traditions, sometimes with the same word having radically different meaning, sometimes different words having the same meaning. Attention, consciousness, self-awareness, higher states, functionally specific states, *tonal, nagual,* ordinary awareness, altered states of consciousness—all are terms used with different meanings at different times by some of the traditions. Again, some schools refer to the content of awareness, some refer to the context of awareness, some refer to awareness of awareness, some refer to the vehicles of awareness (perception), and some refer to the mind as encompassing all of these. Indeed, there is great confusion about these different modes, both within traditions and between traditions. In this section we are going to try to begin to become more precise about description and differentiation of different types of awareness as they are used by various disciplines.

The Content of Awareness and the Context of Awareness

Psychodynamic theory searches for the etiology of the symptom in psychosexual (psychosocial) stages of development for it is believed that the timeless and historic unconscious is the cause of symptomatic behavior. Thus, in the Freudian approach, there is an effort to attain historical insight (awareness) into repressed memories. Because the ego was thought to perform an intellectual, censoring function, techniques for developing awareness attempt to bypass this ego. Thus, Freudian strategies often use free association (with subsequent therapist interpretation) as well as patient dreams (the royal road to the unconscious[6]) to gain this awareness and insight.[65]

Rogers, reflecting the ego psychological viewpoint and theory of human nature, suggests that individuals need to become more aware of the self-actualizing nature within. In this way, Rogers hoped that the individual could let go of external facades, and become more aware of internal experience. As he noted, psychological adjustment existed when the concept of self was such that all the sensory and visceral experiences of the organism could be assimilated and felt as congruent with that "self."[10] Thus, whereas Freud wanted historical insight into the childhood disease etiology, Rogers wanted current awareness and acceptance of present feelings and emotions.

The behavioral approach focuses on what is causing and maintaining the problem behavior in the here and now environment. There is no attempt to probe childhood memories for the etiology of the problem, and the person's past learning and reinforcement history are believed to be important only insofar as they influence present perceptions and subjective expectancies.

Although the focus of awareness is different in the above approaches (i.e., historical memories, perceiving the "real self-actualizing self," here and now functional analysis of the environment), they all are similar in that the focus is on the *content* of experience. Many of the traditions in this book, however, emphasize that focusing on the content of awareness is not as important as focusing on the process of awareness. As Wilber notes, "What inquiry does is disengage attention from the objective displays and turn it on consciousness itself. More precisely, with inquiry, attention turns on attention itself, and on the very *nature* of attention."[32] This point is reflected by Goleman and Epstein[43] who say,

Conventional psychotherapies assume as givens the mechansim underlying perceptual, cognitive, and affective processes, while seeking to alter them at the level of socially conditioned patterns. Asian systems disregard these same socially conditioned patterns, while aiming at the control and self-regulation of the underlying mechanisms themselves.

As an aid to further understanding this distinction between context and content of awareness, it is important that we now look at two different types of awareness, described by several of the traditions in this book—analytic awareness and holistic awareness.

Analytic Awareness and Holistic Awareness

These terms represent two of the many possible different states of consciousness and are often used with slightly different meanings, depending upon the tradition discussing them. Therefore, so that there will be no confusion in the ensuing discussion, let me define what I mean by each of the terms. Analytical awareness refers to the type of awareness which involves precision, with subsequent cause and effect "intellectual" analysis. This type of awareness is reflected in the behavioral technique of self-observation in which one labels a behavior, and then observes how that behavior is influenced by the environment (both internal and external environment) both by antecedent conditions (people, places, events which increase the probability of the behavior occurring) and by consequences (reinforcement and punishment) which sustain the behavior. In this type of awareness, a person can learn the relationship between his own behavior and aspects of the physical, social, and internal environment which condition that behavior. This type of analytical awareness uses words and language to describe experience, focuses on content, and is dichotomous. This is the realm which don Juan calls *tonal,*[44] and what Erhard et al. refer to as consciousness (which has content and is dichotomous).[37]

The second type of awareness is holistic awareness which, as defined here, refers to looking at (1) the whole rather than the parts; (2) *kairos,* a timeless moment, rather than chronological linear time; and (3) awareness which occurs without labeling, categorizing, and/or describing the experience, but just experiencing it (and later, having neither experience nor nonexperience). As referred to in this book, it includes holographic and nonhistorical levels of awareness, "a level wherein the person is the whole, and the whole is of the person."[32] Erhard refers to this as a nondichotomous awareness: "Awareness is consciousness' context; consciousness, its content."[37] Castaneda referred to this as the *nagual,* the area without boundaries, which emerges when we stop the internal dialogue. This transcendent, nondichotomous awareness may allow for a sense of oneness, a merging of subject and object.

Is One Mode of Awareness Higher than the Other?

Almost all traditions discussed in this book suggest that our normal state of awareness is suboptimal. For example, Nasrudin, the wise fool of the Sufi stories, talks about the drunken awareness within which we live.[67] Freud discusses the way we use defenses and repression to avoid seeing what is really happening within us, and Skinner notes that awareness is something that doesn't occur naturally for individuals, but only when social contingencies make it necessary. Thus, Skinner notes that most of us live in an illusion of freedom, with little awareness. Therefore, almost all traditions, whether they place a major emphasis on dichotomous or nondichotomous awareness, believe that our normal state of being involves suboptimal awareness.

The issue then begins to become somewhat cloudier. Many of the traditions in this book appear to be saying that nondichotomous awareness is "higher" along many dimensions. Erhard et al.[37] suggest that this nondichotomous state, awareness, is what makes us whole and what allows us at our fundamental level to be well. They suggest that dichotomous consciousness—i.e., discriminations of health and illness—are second to this:

> We often confuse criteria of well-being drawn from our *consciousness* with criteria drawn from our essential *natures,* and thus confuse being well—which we *are*—with consciousness of experience which we call sickness or wellness, whichever we have at the moment.[37]

The Zen master Renzai said,

> If the heart is still, where do you find the passion? Do not tire yourself by making up discriminations and quite naturally, of itself, you will find the way.[68]

The problems cited with regard to analytical awareness include the following: (1) analytic awareness can only understand itself and can never analyze a nondichotomous state; (2) there are limits to our intellectual capacity and ability to understand reality through reasoning alone;[69] and (3) life needs to be experienced on more than one level. As Martin Buber notes, "To live only in an I/it objective world may cause us to lose the beauty of expressing I/thou relationships."[70]

Given these real limitations, does that necessarily mean that nondichotomous holistic awareness is higher? Although many of us, trained in the West,[71] can clearly see the limitations of precision analysis, it may be important to point out that this type of awareness can be quite valuable in giving us information about the ways in which we interact with the world. From this perspective, it can be a "higher awareness" than acting in a reflexive, conditioned way. Further, somebody that hasn't had training in intellectual and analytical skills may find understanding of the relationship between oneself and the environment—cause and effect understanding—to be an incredibly powerful experience, perhaps no less powerful, no less "high" than someone with nondichotomous altered state experiences which are described in this book.[35,40] How can we decide which is higher?

The term "higher states" used often in this book[2,6] is used in Charles Tart's sense of possessing all the properties and potentials of lower states, plus some additional ones.[72,73] I wrote to Tart about this, posing two questions: (1) Might neither state be "always" higher, but rather higher depending on the situation? and (2) How can a holistic, nondichotomous altered state ever include a dichotomous state?

In reply, he noted as follows:

If you were crossing the street and reality required you to avoid a truck coming down on you but you were immersed in the undifferentiated whole, I suspect this would be a quite "lower" state of consciousness! . . . . Thus the all absorbed "holistic" state . . . might be good for a person [in that] it provides a certain kind of experience that's vital in overall balance, and yet itself is not a state which would be adaptive to be in all the time.[74]

Regarding the second question, he said,

We certainly do get reports of states in which a person feels like they are aware of "everything" and yet don't seem to have any memory of being aware of anything in particular at all.

As Wilber notes,[40] in discussing his altered state experience,

It was both incredibly and profoundly ordinary, so extraordinarily ordinary that it did not even register—there was nobody there to comprehend it, until I fell *out* of it, I guess about three hours later.

Is it possible to have a nondichotomous altered state which can analyze? Or does analysis, by definition, dichotomize? Also, if there are (at least) two different states, might we consider that rather than one state of consciousness being higher—holistic, nondichotomous versus analytical, dichotomous—each state of consciousness may be functionally specific and "higher" depending upon the appropriateness of the situation? Might our task be to understand and utilize both, when appropriate, as well as to learn how each might balance the other? Skillful use of both may help us avoid the problems of suboptimal normal awareness, in which we "nonconsciously" tune out much of the world, and get lost in fantasies and inner dialogue. Either state of awareness could help us learn to differentiate more precisely between experience as such and our mental elaboration about that experience, our active construction of awareness. Perhaps some kind of balance involving the precise and skillful use of both of these states would be the most helpful for us. As the Globuses note, in discussing don Juan, *one* of our tasks is to *break* the *tonal's* unity, the *tonal* which represents dichotomous awareness—the way we make sense out of ordinary reality. When we can break that—which occurs when dialogue stops—we can enter the world of the *nagual.* This allows "extraordinary facets of ourselves to surface as though they had been kept heavily guarded by our words."[75] However, the Globuses point out that it's important not to leave the island of the *tonal,* but rather to use it, and so keep the two in balance.

Thus words, which by definition are dichotomous, divide reality, and make distinctions, discriminations, and separations, certainly can be limiting. However, they may also be quite useful, both in understanding ordinary reality and, interestingly, for some people in facilitating a nondichotomous awareness.

For example, the koan, the intellectual riddle, is often used to get one to see the limits of intellectual awareness. In the Vipasanna tradition, the use of words to label experience is employed to get one to discriminate perceptions more accurately, differentiating emotional "overlays" from the perception itself. Sri Nisargadatta Maharaj describes his experience of perceiving from a nondichotomous place as follows:

I am like a screen—clear and empty—the pictures pass over it and disappear, leaving it as clear and empty as before. In no way is the screen affected by the pictures, nor are the pictures affected by the screen. . . . The feeling: "I am not this or that, nor is anything mine" is so strong in me that as soon as a thing or a thought appears, there comes at once the sense "this I am not."[76]

Although he says he doesn't repeat or verbalize those statements such as "this I am not," it may be that initially he said these cognitions, and that later the conditioning became automatic so that he was able to disidentify, "I am both and neither and beyond." As Wilber says, the form of inquiry can most effectively be stated not as "I must always be aware of my breath," but "Who must be?" It is not "I hold the koan," but "Who holds it?" Thus we can see that often cognitive statements, utilizing words, may be used to help move us beyond a cognitive frame into a nondichotomous state, eventually ending with the dissolution of the "witness."

Some Final Comments on Awareness

Although there are different types of awareness, strategies, and goals within each of the different traditions, there are some areas of overlap and similarities. One in particular which is of interest is the area of "detached observation." This detached observation is an ability to look at oneself and events in one's life without reactivity. An example is described by Sri Nisargadatta Maharaj in the quote above. This detached observation strategy is one which has been utilized by many of the traditions discussed in this book. For example, Freud noted the importance of a type of detached observation in his work with Breuer (*Studies in Hysteria*). He stated that to help the patient overcome resistance, the therapist must help the patient assume an objectivity to his own dilemma, "a crystal ball attitude by the patient toward himself."[77] In this way, Freud noted that the patient learned to see that he had nothing to fear by revealing his true memories and his "customary defenses are shown to be unnecessary." In social learning theory, this detached observation may be attained by systematic desensitization. In effect, systematic desensitization is a process which involves observing aversive stimuli while the person is in a state of relaxation. Thus, the aversive stimuli, through counterconditioning, may become less threatening (i.e., simply observed without any emotional overlay). In Rogerian therapy or client-centered therapy, the therapist, as we have noted, by accurately reflecting the client to himself in a nonjudgmental way, teaches the client to "see his own attitudes, confusions, ambivalences, and perceptions accurately expressed by another but stripped away of their complications of emotion."[78] In Zen, there is an important emphasis on being able to obtain a *perspective on or actions, an immovable wisdom,* a spectator resting in ourselves. Also, in the Vipassana tradition, the transcendent witness (devoid of any sense of exclusive self) may be seen as the goal of the entire practice—the cultivation of detached awareness.

Even though there are similarities in these traditions regarding detached observation, there are also differences. For example, some schools place more emphasis on *decreasing affect* regarding the object or content of experience, whereas other traditions may aim toward more disidentification from the object of awareness. However, the actual effect on affect may be the same.

Summary of Awareness

Most traditions would agree that some efforts to filter reality, and thereby not be overwhelmed by the myriad of inputs with which we are bombarded, is absolutely essential.[32] However, what may be initially adaptive and functional—the active construction of awareness—can eventually become reality corrupting, and therefore be suboptimal and dysfunctional at times.[2,79] There are several ways to develop greater awareness, two of which have been discussed in some detail in this section: holistic (simple, nondichotomous, noninterfering awareness) and analytic (verbal labeling and seeking to understand cause and effect). It may be difficult for these types of awareness to ever understand each other—problems in state dependent and cross state communication. Yet, at times, both may be able to help facilitate the other (e.g., koan; the balance of *tonal* and *nagual*). Thus, what may be important is the ability to skillfully utilize both of these states—having control and flexibility—so that individuals can enter a wide range of states and not be exclusively identified with any.

We may be able to see here a continuum of different states, ranging from precise analytic observation of cause and effect awareness (i.e., how we are conditioned, by the internal and external environments); to focus on affect associated with that cause and effect conditioning; to focusing on the attentional process by which we have the affect; to focusing on our detached selves or watching this process; to focusing on focusing itself. Each of these gives a different understanding and different level of awareness, depending upon where we deploy our attention. At different times, for different reasons, any level of focus may be the "highest" in terms of being most functional.

ROLES AND QUALITIES OF THE THERAPIST/TEACHER

All of the traditions discussed in this book believe, at some level, that a teacher or therapist is necessary as part of the process of change. The actual importance of the teacher in the change process, and the specific role that the therapist performs, vary a great deal, however, depending upon the theory of human nature on which the tradition is based. Relevant dimensions for comparison include how important the therapist is seen as being in the process of change, how active the therapist needs to be, and the exact role that the therapist has to fulfill in the change process. If individuals are seen as evil and resisting, then the teacher or therapist needs to be more active, almost like a parent (Theory 1). If the therapists believe the patient has an innate self-actualizing good nature (Theory 2), they will act differently—more facilitatively—to bring forth that nature. If the therapists believe the person has learned poor skills, then they will want to teach, like an educator, more adaptive skills (Theory 3, behavioral approach). Again in Theory 3 (existential), they may want to share themselves in an authentic, disclosing way. In Theory 4, there is a range of roles for the teacher from "the person has to find the way him/herself and the teacher has nothing to teach" to very explicit statements about the role of the teacher.

Elaboration on Each Theory's View of the Role of the Therapist

Theory 1. The id psychologist, represented by Freud, views the person as struggling against unconscious impulses, utilizing resistance and defenses, and therefore often unaware of why he or she performs certain actions. It is therefore the responsibility of the therapist to pierce through these defenses, to help make the unconscious impulses conscious, and to interpret for the patient the underlying dynamics and motives.[80] The process of therapy is seen as a struggle in which the therapist tries to overcome the patient's resistance. As Freud noted, the therapist has to fight the patient every step of the way, as evidenced in the case of Lucy R., where Freud pitted his will and efforts against her contrary insistence and desires, or in the case of Elizabeth Von R., in which he said, "Tell me what's happening, I know there is more."[77]

Because of patient resistance, the therapist is forced to take what Walter Mischel[81] called an "indirect sign approach." What the patient says either may or may not be true. Usually, it is distorted. The therapist therefore has to interpret what the behavior points to—underlying motives and reasons for the actions—what the patient himself can't understand and is repressing. Freud noted that the qualities of the therapist include the ability to be an "elucidator, sympathizer, father confessor, and teacher." The therapist must be able to shift from participant to observer, from empathy to introspection, from problem solving to intuition, from a more involved to a more detached posture.[82] As Freud noted, the analyst should listen to the patient with evenly suspended attention and be like a mirror to his patients.[83] In order to have empathy, the analyst must "renounce for a time part of his own identity and for this he must have a loose or flexible self-image."[82]

Greenson believed that Freud did not mean by this that the therapist should be cold and unresponsive, but that the therapist should be opaque, reflecting back to the patient nothing but what the patient had said. "The analyst must try to mute his own responses so that he is relatively anonymous to the patient."[82] This was done primarily to effect an analysis of transference. This is defined as the experiencing of feelings, drives, attitudes, fantasies, and defenses which are repetitions of reactions originating in regard to significant persons of early childhood unconsciously displaced onto figures in the present. As Freud noted in the case of Dora (1905), transference which "seems ordained to be the greatest obstacle of psychoanalysis, becomes its most powerful ally if its presence can be detected each time and explained to the patient."[84]

Theory 2. The ego psychologist, represented by Rogers' client-centered therapy, believes the person has an inherent tendency toward self-actualization and that the ego is not a passive creature ruled by the unconscious passions. Therefore, more emphasis is placed on developing conditions of acceptance and nurturance, and less on interpretation and analysis. The therapist not only does not interpret the client's underlying motive, but does very little except provide a warm, trusting environment in which the individual's innate selfactualizing nature can grow and express itself.

Rogers suggested that there are three qualities which a therapist needs in order to help effect change: congruence and genuineness; nonpossessive love and warmth; and nonjudgmental accurate empathy. *Congruence* and genuineness are defined as awareness of one's own attitude toward whatever one is feeling or experiencing. The therapist, in order to help make the client self-aware, must himself be self-aware, with no facades, no fear of admitting to himself how he feels toward the client.[85]

> If I can form a helping relationship to myself, if I can be sensitively aware of and acceptant toward my own feelings—then the likelihood is greater that I can form a helping relationship toward another.[78]

The second quality is *nonpossessive love* and warmth. This involves, according to Rogers, the ability to separate from the client enough so that the therapist is not engulfed by the client and can let himself go more deeply in understanding and accepting because he is not fearful of losing himself. The third quality is *nonjudgmental accurate empathy*. The therapist needs the ability to see the client's feelings, meanings, and hurts—to step into the client's frame of reference without evaluating and judging. Further, the therapist, Rogers noted, should accept the other person as a process of becoming and not be bound by his past or see him as something fixed, classified, or diagnosed.

By genuinely fulfilling the above conditions, Rogers believed the therapist creates an interpersonal situation in which the material may come into the client's awareness and in which the client can see his own attitudes, confusions, ambivalences, and perceptions accurately expressed by another but stripped of their complication of emotion. This allows the client to see himself objectively, to see that his feelings are accepted and are acceptable, and paves the way for acceptance into the self of all those elements which are now more clearly perceived. Thus, in his seminal article "The Necessary and Sufficient Conditions of Therapeutic Personality Change," Rogers[85] listed six items: (1) two people are in psychological contact; (2) the client is in a state of incongruence (i.e., self-concept and experiences are not congruent); (3) the therapist is in a state of congruence vis-à-vis the client; (4) the therapist shows unconditional positive regard for the client; (5) the therapist shows empathetic understanding of the client's internal frame of reference; (6) the client perceives the therapist's empathy and unconditional positve regard.

The therapist is not inducing change, but instead is allowing it, since the individual already has the potential for positive growth. The therapist merely provides the warm, trusting, empathetic climate in which the individual can be his/her true self.

Theory 3.   There are differing views of the Theory 3 (blank slate, existence precedes essence) viewpoint with respect to the role of the teacher. The existential position places great emphasis on the authenticity of the therapist, and on the importance of the therapist sharing him or herself as a critical factor in the process of therapy.[87] The behavioral tradition, as we will see in more detail in the next section, places great emphasis on the techniques of change in the therapy process, and much less on the relationship between the patient and therapist either in terms of transference and countertransference, or empathy, warmth, trust, and authenticity.

The therapist-client relationship is that between teacher and student, expert and apprentice; the therapist is someone who can teach techniques and strategies to the patient which will help the patient manage his or her life better.

Recently, however, more emphasis has been placed on the "teacher." Lazarus[23] and Davidson,[86] among others, have acknowledged that techniques occur within a context, and a certain amount of trust may be necessary before the client is willing to practice the techniques. For example, even shutting one's eyes, for relaxation practice, may be frightening to some people and require a "trusting" relationship with the therapist in order for it to be effective.

Theory 4. The pure theory viewpoint, as we have noted, suggests that individuals are already whole. Therefore, certain traditions, like Zen, suggest that the teacher really has no content to teach for the person already has "Buddha nature" within them. However, in Zen, there are monasteries set up in order to teach this "nonteaching" and to transmit the teaching of "nondogmatic ways" to experience true understanding.

Articles in this Book

Regardless of orientation, all traditions discussed in this book believe that some role is necessary for a teacher and therapist. The exact nature of this role, however, may be quite different depending upon the view of human nature of the respective traditions. Even Theory 2 and Theory 4 viewpoints ascribe an important role to the teacher. While some Theory 4 viewpoints are quite explicit about the teacher's techniques,[42,43] others place relatively more emphasis on the qualities of the therapist/teacher and define the role more as a motivator, model, and educator.

For example, Kornfield[36] talks of masters as reminders, and the Globuses talk about teachers as models and motivators,

> Learning to live like a warrior is an accomplishment which takes years. The teacher, benefactor, and other warriors are of great importance in convincing the apprentice to want to change his ways.[44]

Effective teachers live the values they believe, and therefore, through a process of vicarious modeling, share and teach those values to the apprentice.[88] Rajneesh notes very explicitly that a teacher is necessary, suggesting that the teacher helps the person relax and shows him he is on the right path.

> It's not just gullibility that people become attached to masters; it has a scientific base to it. Moving into the unknown is a tremendous risk. One should move with somebody who has already moved into it. One should move hand-in-hand with somebody who knows the territory—otherwise the thing can happen so shatteringly that you will be at a loss.[35]

Deikman, representing what appears to be a combination Theory 4 and Theory 3 viewpoint, suggests that the development of an intuitive third eye has certain requirements, involving a teacher:

Adequate preparation of suitable students, the correct learning situation, and the activity of a Teacher who has reached the goal and by means of that special knowledge is equipped to teach according to the needs of the particular culture, the particular time, the particular historical period, and the particular person.[42]

Wilber notes that in the lower realms we use our parents who teach us language and egoic self-control, and later the master helps move us further by imposing the special conditions of the higher states.[32]

Summary of Therapists Role

We have seen in this section that there are different views about the role the therapist should take—the Rogerians stress acceptance of the client, and a nonjudgmentalness; Freud stresses the high importance of relationship with respect to overcoming resistance, and analyzing transference and counter-transference; the behaviorist places relatively less importance on the therapist-patient relationship and greater importance on the teaching of techniques; and Theory 4 viewpoints in this book suggest a range of roles, including model, motivator, as well as, in some traditions, an educator teaching specific techniques.

TECHNIQUES

As we saw in the previous section, some schools suggest that only the therapist's authenticity is important, and no "techniques" are necessary (e.g., Rogerian, existential). As Rogers[19] noted,

There was no essential value to therapy of such techniques as interpretation of personality dynamics, free association, analysis of dreams, analysis of transference, and interpretation of lifestyle. (p. 103)

Some schools believe the therapist's role is important, but also utilize some techniques (e.g., Freudian, don Juan). Others say the therapist's role is relatively unimportant other than as a transmittor of techniques (e.g., behavioral). Thus, for example, behaviorists would utilize automated or semiautomated methods of teaching relaxation (e.g., tapes, etc.) in order to effect change. Finally, some viewpoints suggest that really no teacher or techniques are necessary (e.g., Zen). Table 18–7 summarizes each tradition's *stated view* of itself with regard to the role of the teacher and the role of techniques.

Table 18.7. Role of Teacher and Techniques: Different Approaches' Stated Views of Themselves.

		RELATIVELY HIGH IMPORTANCE	RELATIVELY LOW IMPORTANCE
T E C H N I Q U E S	Relatively high importance	don Juan Sufi	Behavioral
	Middle	Freud	
	Relatively low importance	Existential Rogerian	Zen

The "Technique" Traditions

As we can see from the Table 18–7, there are certain schools (e.g., behavioral, don Juan, Sufi) which place a high importance on techniques and are quite explicit about their views. The techniques may help the student/patient/client overcome resistances, barriers, and obstacles along the way and thereby provide the means which enable individuals to change (evolve) from the tradition's view of human nature (who they are) to the vision and goal of therapy (who they can become). Deikman, for example, notes that we need a larger view of human nature, and suggests that the Sufis have the vision and techniques to reach it; he talks about techniques in terms of the Sufi stories:

> The stories provide templates to which we can match our own behavior. ... The story slides past our vigilant defenses and ... we "see," as in a mirror, the shape and meaning of what we are actually doing.... the development of this channel of knowing directly adds a new dimension to ordinary consciousness.[42]

Don Juan is also quite specific about the fact that there *are* steps (techniques) to the path of knowledge.

> We must follow certain steps, because it is the steps where man finds strength. Without them we are nothing.[89]

Some of these techniques are perceptual strategies, detaching oneself from all that is familiar so that everything is new—not-doing techniques. Some of these strategies are cognitive in that the warrior takes what comes to him as a challenge and as neither good nor bad—controlled folly. These techniques—ranging from erasing one's past and creating a fog, to stalking personal habits, losing self-importance, and reducing wants and desires—are discussed in detail in Chapter 14.[44] Some Eastern approaches are also specific about the importance of learning techniques. There are techniques of identification with everything, "I am that also," and there is a path where one disidentifies with everything (neti-neti), "I am not this, not this."

The "No Technique" Traditions

The other school of thought is the "no technique" school, the school which believes that change strategies and techniques are unnecessary. For example, Theories 2 and 4 say that people are already perfect, but just don't recognize it.

The no technique school is evidenced by the comments of Rogers at the start of this section as well as by several traditions discussed below. For example, Rajneesh, citing Chenzenji, notes that "amending my nature is needless" because the nature is already there.[35] Wilber[32] talks about letting one's true self come forth naturally: "One does not learn to become a Buddha. One discovers it. . . . The flight from the self to the Self is a flight from *personal manipulation to transcendent witnessing*" (italics mine). Kornfield[36] says that we need to let problems naturally drop away:

Selfish thoughts and limiting perspectives such as fear and doubt are not seen as qualities which must be actively fought, uprooted, or overcome. Instead they *drop away naturally* as the limited identification with body, mind, and smaller parts of the world ceases. (italics mine)

Rajneesh[35] suggests, "Enlightenment is a process of unlearning. It is utter ignorance . . ." and, regarding meditation, "Meditation cannot be created by human effort; . . . . *You cannot manipulate it*. It only happens when you are in a tremendous surrender"[35] (italics mine).

Are No Techniques Really Techniques?

How are the above statements of the no technique school to be understood? Are there really no techniques being utilized? In the subsequent paragraphs I would like to raise several questions about the no technique schools. As a preface, I would like to state that perhaps the questions that I raise are merely semantic distinctions and therefore not of high relevance. Further, it may be that because of my background and training as a social learning theorist and behavior therapist, I see the laws of conditioning everywhere, and therefore it is very difficult for me to understand change occurring without a technique (i.e., without laws of conditioning being in effect). Therefore, I think we may gain a certain amount of clarity if we look at "no technique" as really *different types* of techniques.

For example, Rogers suggests the therapist should avoid advice, reassurance, interpretation, and praise. He notes that comments should be primarily reflection, restatement of general comment, structuring, clarification of feeling, and simple acceptance.[90] Yet aren't these techniques themselves, albeit of a different sort? Couldn't unconditional positive regard (i.e., the therapist should reinforce all the person with all his existing potentialities) be seen as a change strategy? By using "nonjudgmental" verbal strategies, doesn't a Rogerian therapist teach the client to become free from the threat of external evaluation, both good and bad, and also teach him to recognize that the locus of evaluation and the center of responsibility can be (and should be) within himself?

Similarly, when Rajneesh says the self has to let go in order to have meditation occur—"You cannot manipulate it," and "First you have to do all that you can do, and then you have to learn nondoing"[35]—isn't this in fact a strategy, i.e., to produce effort and then let go of effort? Couldn't the effort that Rajneesh discusses, or personal manipulation which Wilber comments upon, be referred to as active change strategies (active control)?[62] Also, might these strategies be contrasted with letting-go change strategies (letting-go control) which could then include what Wilber refers to as transcendent witnessing and what Rajneesh calls learning to do nothing? *Learning* to be accepting, to "let it be," to just watch without interfering or making affective judgments is, we might suggest, a change strategy, though of a different sort. Perhaps the *process* of learning to "discover" Buddha is different from an analytical approach, but doesn't it represent a learning nonetheless? *Both* modes (personal manipulation and transcendent witnessing; active effort and letting-go effort) might be considered to be brought about by techniques; both might be viewed as "manipulations" to effect change, whether active change or letting-go acceptance.

In the latter type of change strategy, we might suggest that there is a cognitive restructuring of one's beliefs, attitudes, and feelings to enable an individual to become more detached and disidentified from the personal self. As Wilber himself notes, "Since major characteristics of the higher realms include timelessness, love, no avoidance, total acceptance, and the subject/object unity, these are most often the special conditions of meditation." He then offers certain cognitions, which might be beneficial to actualize these characteristics: "Stay in the now always; recognize your avoidances; the only condition is love; become one with your meditation and your world; accept everything since everything is Buddha."[32]

However, it seems important to make the distinction between passive acceptance as a goal and the effort of techniques that may be necessary in order to reach that goal. To state that there are no techniques (except as a technique itself to encourage people to let go more!) may cause individuals to feel that there really isn't anything they can do and may be doing a disservice to the clients or patients. For example, as we have noted, the existentialist suggests that people are born free. Existentialists eschew techniques in favor of interpersonal authenticity. However, the existentialist may be doing us a disservice by saying that we are born free (view of human nature) rather than that we can learn to become free (vision of health). Does everyone naturally and a priori have the skills and abilities to become free? If they don't, then it may be that we need to learn techniques to develop the skills of freedom. To eschew techniques based on a theory of human nature may be therapeutically unhelpful.

Some Summary Comments on Techniques

Techniques may be seen as a critical variable which can be utilized to help individuals change from who they are (view of human nature) to who they can become (goal of therapy). I use the word technique here not in the pejorative sense of a "gimmick" or cookbook recipe, but as a means by which change is effected. Insofar as the traditions in this book are involved in some kind of teaching or educational process, a teacher then becomes a vehicle for transmitting knowledge. The therapist or teacher is usually the one that presents these techniques, and they can be presented either formally or informally. When presented formally, through modeling, or demand characteristics (i.e., differential, verbal, or nonverbal cues and consequences for the desired behavior in the person/client), the actual quality and nature of the therapist may be considered to be a "technique" of change. Although some schools suggest that they utilize "no technique," it is being suggested here that there are in fact strategies which are utilized among almost all traditions (even the technique of no technique) in order to achieve the state of psychological health as defined by that particular tradition. On a process level, these techniques may range from very specific concrete instructions— verbal, symbolic, behavioral—which are transmitted formally through a combination of writings and/or regular teachings; or they may be transmitted informally by placing the "therapist/teacher" in close proximity to the client so that the skills and techniques can be modeled. On a content level, these strategies include cognitive strategies (changing thoughts and self-statements); awareness strategies, including identification, disidentification, detached observation; different types of strategies for stopping thoughts or reducing affect about thoughts; imagery strategies; perceptual strategies; kinesthetic strategies; content and context focusing strategies; affective strategies to change from unhealthy to healthy mental factors; and acceptance strategies to decrease the amount of affect and desire.

One interesting thing is that although the nature of the techniques, as well as the goals for which the techniques are utilized, may be different in these traditions, all of these approaches—on a meta level—are quite similar. All of these traditions believe fundamentally in an educational process either explicitly through teaching or implicitly through modeling the skills. Eventually, more often than not, the traditions teach that no teacher is necessary.

Because people are incredibly complex, with varied goals, I believe it is important that we be quite precise in our discussion of techniques. In this way, hopefully, we can begin to develop a precision in our use of change strategies, and see how those change strategies are related to the view of human nature, the goal of therapy, and the role of the therapist. These issues are summarized in Table 18-8. We can begin to see that no one technique may be appropriate for every person at all times and thus can begin to develop a more skillful and functional matching of a particular strategy to a particular person for a particular goal.

CONCLUDING REMARKS

The bias of this chapter has been toward precision and analysis. Its intent has been to provide a framework, and then to look as carefully and exactly as possible at the statements and claims of the various disciplines, so that each may be compared to each other. This lays the groundwork for determining their probable accuracy and acceptability, and the nature of their evidence, and for separating beliefs from pseudoscience.

In these concluding paragraphs I would like to make some summary statements which I believe may provide useful cautions when exploring many of the traditions in this book. First, we need to make sure that the concept of ennobling vision and "global growth" is not set forth without trying to tie it down to more specific goals. Growth is such an amorphous word that unless we are more specific, it becomes nearly impossible to evaluate our progress. In fact, if we look to the Eastern traditions, we see that some of them have very clear demarcations of internal states of consciousness so that one can evaluate where one is.[43,91]

Second, we should be aware of our own preconceptions and biases toward what "growth" is. For example, although it may be important for those of us who are therapists and health science professionals to posit alternative

Table 18–8. Motivation, Awareness, Techniques, Role of Teacher.

AUTHOR/ARTICLE	MOTIVATION	AWARENESS	TECHNIQUES	ROLE OF TEACHER
		PART I		
Walsh	Not discussed	Eastern awareness includes "higher"	Meditation is a technique for that awareness	Not discussed
		PART II		
Wilber	Higher levels	"Higher" awareness involves disidentification with the content of actions; content becoming context	Not discussed	Not discussed
Erhard, Gioscia, and Anbender	Mastery	Awareness equals context and is nondichotomous; consciousness equals content and is dichotomous	Not discussed	Not discussed
Heath	Survival	Symbolization as awareness; first step in change	Not discussed	Not discussed
Shapiro and Shapiro	Intimacy	Both types needed, as appropriate	Not discussed	Not discussed
		PART III		
Walsh	Selfless service	Not discussed	Meditation as a means for transformation	Models
Goleman and Epstein	Healty factors relieve suffering	Buddhist tradition emphasizes the importance of context of consciousness, not content	Meditation as a means for developing healthy mental factors and eradicating unhealthy ones	Models
Shapiro	Not discussed	Mind as mirror; holistic awareness	Meditation as a technique for developing this awareness	To teach that there's nothing to teach

			Techniques for "cleaning" perceptions	Models
Smith	Not discussed	We have "colored" perceptions of reality; need to develop higher awareness		
Deikman	Finding meaning	Intuitive awareness is higher; however, also mentions need for cause-effect understanding	Sufi stories	High need
Globus and Globus	Will, path of heart	*Tonal* is ordinary awareness and *nagual* is altered state; need for stopping thoughts to gain access to the *nagual*; but both states are necessary	Many different types of cognitive focusing strategies discussed; stop the world; disrupt routines, etc.	High need
Kornfield	Selfless service	holistic, compassionate awareness is higher	Meditation is a technique for this transformation, but no discipline is necessary	High need
		PART IV		
Wilber	Multilevels	The detached witness and the witness disappearing are the highest steps of awareness	Meditation is developmental and occurs along many different areas of the unconscious	Not discussed
Shapiro	Multilevels	Precision awareness and holistic awareness	Variety of techniques discussed; depending upon the context	Not discussed
Walsh and Vaughan	Selfless service and multilevels	Eastern "holistic" awareness is higher; perception is clouded normality; identity; defenses; a function of identification with content of awareness	Meditation is a path for transformation; identification and disidentification	Models
Shapiro	Summary model	Summary position; argues that Eastern and Western may be higher	Summary	Summary

NOTE: The view of "intimate" relationships and control issues is not discussed here because it is discussed in detail in other chapters in this book.

Table 18-9. Comparison and Contrast: Four Schools of Psychotherapy.

SUBJECT	PSYCHODYNAMIC (ID PSYCHOLOGY: FREUD)	CLIENT-CENTERED THERAPY (EGO PSYCHOLOGY: ROGERS)	SOCIAL LEARNING THEORY (BEHAVIORAL PSYCHOLOGY)	ZEN BUDDHISM
Motivation	Motivation based primarily on id energy and impulses; a tension reduction model	A hierarchy of motivation ranging from security needs to self-actualizing needs (from Maslow)	Social and environmental contingencies; models; reinforcement	A harmony with oneself and the world around; learning to hear the sound of one's heart
Awareness	Know thy unconscious past; self-awareness is defined as insight into childhood; the crucial element in therapeutic cure	Know thy self-actualizing ego; insight is fresh understanding and experience of the self; this is the crucial element in making self-concept and self-experiences congruent	Know thy controlling variables; self-observation is method of defining problem; and a potential intervention strategy (reactive effect)	Know the bird's song; nonreactive observation is a means and end in itself; self-evaluation and self-reinforcement are extraneous
Origin of self-awareness	Not discussed fully; only mention is id cathecting ego, in *On Narcissism* (1914)	Both from evaluation of others and from within oneself	Socially conditioned by verbal community	Socially conditioned by language, culture; logic
Techniques to increase self-awareness	Verbal, intellectual, rational only; interpretation by therapist	Verbal, experiential, rational; reflection rather than interpretation; no interpretation	Verbal, intellectual, rational; use by client of charts, wrist counters, self-quantification; antecedents, consequences	Some verbal; mainly nonverbal; doing, not talking; non-intellectual; nonrational

		Past; childhood memories	Present feelings	Present perceptions and controlling environment	Now
Focus	Detached observation; self-objectification as goal of self-awareness	Freud: patient must assume a crystal ball attitude toward himself; not to be afraid of revealing his true memories	Rogers: client, by therapist reflection, can come to see himself objectively; his feelings stripped of complications of emotion and evaluation	Desensitization is an attempt to get client to see himself in fear-arousing situation, be objective to self, and not become tense	Self-observation without self-evaluation is the goal of life
Techniques		Techniques are used to overcome patient resistance	Ostensibly, none are used; other than "authenticity" of therapist	High use of techniques	Ostensibly no techniques needed, but many are used; Koan meditation etc.
Role/qualities of the therapist		High for therapist; his role is critical; analysis of transference/countertransference; Greenson[65] says that for an analyst to have empathy, "he must renounce for a time part of his own identity; and for this he must have a loose or flexible self-image"	Therapist role important; no analysis of relationship; dynamics, however; Rogers says the therapist must be able to see the client without reacting emotionally or judgmentally; to be strong enough to be a separate person; and at the same time to see clearly and accurately what the client is saying	Therapist role important only as a teacher or coach; not much attention to qualities of the therapist; Lazarus[23] states, though, that the therapist should be compassionate and empathetic	Zen says that the highest ego is no-ego; empty; like a mirror; this gives flexibility; strength; accurate reflection; the teacher models "right action," but ultimately teaches no teaching

models for our clients, it is also important to hear and listen to the client's concern as he/she sees it. Not everyone who comes to us with a specific hurt (e.g., loneliness) may need to first experience facing existential angst. It should not be beneath us to teach our clients practical skills (e.g., social skills) to help them deal with their everyday hurts. Also, for many people, transcendence, or nonreactive awareness, may not be a sufficient answer.

Third, although I believe (1) that Eastern spiritual values can provide a useful adjunct to our technology and science, and (2) that Eastern emphasis on spirituality, holistic perception of the world, and altered states of consciousness can provide us with valuable knowledge and wisdom, I also believe we make a mistake if we unquestioningly embrace all aspects of Eastern tradition, eschewing logic and analysis, or even placing them "lower" in value. As Alan Watts has noted, Eastern disciplines such as Zen may become rigidified in the dogma of nondogma, therely developing static qualities and blinders of their own. By using tools of intellect and analysis, we can come to see some of the blinders and the static qualities that may have developed in formal traditions (East or West, scientific or religious). Further, a balanced approach, which also emphasizes intellect, reason, and analysis, may help provide us with certain tools that are useful in translating the descriptive terminology of Eastern spiritual disciplines into terms more understandable to Western readers. These tools "demythologize" Eastern mysticism and help us get at the heart of why techniques such as meditation work. Further, this approach may help us show which techniques can be useful and which not, and for whom.

Finally, although we need to acknowledge that many of the traditions discussed in this book provide us with a pleasing vision of our human potential, it may be just a *descriptive* vision and not a priori true. We may in fact not be innately self-actualizing creatures; we may not be innately born with free will. We may need the skills to attain these qualities of existential freedom—of developing warm and compassionate human relationships. We may need to believe in the vision, but as noted, it may be important not to let it blind us to the skills which may be necessary to make the vision a reality.

Finally, it should be acknowledged in conclusion that an attempt to cover the breadth of material reflected in this chapter may inevitably lead to errors—of omission, if not commission. My hope is that such errors, in terms of depth of coverage, have not done a disservice to the traditions discussed, and that the systematic comparison of these different traditions may provide the soil and impetus for more thorough and complete integrations in the future.

Acknowledgment.   I wish to thank Dr. Richard Chapman, Dr. Gordon Globus, Dr. Ken Anderson, Dr. Johanna Shapiro, my coeditor, and residents in my first year core seminar in psychiatry for their comments and feedback on previous drafts of this manuscript.

REFERENCES

1. See for example Tart, C. States of consciousness and state specific sciences. *Science,* 1972, *186,* 1203–10; also Globus, G. Personal communication, January, 1981.
2. Walsh, R.N. and Vaughan, F. Toward an integrative psychology of well-being. This book.
3. Walsh, R.N. and Vaughan, F. Beyond ego: toward transpersonal models of the person and psychotherapy. *Journal of Humanistic Psychology,* 1980, *20,* 5–32.
4. Freud, S. *The Ego and the Id.* New York: Norton Library, 1923, p. 27.
5. Freud, S. *Civilization and Its Discontents.* New York: Norton, 1961, p. 57–58.
6. Freud, S. *Interpretation of Dreams* (1903). New York: Avon, 1970.
7. Freud, S. Analysis terminable and interminable. *The Standard Edition of the Complete Psychological Works of Sigmund Freud* (J. Strachey, Ed.), Vol. 23. London: Hogarth, 1953–1966, p. 250.
8. See Freud, S. *The Problem of Anxiety.* New York: Norton, 1936; and Breur, J. and Freud, S. Studies in hysteria. In *The Standard Edition of the Complete Psychological Works of Sigmund Freud,* Vol. 2, (J. Strachey, Ed.). London: Hogarth, 1955.
9. Hartman, H. *Essays on Ego Psychology: Selected Problems in Psychoanalytic Theory.* New York: International University Press, 1964.
10. See Carl Roger's classic work, *Client-centered therapy.* Boston: Houghton Mifflin, 1951.
11. See for example Maslow, A. *Motivation and Personality* (2nd ed.). New York: Harper & Row, 1970; and Maslow, A. *Toward a Psychology of Being.* Princeton: Van Nostrand, 1968.
12. Angyal, A. *Neurosis and Treatment: A Holistic Theory.* New York: Wylie, 1965.
13. Goldstein, K. *The Organism.* New York: American Book Company, 1939.
14. Jung, C.G. The structure and dynamics of the psyche. In *Collected Works,* Vol. 8. Princeton: Princeton University Press, 1960. See also Jung, C. Conscious, unconscious, and individuation. In *Collected Works,* Vol. 9, Part I.
15. White, R. Motivation reconsidered: the concept of competence. In *Functions of Varied Experiences.* (D.W. Fiske and S.R. Maddi, Eds.). Homewood, Ill: Dorsey, 1961, Ch. 10; see also White, R. Ego and reality in psychoanalytic theory: a proposal regarding independent ego energies. *Psychological Issues,* 1963, *3,* 1–210.
16. Humanist Manifesto II. *The Humanist,* 1973, 33, 4–9.
17. See reference 10, p. 491.
18. Ibid., p. 517.
19. Rogers, C. Necessary and sufficient conditions for therapeutic personality change. *Journal of Consulting Psychology,* 1957, *21*(2), 95–103.
20. Skinner, B.F. *Science and Human Behavior.* New York: Macmillan, 1953.
21. Bandura, A. *Principles of behavior modification.* New York: Holt, Rinehart, and Winston, 1969; and Bandura, A. *Social learning theory.* Englewood Cliffs, N.J.: Prentice Hall, 1977.
22. Wolpe, J. *The Practice of Behavior Therapy.* New York: Pergamon Press, 1969.
23. Lazarus, A. *Behavior Therapy and Beyond.* New York: McGraw-Hill, 1971.
24. Watson, J.B. Psychology as a behaviorist views it. *Psychological Review,* 1913, *20,* 158–177.
25. Skinner, B.F. *Beyond Freedom and Dignity.* New York: Bantam Books, 1971.
26. Skinner, B.F. Behaviorism at fifty. In *Behaviorism and Phenomenology: Contrasting basis*

for Modern Psychology (W.T. Wann, Ed.). Chicago: University of Chicago Press, 1964, pp. 79–108.

27. Mahoney, M.J., Thoresen, C.E. and Danher, B.G. Covert behavior modification: an experimental analogue. *Journal of Behavior Therapy and Experimental Psychiatry,* 1972, *3,* 7–14.

28. Meichenbaum, D. *Cognitive behavior modification: an integrative approach.* New York: Plentum, 1977.

29. Beck, A. *Cognitive Therapy and the Emotional Disorders.* New York: International University Press, 1976.

30. Bandura, A. The self system in reciprocal determinism. *American Psychologist,* 1978, *33*(4), 344–58.

31. See Owens, C. Zen Buddhism. In *Transpersonal Psychologies* (C. Tart, Ed.). New York: Harper & Row, 1975.

32. Wilber, K. The evolution of consciousness. This book.

33. Wilber, K. Where It was, there I shall become. This book.

34. Walsh, R. Beyond belief. *Journal of Pastoral Counseling,* in press.

35. Rajneesh, B.S. Way of the white cloud. Rajneesh Foundation, Poona, India.

36. Kornfield, J. Higher consciousness: an inside view. This book.

37. Erhard, E., Gioscia, V. and Anbender, K. Being well. This book.

38. Smith, H. The sacred unconscous. This book.

39. Teilhard de Chardin, P. *The Future of Man.* New York: Harper & Row, 1964.

40. Wilber, K. Odyssey. *Journal Humanistic Psychology,* in press.

41. Walsh, R.N. The ten perfections: qualities of the fully enlightened individual as described in Buddhist psychology. This book.

42. Deikman, A. Suffism and psychiatry. This book.

43. See Goleman, D. and Epstein, M. Meditation and well-being: an Eastern model of psychological health. This book. And Goleman, D. Varieties of the Meditation experience. New York: Dutton, 1977.

44. Globus, M. and Globus, G. The man of knowledge. This book.

45. Needleman, J. *Lost Christianity.* New York: Doubleday, 1980.

46. Heath, D. The maturing person. This book.

47. Castaneda, C. *The Teachings of Don Juan: A Yaqui Way of Knowledge.* New York: Ballentine Books, 1969.

48. Lao-tse, *The Tao Teaching* (G. Fing and J. English, translators). New York: Vintage, 1973.

49. Shah, I. *The Pleasantries of the Incredible Mulla Nasrudin.* New York: Dutton, 1971.

50. See, for example, references 20 and 25.

51. Rogers, C. *Freedom to Learn.* Columbus, Ohio: Merrill, 1969.

52. Homme, L.E. and Tosti, D. *Behavior Technology: Motivation and Contingency Management.* San Raphael, Calif.: Individual Learning Systems, 1971; see also Homme, L.E. Perspectives in psychology: 14. Control of coverants, the operants of the mind. *Psychological Record,* 1965, *15,* 501–511.

53. Dollard, J. and Miller, N. *Personality and Psychotherapy: An Analysis in Terms of Learning, Thinking, and Culture.* New York: McGraw-Hill, 1950.

54. Freud, S. *New introductory lectures on psychoanalysis.* Standard Edition, Vol. 22. London: Hogarth, 1955, pp. 454–55.

55. See reference 15, Robert White.

56. Ibid.

57. Fromm, E. *The Art of Loving.* New York: Harper & Row, 1962.

58. Horney, K. *Neurosis and Human Growth.* New York: Norton, 1950.

59. Roberts, T. On self-actualization. *ReVision,* 1978, *1,* 42–46.

60. Goldiamond, I. Self control procedures in personal behavior problems. *Psychological Reports,* 1965, *17,* 851–868.
61. See, for example, Wachtel, P.L. Psychoanalysis and Behavior Therapy New York: Basic Books, 1977.
62. Shapiro, D. Self control and positive health: multiple perspectives of balance. This book.
63. See for example Shapiro, J. and Shapiro, D. Well-being and relationship. This book; also McGrath, E. Power and intimacy, in preparation.
64. Mischel, W. *Personality and Assessment.* New York: Wylie, 1986.
65. Greenson, R. *The Technique and Practice of Psychoanalysis,* Vol. 1. New York: International University Press, 1968.
66. Walsh, R. The psychologies of East and West. This book.
67. Shah, I. *The Exploits of the Incomparable Mulla Nasrudin.* New York: Dutton, 1972.
68. Renzai. *The Zen Teachings of Renzai.* Berkeley: Shambala, 1976.
69. Kline, M. *Mathematics: A Loss of Certainty.* New York: Oxford Press, 1980; see also Capra, F. *The Tao of Physics.* Berkeley: Shambala, 1975.
70. Buber, M. *I/Thou* (W. Kaufmann, translator). New York: Scribner, 1970.
71. Note, for example, in this book, Wilber says, "My mental youth was an idol of precision and accuracy, a fortress of the clear and evident"; (see ref. 40) and Walsh describes himself as part of a resident group which was "a somewhat homogenous group of obsessive nature." (see ref. 34)
72. See for example Tart, C. *States of Consciousness.* New York: Dutton, 1975.
73. Tart, C. States of consciousness and state specific sciences. *Science,* 1972, *176,* 1203–1210.
74. Tart, C. Personal communication. March 6, 1981.
75. Castaneda, C. *The Tales of Power.* New York: Simon and Schuster, 1974.
76. Cited in Kornfield, J. Higher consciousness. This book.
77. Breuer, J. and Freud, S. *Studies on hysteria* (first German edition, 1895). *Standard Edition,* Vol. 2. London: Hogarth, 1955.
78. Rogers, C. *On Becoming a Person.* Boston: Houghton Mifflin, 1961.
79. Smith, H. The sacred unconscious. This book.
80. Freud, S. *Dynamics of Transference* (1912). *Standard Edition.* London: Hogarth, 1955.
81. See reference 64; also Mischel, W. *Introduction to Personality.* New York: Holt, Rinehart and Winston, 1971.
82. Reference 65, p. 366.
83. Freud, S. *Recommendations to physicians practicing psychoanalysis* (1912a). *Standard Edition.* London: Hogarth, 1955.
84. Reference 65, p. 13.
85. See reference 19.
86. Davidson, G. Counter control and behavior modification. In (Hamerlynck D. et al., Eds.). *Behavior Change, Methodology, Concepts, Practice* Champaign, Ill: Research Press, 1973.
87. May, R. (Ed.). *Existential Psychology.* New York: Random House, 1961.
88. Bandura, A. Vicarious and self-reinforcement processes. In *The Nature of Reinforcement.* (R. Glaser, Ed.). New York: Academic Press, 1971. pp. 228–278.
89. Castaneda, C. *The Teachings of don Juan.* New York: Ballantine Books, 1969.
90. See for example Truax, C. Reinforcement and nonreinforcement in Rogerian psychotherapy. *Journal of Abnormal Psychology,* 1966, *71* 1–9.
91. Freud, S. *The problem of anxiety,* the Psychoanalytic Quarterly Press, (Henry Bunker, tr.) W.W. Norton, 1936.
92. Freud, S. Introductory lectures (1916–1917) Standard Edition, London: Hogarth, 1955.

V
EPILOGUE

Most of us try to make the world serve us,
The sages try to serve the world.

This book has surveyed some of the world's major maps of the farthest
reaches of the human potential. Drawn from diverse cultures, languages,
and centuries, they are unanimous in agreeing that there is indeed more to
the human condition than is usually appreciated, and also agree in many
ways as to what this more is.

All of them point to the possibility of realizing and becoming this potential
through intensive mental training. This training may take many forms, but
all involve bringing formerly subliminal and involuntary mental processes
under increasingly greater voluntary control. All traditions argue that our
state of consciousness and sense of identity are considerably more fluid than
are usually appreciated. As a result of mental training, they claim, radical
shifts in consciousness and identity may occur of such magnitude that they
have traditionally been viewed as transcendent or religious. And the source
of this experience is said to be none other than the recognition of the true
nature of our mind and self.

An examination of these maps points to a number of syntheses of what
have for long seemed like irreconcilable schisms. Integrations between apparently divergent Eastern systems are clearly possible. Thanks to the
development of concepts such as state dependency, cognitive behavior
modification, and peak experiences we can also see the emergence of initial
syntheses between Eastern and Western psychologies. Even psychologies
and religions may not be the irreconcilably different systems that they were
once thought to be. At the esoteric core of all the great religions it seems that
one can find practical disciplines for inducing higher states of consciousness,
and certain aspects of the great religions may be viewed as state specific
technologies. Indeed, at the heights of human experience there appears to
occur a transcendental fusion of a range of dualisms, a fact pointed out by
Abraham Maslow among others.

The implications of these maps are awesome. For if they are correct, then
most of us are as much asleep as awake, automated unconscious shadows of
what we could be, closer to our animal than our God-like nature, yet capable
of awakening at any time if we are willing to undertake the necessary mental
training.

To what extent are these claims correct? How do we find out whether they
are or not? And if they are correct, then how do we actualize the potentials
they describe? These are questions which may be among some of the most
important we can ask. For if they are even partially correct, shouldn't we

494

urgently mobilize our energies, personally, scientifically, and socially to explore and actualize these realms?

Apart from the individual satisfactions such explorations might bring, might they not hold solutions to many of the global problems which now threaten us? Would a society composed of significant numbers of people moving towards the visions described in this book tolerate a world in which 20 million people die each year of starvation, another 750 million live in dire poverty and malnutrition, in which pollution, ecological imbalance, and nuclear contamination and warfare pose increasing risks to health and even planetary survival, and in which the human family meanwhile squanders an inconceivable one and a half billion dollars on weapons each day?

Gordon Allport wrote that "by their own theories of human nature, psychologists have the power of elevating or degrading that same nature. Debasing assumptions debase human beings; generous assumptions exalt them." By their own beliefs individuals and societies may also elevate or degrade human nature. The importance of adopting more healthful beliefs about our own nature and that of others, both those we call friends and those we call enemies, seems hard to overestimate. Our individual welfare as well as our collective survival and civilization may depend upon it.

How are we to begin this exploration? We possess scientific and technical skills which were undreamed of only decades ago but as yet they have been infrequently employed in these areas. Research such as that of Douglas Heath and studies of advanced practitioners of the consciousness disciplines are at present exceptional but must become commonplace.

Yet meaningful exploration and transformation must begin within. No amount of objective experimental research can ever be wholly satisfying or transformative. There is a vast gap between the personal experience of joy and wellbeing and a research paper on it. The ultimate testing ground and goal lie within us and are us. Each of us possesses everything that is necessary to explore our deepest nature, and in so doing to test the validity of many of the claims presented in this book. The primary tool is our own trained awareness. The question is whether we are prepared to train it. In the words of an ancient Buddhist sage, "To see if this be true, look within your own mind."

No one else in all human kind can do it for us. The responsibility and opportunity for becoming aware of all that we most truly are and sharing it with others is ultimately our own.

Glossary of Terms

ABHIDHAMMA: literally "the ultimate doctrine", a systematic Buddhist description and taxonomy of the nature of mind and its components and states.

ADEQUATIO: the philosophical principle of adequacy, which postulates that the understanding of the knower must be adequate to the thing to be known.

ADVAITA VEDANTA: a systematized theology of radical monism based on the Upanishads and affirming the existence of a single, ubiquitous, spiritual principle—the neutral Brahman; all else in the universe is said to be a derived manifestation.

AJNA CHAKRA: the center of consciousness located between the eyebrows and claimed to be awakened by Kundalini energy.

ALAYAVIJNANA: "store consciousness"; Mahayana Buddhist term denoting the causal region of consciousness.

ALLOCENTRIC: having one's interest and attention centered on other persons.

ANANDAMAYAKOSA: literally "sheath made of bliss"; Hindu term denoting the causal region of consciousness.

ANATTA: the insight that there is no permanent and unchanging self or ego; one of the three Buddhist marks of existence.

ANGST: existential anxiety; a feeling of anguish or dread.

ANICCA: the recognition of the impermanence and state of constant flux in the world; one of the three Buddhist marks of existence.

ANNAMAYAKOSA: literally "sheath made of food"; Vedanta Hindu term denoting the level of "hunger", one of the lowest and most basic levels of human development.

ANUSAYAS: Buddhist term describing the latent capacity for unhealthy mental factors and states to recur in the unenlightened mind.

ANUTTARA SAMYAK SAMBODHI: literally "supreme unexcelled enlightenment"; the final transformation of consciousness in which an individual transcends the "I-ness" of the causal realm and experiences being both nothing and every-thing.

ARAHAT (also ARAHANT): a saint or perfected being; the highest level of enlightenment recognized in Theravadin Buddhism

ARETE: the sum of good qualities said to comprise character: excellence, value, virtue, and manliness.

ASHRAM: a religious center or retreat

ATMAN: the supreme universal self or spirit in the Hindu tradition; the innermost essence of each individual.

ATTA: self, what Westerners commonly denote by the word "personality".

AVIDYA: metaphysical ignorance simultaneously concealing the true non-dual nature of Brahman and projecting the universe of multiplicity.

BEHAVIORISM: a branch of psychology which places emphasis on studying overt behavior and the role of conditioning and reinforcement in determining behavior.

BHAKTI YOGA: a yoga emphasizing love and devotion as a means for self-realization; a state of intense devotional love for God, grace, or any divine principle.

BHAVANGA: "life-continuum" consciousness; the concept that each moment of awareness is shaped by the previous instant and in turn determines the following moment.

BHIKKU: a Buddhist monk; a mendicant (one who begs food).

BIJA-MANTRA: "root mind form"; archetypal forms of existence.

BIOENERGETIC ANALYSIS: analysis based on understanding and interpreting personality in terms of the body and its energetic processes; i.e., mental qualities are reflected by the body and vice versa.

BIOENERGETIC THERAPY: therapy aimed at releasing emotional blocks manifested in the body so as to facilitate an individual's potential for joy and effective living.

BODHIDHARMA: the Buddhist sage credited with introducing Buddhism to China.

BODHISATTVA: an individual committed to achieving enlightenment; especially one who has vowed to work for the enlightenment of all sentient beings, renouncing personal liberation until that goal is accomplished.

BRAHMA (also BRAHMAN): Hindu term meaning universal self; absolute reality or all-pervading consciousness.

CATATONIA: a form of schizophrenia manifested as a state of extreme immobility.

CATHECT: to invest with libidinal energy.

CATHEXIS: the investment of libidinal energy in a person, object, idea, or activity.

CHAKRA: in yoga, a center of awareness said to be associated with a specific state of consciousness.

CONFUCIANISM (also CONFUCIAN): a Chinese system of philosophy and ethics, introduced by Confucius.

COSMOGONY: a theory about the origin of the universe.

CROSS-STATE COMMUNICATION: communication occurring between persons who are experiencing different states of consciousness.

CROSS-STATE RETENTION: comprehension of insights or knowledge gained in a specific state of consciousness while one is no longer in that state.

CYBERNETIC THEORY: a hypothesis about the similarity between the human central nervous system and mechanoelectrical communication devices (e.g. computing machines or thermostats).

DASEIN: literally "existence"; factual reality or being within the time/space realm.

DHAMMA: a difficult Buddhist term to translate owing to its many connotations, including the way, the path, the teaching, wisdom; an ultimate constituent of phenomenal reality.

DHARMAKAYA: "the truth body"; the causal or unmanifest realm of consciousness, attained in advanced meditation.

DHIKR: Islamic/Sufi term denoting a rhythmic chant; recitation of a phrase, verse, or name.

DUKKHA: the recognition of the unsatisfactoriness and inevitability of suffering; one of the three Buddhist marks of existence.

EPIPHENOMENON: a secondary phenomenon accompanying a first and thought of as caused by it.

ESCAPE/AVOIDANCE LEARNING: conditioning motivated by the desire to escape from or avoid an aversive stimulus.

EXISTENTIALISM: an introspective theory positing that human existence is not exhaustively describable or understandable in either scientific or idealistic terms and emphasizing the analysis of intensely subjective phenomena in critical situations (e.g., anxiety, suffering, and guilt) occurring in an apparently purposeless world.

FANA: Islamic term denoting the Sufi concept of annhilation of individual human will before the will of God.

FIELD THEORY: a systematic psychological theory mathematically describing the interrelatedness between a concrete event and the influences of an individual's personality and environment; one must treat a situation as a field to view it in its totality.

GESTALT: an integrated configuration of physical, biological, or psychological phenomena constituting a functional unit with properties not derivable from its parts.

GESTALT PSYCHOLOGY: the study of behavior based on an organism's response to configurational wholes and placing stress on psychological and physiological events while rejecting atomistic or elemental analyses.

GNOSTIC: the thought and practice of early Christian groups distinguished by mystical esoteric religious insights and emphasis on direct personal knowledge and wisdom as opposed to faith.

GURU: a religious teacher, often implied to be enlightened.

HASIDIC (also CHASIDIC): a pious Jewish sect devoted to the strict observance of purification rituals and to mysticism (the word "Hasid" literally means "pious").

HATHA YOGA: a branch of yoga placing emphasis upon the use of physical postures and breathing exercises (pranayama).

HINAYANA: see THERAVADIN.

HOLISM: the philosophical theory postulating that the determining factors in the universe are wholes (i.e., organisms), irreducible to the sum of their parts.

HOLISTIC: term referring to an emphasis on the functional relationships between parts and wholes, tending to view phenomena as wholes rather than reducing them to their component parts.

HUMAN POTENTIAL MOVEMENT: a social movement aimed at fostering psychological development and self actualization in both individuals and society.

HUMANISTIC PSYCHOLOGY: a branch of Western psychology focussing on uniquely human experiences such as meaning, love, will, psychological maturity, and self actualization.

INDIVIDUATION: a Jungian term describing the process and state of adult psychological maturation.

ISHTAM: the particular deity chosen by an individual in accordance with his or her religious inclinations; desired, cherished, or beloved aspects.

ISHVARA: personal deity or God (as opposed to the abstract nonpersonal Godhead).

JHANA: Buddhist term for states of consciousness marked by extreme concentration and mental imperturbability.

JIVA: Hindu term meaning literally "soul"; as in "jivanmukti", a fully realized person (enlightened soul)

JIVANMUKTI: a person who is liberated though still inhabiting a physical body.

JNANA YOGA: a yoga which emphasizes wisdom as a means for self-realization.

KABBALAH: literally "received"; in Judaism, the Kabbalah is the handed-down inspired tradition of mystical understanding of God and the universe.

KARMA YOGA: the yoga of selfless service; the performance of all actions without the desire for reward.

KI: Japanese term meaning sensitivity to another's feelings and intentions.

KOAN: a Zen Buddhist technique consisting of a riddle unsolvable by rational logic alone, but demanding insight and intuitive wisdom as well.

KRIYA YOGA: the yoga of purifying the body and mind through spontaneous bodily movements in turn initiated by the awakening of Kundalini energy.

KUNDALINI YOGA: the path of awakening the primordial shakti or cosmic energy in an attempt to bring about self purification; upon entering the final chakra, the individual is said to attain the state of Self-realization.

LAMA: a Tibetan Buddhist priest or monk.

LIBIDO: Freudian term for a force related to sexual excitation; the drive towards or instinct of love.

LIMBIC: an area of the brain said to be associated with emotion.

MAHABHARATA: a Hindu epic.

MAHAYANA BUDDHISM: a major division of Buddhism which has evolved continuously rather than rigidly adhering to the original Buddhist teachings; predominant especially in Japan and Tibet and inclusive of Zen.

MAKYO: Zen term for inferior mental products of meditation; images, visions, hallucinations.

MANAS: literally "higher mind"; Mahayana Buddhist term denoting the high-subtle realm of consciousness.

MANIPURA: the aggressive-power level of the lower three chakras; one of the lowest and most basic levels of human development.

MANOMAYAKOSA: literally "sheath made of mind"; Hindu term for the verbal ego-mind.

MANOVIJNANA: literally "discursive mind"; Mahayana Buddhist term for the verbal ego-mind.

MANTRA: sacred word or sound used as a focus in meditation.

MAYA: illusion

META: more sophisticated organization or specialized form; of a higher logical type.

MONDO: a discourse between master and monk, used as a teaching tool in the Zen tradition.

MUDRA: specific hand postures, usually used as part of meditation practice.

MULADHARA: the root material and pleromatic level of the lower three chakras; one of the lowest and most basic levels of human development.

NADA: divine sounds or music said to be heard in a particular state of meditation; sometimes made the object of meditation.

NETI–NETI: literally "not this, not this"; term signifying that the Absolute is beyond any and all qualifications.

NIBBANA: see NIRVANA.

NIRMANAKAYA: the manifest physical realm of consciousness.

NIRODH: Buddhist term denoting a high-causal realm of consciousness in which all mental functioning and awareness is said to cease.

NIRVANA: the state of consciousness regarded as the goal of Buddhist practice.

NIRVIKALPA SAMADHI: "formless absorption"; Hindu term denoting the high causal realm of consciousness.

PAIDEIA: the specific training of physical and mental faculties designed to produce a harmonious combination of broad enlightened outlook and maximum cultural development.

PARADIGM: a large theory or model which encompasses a wide range of data and smaller theories.

PARAMITAS: literally "perfections" in the Buddhist tradition, mental qualities and attributes said to characterize the highest levels of psychological development.

POTENTIA: potency or power.

PRANA: literally "life breath", the vital life-sustaining force of the body and universe holding the power of animation according to Vedic and Hindu traditions.

PRANAMAYAKOSA: literally "sheath made of life force"; Vedanta Hindu term denoting the level of emotional sexuality; one of the lowest and most basic levels of human development.

PRANAYAMA: a yoga form of the Nirmanakaya meditative class, dealing with bodily or typhonic energies and their transmutation into the lower-subtle region.

PRE-EGOIC: a primitive stage, state, or condition existing before the development of the ego.

PRETAS: a Buddhist term meaning literally "hungry ghosts", referring to insatiable appetite or needfulness.

PSI: refers to extrasensory or parasensory phenomena.

RADICAL BEHAVIORISTS: adherants to a strict perspective which considers only external observable behavior to be worthy of scientific investigation.

RECIPROCAL DETERMINISM: condition in which two or more phenomena effect one another.

SAHASRARA: the uppermost chakra, said to be located at the crown of the head.

SAMADHI: literally "bringing together"; a state of meditative union with the Absolute.

SAMBHOGAKAYA: "the bliss body"; Buddhist term for the major realm of consciousness dealing with the subtle regions.

SAMSARA: the continuing successive cycles of worldly existence and illusion; see also MAYA.

SANGHA: the Buddhist brotherhood or group of people who practice the Buddhist teaching.

SAT–CHIT–ANANDA: literally total unbounded unlimited being, awareness, and bliss.

SATORI: sudden enlightenment and a state of consciousness attained by intuitive illumination representing the spiritual goal of Zen Buddhism.

SAVIKALPA SAMADHI: "absolution with form"; Hindu term denoting the state of consciousness in which the low-causal level is revealed, representing the pinnacle of God-consciousness.

SELF ACTUALIZATION: the process of the development and realization of one's potential.

SHIKAN–TAZA: a form of Zen meditation involving choiceless awareness or examination of all that arises into consciousness.

SIDDHA: an individual who has attained self realization, unity awareness, and mastery over his senses and their objects.

SIDDHA YOGA: the yoga of devotion to a Siddha or perfect master.

SIDDHIS: paranormal powers said to sometimes develop as a result of meditative/yogic training; e.g., extrasensory perception or telekinesis.

SIKH: a follower of Sikhism, a syneretic religious movement combining elements of Sufism and Hindu Bhakti.

SKANDHAS: the five Buddhist transitory elements—body, perception, conception, volition, and consciousness—whose temporary concatenation is the basis for the experience of the existence of ego or individuated self.

SMRTI: a Hindu text.

SOCIAL LEARNING THEORY: a psychology derived from behaviorism emphasizing the importance of social influences and conditioning in the determination of behavior.

SOTERIOLOGICAL: of or pertaining to soteriology; liberation or salvation.

STATE–DEPENDENT: any situation where experiences, understanding, or memories are at least partially restricted to the state of consciousness in which they were experienced and less available in other states.

SUFISM (also SUFI): Islamic mysticism whose goal is communion with the deity through contemplation.

SUPEREGO: the mostly unconscious sector of the psyche that develops through internalization of 'and in response to' advice and punishment and serves as the protector of the ego from overwhelming id impulses.

SUTRA: a collection of aphorisms forming a text that deals with some area of knowledge such as philosophy, ritual, or grammer; in Buddhism, one of the talks of the Buddha.

SVABHAVIKAKAYA: "the body of suchness"; the prior condition or reality of all realms; the fundamental ground of being.

SVADHISTHANA: the emotional-sexual level of the lower three chakras; one of the lowest and most basic forms of human development.

TANTRIC: term given to a wide range of Buddhist and Hindu practices which, unlike many religious disciplines, tend to include sensual and sexual experiences and practices.

TAOISM (also TAO): a Chinese philosophy/religion teaching conformity to the Tao through unassertive action (surrender), the highest aim of which is identification with and absorption by the Tao.

TAT TVAM ASI: literally "Thou art That", meaning "I am that also"; the sense that results when the self transcends all dualisms.

THERAVEDA BUDDHISM (also HINAYANA BUDDHISM): the original orthodox sect of Buddhism, practiced primarily in Sri Lanka, Burma, Thailand, Cambodia, and Laos ("Theraveda means "the teaching of the elders").

TRANSCENDENCE: going beyond or exceeding usual limits.

TRANSFERENCE: a term used in psychoanalysis to describe the phenomenon of redirecting feelings and desires (especially those unconsciously retained from childhood) towards a new object.

TRANSPERSONAL: literally trans (beyond) the personal (persona, personality, or ego); experiences which extend beyond usual egoic boundaries and identity.

TRANSPERSONAL PSYCHOLOGY: the study of experiences such as psychological wellbeing along with the disciplines said to develop them.

UPANISHADS: the Vedic teaching at the source of orthodox Hindu philosophy; its central tenet posits that all phenomena of both nature and the individual human soul are one with the Absolute or Brahman.

VEDANTA: certain philosophical teachings embodied in the Vedas and including the Upanishads, the Bhagavad Gita, and the Brahma Sutras, the doctrine of which is the non-dualism of the Supreme Soul or Brahman.

VIJNANAMAYAKOSA: literally "the sheath made of higher intellect"; Hindu term denoting the high-subtle realm of consciousness.

VIJNANAS: the realm of the five senses in Mahayana Buddhism, representing the lowest levels of human development.

VIPASSANA: a Buddhist term for insight resulting from refined perceptual sensitivity; awareness of the arising and passing away of each moment of experience.

VISUDDHA CHAKRA: the fifth chakra, representing the discursive verbal mind.

VISUDDHIMAGGA: an ancient Buddhist text containing most of the early Buddhist teachings.

WEI-JI: Chinese term meaning literally "turning point" and often translated as "crisis".

YOGA (also YOGA CARA):   literally "yoke", a state of union with God; the disciplines employed to develop such union or attain enlightenment.

YOGI: one who practices yoga or has attained the goal of yogic practices.

ZADDICK: the spiritual leader of a Hasidic community.

ZAZEN: a Zen form of meditation.

ZEITGEIST: the cultural trends of an era; the intellectual/moral state and taste characteristics of the times.

ZEN BUDDHISM (also ZEN):   a Japanese school of Mahayana Buddhism teaching self-discipline, deep meditation, and the attainment of enlightenment through direct intuitive insight and characteristically expressing its teachings in paradoxical and nonlogical forms.

Index